Analyzing Longitudinal Clinical Trial Data

A Practical Guide

Chapman & Hall/CRC Biostatistics Series

Published Titles

Adaptive Design Methods in Clinical Trials, Second Edition
Shein-Chung Chow and Mark Chang

Adaptive Designs for Sequential Treatment Allocation
Alessandro Baldi Antognini and Alessandra Giovagnoli

Adaptive Design Theory and Implementation Using SAS and R, Second Edition
Mark Chang

Advanced Bayesian Methods for Medical Test Accuracy
Lyle D. Broemeling

Analyzing Longitudinal Clinical Trial Data: A Practical Guide
Craig Mallinckrodt and Ilya Lipkovich

Applied Biclustering Methods for Big and High-Dimensional Data Using R
Adetayo Kasim, Ziv Shkedy, Sebastian Kaiser, Sepp Hochreiter, and Willem Talloen

Applied Meta-Analysis with R
Ding-Geng (Din) Chen and Karl E. Peace

Basic Statistics and Pharmaceutical Statistical Applications, Second Edition
James E. De Muth

Bayesian Adaptive Methods for Clinical Trials
Scott M. Berry, Bradley P. Carlin, J. Jack Lee, and Peter Muller

Bayesian Analysis Made Simple: An Excel GUI for WinBUGS
Phil Woodward

Bayesian Designs for Phase I–II Clinical Trials
Ying Yuan, Hoang Q. Nguyen, and Peter F. Thall

Bayesian Methods for Measures of Agreement
Lyle D. Broemeling

Bayesian Methods for Repeated Measures
Lyle D. Broemeling

Bayesian Methods in Epidemiology
Lyle D. Broemeling

Bayesian Methods in Health Economics
Gianluca Baio

Bayesian Missing Data Problems: EM, Data Augmentation and Noniterative Computation
Ming T. Tan, Guo-Liang Tian, and Kai Wang Ng

Bayesian Modeling in Bioinformatics
Dipak K. Dey, Samiran Ghosh, and Bani K. Mallick

Benefit-Risk Assessment in Pharmaceutical Research and Development
Andreas Sashegyi, James Felli, and Rebecca Noel

Published Titles

Benefit-Risk Assessment Methods in Medical Product Development: Bridging Qualitative and Quantitative Assessments
Qi Jiang and Weili He

Bioequivalence and Statistics in Clinical Pharmacology, Second Edition
Scott Patterson and Byron Jones

Biosimilars: Design and Analysis of Follow-on Biologics
Shein-Chung Chow

Biostatistics: A Computing Approach
Stewart J. Anderson

Cancer Clinical Trials: Current and Controversial Issues in Design and Analysis
Stephen L. George, Xiaofei Wang, and Herbert Pang

Causal Analysis in Biomedicine and Epidemiology: Based on Minimal Sufficient Causation
Mikel Aickin

Clinical and Statistical Considerations in Personalized Medicine
Claudio Carini, Sandeep Menon, and Mark Chang

Clinical Trial Data Analysis using R
Ding-Geng (Din) Chen and Karl E. Peace

Clinical Trial Methodology
Karl E. Peace and Ding-Geng (Din) Chen

Computational Methods in Biomedical Research
Ravindra Khattree and Dayanand N. Naik

Computational Pharmacokinetics
Anders Källén

Confidence Intervals for Proportions and Related Measures of Effect Size
Robert G. Newcombe

Controversial Statistical Issues in Clinical Trials
Shein-Chung Chow

Data Analysis with Competing Risks and Intermediate States
Ronald B. Geskus

Data and Safety Monitoring Committees in Clinical Trials
Jay Herson

Design and Analysis of Animal Studies in Pharmaceutical Development
Shein-Chung Chow and Jen-pei Liu

Design and Analysis of Bioavailability and Bioequivalence Studies, Third Edition
Shein-Chung Chow and Jen-pei Liu

Design and Analysis of Bridging Studies
Jen-pei Liu, Shein-Chung Chow, and Chin-Fu Hsiao

Design & Analysis of Clinical Trials for Economic Evaluation & Reimbursement: An Applied Approach Using SAS & STATA
Iftekhar Khan

Design and Analysis of Clinical Trials for Predictive Medicine
Shigeyuki Matsui, Marc Buyse, and Richard Simon

Design and Analysis of Clinical Trials with Time-to-Event Endpoints
Karl E. Peace

Design and Analysis of Non-Inferiority Trials
Mark D. Rothmann, Brian L. Wiens, and Ivan S. F. Chan

Difference Equations with Public Health Applications
Lemuel A. Moyé and Asha Seth Kapadia

DNA Methylation Microarrays: Experimental Design and Statistical Analysis
Sun-Chong Wang and Arturas Petronis

DNA Microarrays and Related Genomics Techniques: Design, Analysis, and Interpretation of Experiments
David B. Allison, Grier P. Page, T. Mark Beasley, and Jode W. Edwards

Dose Finding by the Continual Reassessment Method
Ying Kuen Cheung

Dynamical Biostatistical Models
Daniel Commenges and Hélène Jacqmin-Gadda

Elementary Bayesian Biostatistics
Lemuel A. Moyé

Empirical Likelihood Method in Survival Analysis
Mai Zhou

Published Titles

Essentials of a Successful Biostatistical Collaboration
Arul Earnest

Exposure–Response Modeling: Methods and Practical Implementation
Jixian Wang

Frailty Models in Survival Analysis
Andreas Wienke

Fundamental Concepts for New Clinical Trialists
Scott Evans and Naitee Ting

Generalized Linear Models: A Bayesian Perspective
Dipak K. Dey, Sujit K. Ghosh, and Bani K. Mallick

Handbook of Regression and Modeling: Applications for the Clinical and Pharmaceutical Industries
Daryl S. Paulson

Inference Principles for Biostatisticians
Ian C. Marschner

Interval-Censored Time-to-Event Data: Methods and Applications
Ding-Geng (Din) Chen, Jianguo Sun, and Karl E. Peace

Introductory Adaptive Trial Designs: A Practical Guide with R
Mark Chang

Joint Models for Longitudinal and Time-to-Event Data: With Applications in R
Dimitris Rizopoulos

Measures of Interobserver Agreement and Reliability, Second Edition
Mohamed M. Shoukri

Medical Biostatistics, Third Edition
A. Indrayan

Meta-Analysis in Medicine and Health Policy
Dalene Stangl and Donald A. Berry

Mixed Effects Models for the Population Approach: Models, Tasks, Methods and Tools
Marc Lavielle

Modeling to Inform Infectious Disease Control
Niels G. Becker

Modern Adaptive Randomized Clinical Trials: Statistical and Practical Aspects
Oleksandr Sverdlov

Monte Carlo Simulation for the Pharmaceutical Industry: Concepts, Algorithms, and Case Studies
Mark Chang

Multiregional Clinical Trials for Simultaneous Global New Drug Development
Joshua Chen and Hui Quan

Multiple Testing Problems in Pharmaceutical Statistics
Alex Dmitrienko, Ajit C. Tamhane, and Frank Bretz

Noninferiority Testing in Clinical Trials: Issues and Challenges
Tie-Hua Ng

Optimal Design for Nonlinear Response Models
Valerii V. Fedorov and Sergei L. Leonov

Patient-Reported Outcomes: Measurement, Implementation and Interpretation
Joseph C. Cappelleri, Kelly H. Zou, Andrew G. Bushmakin, Jose Ma. J. Alvir, Demissie Alemayehu, and Tara Symonds

Quantitative Evaluation of Safety in Drug Development: Design, Analysis and Reporting
Qi Jiang and H. Amy Xia

Quantitative Methods for Traditional Chinese Medicine Development
Shein-Chung Chow

Randomized Clinical Trials of Nonpharmacological Treatments
Isabelle Boutron, Philippe Ravaud, and David Moher

Randomized Phase II Cancer Clinical Trials
Sin-Ho Jung

Sample Size Calculations for Clustered and Longitudinal Outcomes in Clinical Research
Chul Ahn, Moonseong Heo, and Song Zhang

Published Titles

Sample Size Calculations in Clinical Research, Second Edition
Shein-Chung Chow, Jun Shao, and Hansheng Wang

Statistical Analysis of Human Growth and Development
Yin Bun Cheung

Statistical Design and Analysis of Clinical Trials: Principles and Methods
Weichung Joe Shih and Joseph Aisner

Statistical Design and Analysis of Stability Studies
Shein-Chung Chow

Statistical Evaluation of Diagnostic Performance: Topics in ROC Analysis
Kelly H. Zou, Aiyi Liu, Andriy Bandos, Lucila Ohno-Machado, and Howard Rockette

Statistical Methods for Clinical Trials
Mark X. Norleans

Statistical Methods for Drug Safety
Robert D. Gibbons and Anup K. Amatya

Statistical Methods for Healthcare Performance Monitoring
Alex Bottle and Paul Aylin

Statistical Methods for Immunogenicity Assessment
Harry Yang, Jianchun Zhang, Binbing Yu, and Wei Zhao

Statistical Methods in Drug Combination Studies
Wei Zhao and Harry Yang

Statistical Testing Strategies in the Health Sciences
Albert Vexler, Alan D. Hutson, and Xiwei Chen

Statistics in Drug Research: Methodologies and Recent Developments
Shein-Chung Chow and Jun Shao

Statistics in the Pharmaceutical Industry, Third Edition
Ralph Buncher and Jia-Yeong Tsay

Survival Analysis in Medicine and Genetics
Jialiang Li and Shuangge Ma

Theory of Drug Development
Eric B. Holmgren

Translational Medicine: Strategies and Statistical Methods
Dennis Cosmatos and Shein-Chung Chow

Chapman & Hall/CRC Biostatistics Series

Analyzing Longitudinal Clinical Trial Data

A Practical Guide

Craig Mallinckrodt

Eli Lilly Research Laboratories

Indianapolis, Indiana, USA

Ilya Lipkovich

Quintiles

Durham, North Carolina, USA

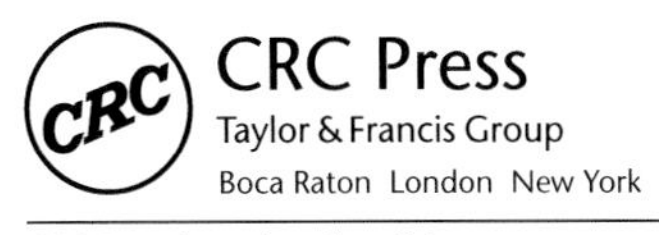

CRC Press is an imprint of the
Taylor & Francis Group, an **informa** business
A CHAPMAN & HALL BOOK

CRC Press
Taylor & Francis Group
6000 Broken Sound Parkway NW, Suite 300
Boca Raton, FL 33487-2742

First issued in paperback 2020

ISBN-13: 978-1-4987-6531-2 (hbk)
ISBN-13: 978-0-367-73658-3 (pbk)

Library of Congress Cataloging-in-Publication Data

Names: Mallinckrodt, Craig H., 1958- | Lipkovich, Ilya.
Title: Analyzing longitudinal clinical trial data / Craig Mallinckrodt and Ilya Lipkovich.
Description: Boca Raton : CRC Press, 2017. | Includes bibliographical references.
Identifiers: LCCN 2016032392 | ISBN 9781498765312 (hardback)
Subjects: LCSH: Clinical trials--Longitudinal studies.
Classification: LCC R853.C55 M33738 2017 | DDC 615.5072/4--dc23
LC record available at https://lccn.loc.gov/2016032392

Visit the Taylor & Francis Web site at
http://www.taylorandfrancis.com

and the CRC Press Web site at
http://www.crcpress.com

Contents

Section II Modeling the Observed Data

Section III Methods for Dealing with Missing Data

Section IV A Comprehensive Approach to Study Development and Analyses

Preface

The statistical theory relevant to analyses of longitudinal clinical trial data is extensive, and applying that theory in practice can be challenging. Therefore, this book focuses on the most relevant and current theory, using practical and easy-to-implement approaches for bringing that theory into routine practice. Emphasis is placed on examples with realistic data, and the programming code to implement the analyses is provided, usually in both SAS and R.

While this book focuses on analytic methods, analyses cannot be considered in isolation. Analyses must be considered as part of a holistic approach to study development and implementation. An industry working group recently proposed a study development process chart that begins with determining objectives, followed by choosing estimands, design, and analyses and assessing sensitivity (Phillips et al. 2016). This book is oriented in accordance with that process. Early chapters focus on objectives, estimands, and design. Subsequent chapters go into detail regarding analyses and sensitivity analyses. The intent of this book is to help facilitate an integrated understanding of key concepts from across the study development process through an example-oriented approach. It is this holistic approach to analysis planning and a focus on practical implementation that sets this text apart from existing texts.

Section I includes an introductory chapter along with chapters discussing estimands and key considerations in choosing them, study design considerations, introduction of the example data sets, and a chapter on key aspects of mixed-effects model theory. Section II covers key concepts and considerations applicable to modeling the observed data, including choice of the dependent variable, accounting for covariance between repeated measurements, modeling mean trends over time, modeling covariates, model checking and validation, and a chapter on modeling categorical data. Section III focuses on accounting for missing data, which is an inevitable problem in clinical trials. Section IV integrates key ideas from Sections I to III to illustrate a comprehensive approach to study development and analyses of realistic data sets.

Throughout this book, example data sets are used to illustrate and explain key analyses and concepts. These data sets were constructed by selecting patients from actual clinical trial data sets and manipulating the observations in ways useful for illustration. By using small data sets, readers can more easily understand exactly what an analysis does and how it does it. For the comprehensive study development and analysis example in Section IV, two data sets contrived from actual clinical trial data are used to further illustrate key points for implementing an overall analytic strategy that includes sensitivity analyses and model checking.

Craig Mallinckrodt
Eli Lilly Research Laboratories, Indianapolis, Indiana

Ilya Lipkovich
Quintiles, Durham, North Carolina

Acknowledgments

We would like to thank the Drug Information Association Scientific Working Group on missing data. We have benefited significantly from many discussions within the group and from our individual discussions with other group members. In this book, we have frequently cited work from the group and from its individual members. We especially thank Lei Xu, James Roger, Bohdana Ratitch, Michael O'Kelly, and Geert Molenberghs for their specific contributions to this book.

List of Tables

List of Figures

List of Code Fragments

Section I

Background and Setting

Section I begins with an introductory chapter covering the settings to be addressed in this book. Chapter 2 discusses trial objectives and defines and discusses estimands. Study design considerations are discussed in Chapter 3, focusing on methods to minimize missing data. Chapter 4 introduces the data sets used in example analyses. Chapter 5 covers key aspects of mixed-effects model theory.

Some readers may at least initially skip Chapter 5 and refer back to it as needed when covering later chapters. Other readers may benefit from this review of mixed-effect models prior to moving to later chapters.

1

Introduction

The evidence to support new medicines, devices, or other medical interventions is based primarily on randomized clinical trials. Many of these trials involve assessments taken at the start of treatment (baseline), followed by assessments taken repeatedly during the treatment period. In some cases, such as cancer trials, the primary outcome is whether or not some important event occurred during the assessment intervals. These outcomes can be summarized by the time to the event, or as a percentage of patients experiencing the event at or before some landmark time point. Alternatively, the multiple post-baseline assessments can all be used in a longitudinal, repeated measures framework, which can either focus on a landmark time point or consider outcomes across time points. This book focuses on the longitudinal, repeated measures framework.

With multiple post-baseline assessments per subject, linear mixed-effects models and generalized linear mixed-effect models provide useful analytic frameworks for continuous and categorical outcomes, respectively. Important modeling considerations within these frameworks include how to model the correlations between the measurements; how to model means over time; if, and if so, how to account for covariates; what endpoint to choose (actual value, change from baseline, or percent change from baseline); and how to specify and verify the assumptions in the chosen model. In addition, missing data is an incessant problem in longitudinal clinical trials. The fundamental problem caused by missing data is that the balance provided by randomization is lost if, as is usually the case, the subjects who discontinue differ in regards to the outcome of interest from those who complete the study. This imbalance can lead to bias in the comparisons between treatment groups (NRC 2010).

Data modeling decisions should not be considered in isolation. These decisions should be made as part of the overall study development process, because how to best analyze data depends on what the analysis is trying to accomplish and the circumstances in which the analysis is conducted. Therefore, study development decisions and data modeling decisions begin with considering the decisions to be made from the trial, which informs what objectives need to be addressed. Study objectives inform what needs to be estimated, which in turn informs the design, which in turn informs the analyses (Garrett et al. 2015; Mallinckrodt et al. 2016; Phillips et al. 2016).

The decisions made from a clinical trial vary by, among other things, stage of development. Phase II trials are typically used by drug development decision makers to determine proof of concept or to choose doses for subsequent studies. Phase III, confirmatory, studies typically serve a diverse audience and therefore must address diverse objectives (Leuchs et al. 2015). For example, regulators render decisions regarding whether or not the drug under study should be granted a marketing authorization. Drug developers and regulators must collaborate to develop labeling language that accurately and clearly describe the risks and benefits of approved drugs. Payers must decide if/where a new drug belongs on its formulary list. Prescribers must decide for whom the new drug should be prescribed and must inform patients and care givers what to expect. Patients and care givers must decide if they want to take the drug that has been prescribed.

These diverse decisions necessitate diverse objectives and therefore diverse targets of estimation, and a variety of analyses. For example, fully understanding a drug's benefits requires understanding its effects when taken as directed (efficacy) and as actually taken (effectiveness) (Mallinckrodt et al. 2016). As will be discussed in detail in later chapters, different analyses are required for these different targets of estimation.

It is important that the study development process be iterative so that considerations from downstream aspects can help inform upstream decisions. For example, clearly defined objectives and estimands lead to clarity in what parameters are to be estimated, which leads to clarity about the merits of the various analytic alternatives. However, an understanding of the strengths and limitations of various analytic methods is needed to understand what trial design and trial conduct features are necessary to provide optimum data for the situation at hand. Moreover, for any one trial, with its diverse objectives and estimands, only one design can be chosen. This design may be well-suited to some of the estimands and analyses but less well-suited to others.

Therefore, an integrated understanding of objectives, estimands, design, and analyses are required to develop, implement, and interpret results from a comprehensive analysis plan. The intent of this book is to help facilitate this integrated understanding among practicing statisticians via an example-oriented approach.

2

Objectives and Estimands—Determining What to Estimate

2.1 Introduction

Detailed discussion of estimands is relatively new to clinical trial literature, but very important. Estimands bridge the gap between study objectives and statistical methods (Phillips et al. 2016). The importance of estimands was highlighted in the National Research Council's (NRC) expert panel report that was commissioned by the Food and Drug Administration (FDA) (NRC 2010). Although the report focused on the problem of missing data, their recommendations set forth an overarching framework for the analysis of longitudinal clinical trial data.

Until recently, many protocols had general objectives such as "To compare the efficacy and safety of…." Such statements give little guidance to the designers of the studies and can lead to statistical analyses that do not address the intended question (Phillips et al. 2016). Estimands link study objectives and the analysis methods by more precisely defining what is to be estimated and how that quantity will be interpreted (Phillips et al. 2016). This provides clarity on what data needs to be collected and how that data should be analyzed and interpreted.

Conceptually, an estimand is simply the true population quantity of interest (NRC 2010); this is specific to a particular parameter, time point, and population (also sometimes referred to as the intervention effect).

Phillips et al. (2016) used an example similar to the one below to illustrate the key considerations in defining the intervention effect component of estimands. Consider a randomized, two-arm (Drug A and Drug B) trial in patients with type 2 diabetes mellitus. The primary endpoint is mean change from baseline to Week 24 in HbA1c levels. Assessments are taken at baseline and at Weeks 4, 8, 12, 16, and 24. For ethical reasons, patients are switched to rescue medication if their HbA1c values are above a certain threshold. Regardless of rescue medication use, all patients are intended to be assessed for the 24-week study duration.

TABLE 2.1

Three Estimands of Interest in an Example Trial

Estimand	Intervention Effect
1	Population-average effect regardless of what treatment was actually received; i.e., effect of treatment policy. Includes data after initiation of rescue treatment
2	Population-average effect attributable to the initially randomized medications; i.e., free from the confounding effects of rescue medication, and which accounts for reduction or loss of effect after discontinuation of the randomized treatment
3	Population-average effect if all patients remain on the initially randomized treatment throughout the study; i.e., effect if patients who switched to rescue would have remained on their randomized treatment

Table 2.1 outlines three of the estimands that can be defined for this trial. Each estimand is based on all randomized patients at the planned endpoint of the trial. However, as detailed in subsequent sections, each estimand implies different data to be included and potentially different analysis methods. Simply specifying the objective as assessing mean change from baseline to Week 24 does not distinguish between these three estimands.

Although estimands are often discussed in the literature as part of dealing with missing data, the above considerations exist even if all the data intended to be collected were indeed observed. However, further complexity does arise from the missing data caused by patients failing to adhere to the protocol specified procedures. Patients may fail to adhere on an intermittent basis, being compliant with protocol procedures and having outcome assessments during some treatment intervals, but not all. Early discontinuation (dropout) from the trial and the missing data that can result from it is a more frequent and more troublesome problem. Missing data issues are covered in detail in Section III.

With the diversity in medical research and the many clinical trial scenarios that exist, consensus on a universally best estimand is neither realistic nor desirable. Therefore, attention has turned to how to choose estimands (Mallinckrodt et al. 2016). Phillips et al. (2016) proposed a study development process chart similar to the one depicted in Figure 2.1. As the chart illustrates, choice of the primary estimand is informed by the decisions to be made from the trial and the objectives needed to inform these decisions. Although the general approach is to move from the top of the chart to the bottom, the arrows point in both directions. The study development process proceeds in an iterative manner so that interactions between the various components can be considered (Phillips et al. 2016). Importantly, the chart makes clear that in order to determine how best to analyze clinical trial data, it is important to first consider the trial objectives and the estimands needed to be estimated in order to address those objectives.

Trial objectives are typically driven by the decisions to be made from the trial results (Mallinckrodt et al. 2016). In Chapter 1, it was noted that the decisions to be made from a trial depend in part on stage of development. Phase II trials

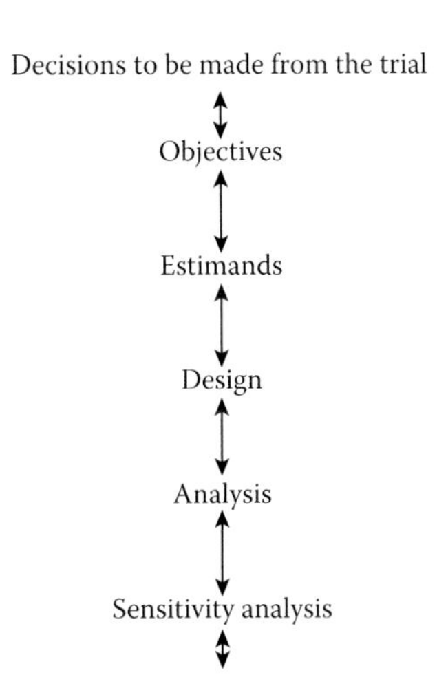

FIGURE 2.1
Study development process chart.

typically inform drug development decisions. Phase III, confirmatory studies typically inform a diverse audience, including the sponsor, multiple regulatory agencies, dozens of disparate health technology assessment groups (payers), prescribers, patients, journal editors and reviewers, along with other researchers (Leuchs et al. 2015; Mallinckrodt et al. 2016).

Specific estimands are as numerous and varied as the clinical trials scenarios in which they are applied. However, estimands can be grouped in several meaningful ways. For example, at the most conceptual level, estimands can be divided into two general categories based on adherence to protocol-defined interventions: (1) Efficacy is the effects of the drug if taken as directed; that is, the effects if patients adhere to the protocol-defined interventions. (2) Effectiveness is the effects of the drug as actually taken; that is, the effects without regard to adherence to the protocol-defined interventions (Mallinckrodt et al. 2012, 2014; Leuchs et al. 2015). However, the efficacy and effectiveness nomenclature does not make sense for safety outcomes. Therefore, a more general terminology is de jure (if taken as directed) and de facto (as actually taken) (Carpenter et al. 2013). The estimands introduced in Table 2.1 can be categorized according to this nomenclature. Again, each of these estimands involves the difference versus control in change to the planned endpoint of the trial, in all randomized patients.

- *Estimand 1* is the change due to the treatments as actually taken, a de facto (effectiveness) estimand. The inference target is the treatment regimens; that is, Drug A plus rescue versus Drug B plus rescue.
- *Estimand 2* is the change due to the initially randomized treatments as actually taken, a de facto (effectiveness) estimand. The inference

target is the initially randomized treatments; that is, Drug A versus Drug B.

- *Estimand 3* is the change due to the initially randomized treatments if taken as directed, a de jure (efficacy) estimand. The inference target is the initially randomized treatments.

It is important to differentiate estimand 3, which is based on all randomized patients, from a similar de jure estimand that is based on completers—that is, conditional on having been adherent. The completers estimand is limited for inference because it does not preserve the initial randomization. In contrast, estimand 3 includes all randomized patients. Therefore, inferences and parameter estimates apply to all patients in the population, not merely to those who were doing well enough to remain adherent, as is the case for compeleters analyses.

2.2 Fundamental Considerations in Choosing Estimands

Given the diversity in clinical settings and decisions to be made from clinical trial data, no universally best primary estimand exists, and therefore multiple estimands are likely to be of interest for any one trial (Mallinckrodt et al. 2012, 2014, 2016; Garrett et al. 2015; Leuchs et al. 2015; Phillips et al. 2016).

Each of the three estimands defined in Section 2.1 have strengths and limitations. Estimand 3, the de jure estimand, can be considered hypothetical (i.e., counterfactual) for groups of patients because treatment effects are assessed as if taken as directed when in any meaningfully sized group some patients will not adhere (NRC 2010). Therefore, de jure estimands assess what is possible to achieve in a group of patients, not what actually was achieved. However, de jure estimands assess what to expect if patients are adherent—and in most clinical settings the majority of patients are adherent (Mallinckrodt et al. 2014). In addition, patients are advised to take their medication as directed; therefore, it is important to assess what would happen if a medication were taken as directed so that optimal directions can be developed (Mallinckrodt et al. 2016).

De facto estimands can be considered counterfactual for individual patients because treatment effects are assessed from a mix of adherent and nonadherent patients, but each patient is either adherent or not adherent, no patient is both. On the other hand, de facto estimands can provide useful estimates of what to expect from the group as a whole (CHMP 2010; NRC 2010).

Most of the discussion on de jure and de facto estimands has been in the context of assessing drug benefit. However, estimands for assessing drug risk are also important. Consider a drug that has the adverse effect of increasing blood pressure. Some patients may become hypertensive and discontinue study medication and/or take medication to treat the high blood pressure, with subsequent return to normal blood pressure. De facto estimands would reflect the patients' return to normal, thereby suggesting no change at the planned endpoint of the trial. De jure estimands would not reflect a return to normal and would reflect increases at endpoint because had the patients been adherent they would likely have continued to be hypertensive (Mallinckrodt et al. 2016).

2.3 Design Considerations in Choosing Estimands

2.3.1 Missing Data Considerations

Universal agreement exists that clinical trials should aim to minimize missing data, thereby maximizing the portion of the intended data that was actually collected. The intent is to maximize adherence to the initially assigned treatments in order to minimize reliance of inferences on untestable assumptions about the missing data (Verbeke and Molenberghs 2000; Molenberghs and Kenward 2007; CHMP 2010; NRC 2010; Mallinckrodt 2013; Ratitch and O'Kelly 2014). These considerations have often been in the context of de jure estimands. However, the impact of maximizing retention on de facto estimands is also important (Leuchs et al. 2015; Mallinckrodt et al. 2016).

Increasing adherence is likely to increase benefit from the drug as actually taken, thereby resulting in more favorable outcomes for de facto estimands. If the measures used to engender adherence in the clinical trial are not feasible in clinical practice the trial could yield biased estimates of effectiveness relative to the conditions under which the drug would be used.

Specifically, assessment of de facto estimands often entail using adherence as part of the primary outcome. For example, patients that discontinue study drug can be considered a treatment failure regardless of the observed outcomes. Therefore, it is important to consider the degree to which treatment adherence decisions in the clinical trial match adherence decisions in clinical practice. These generalizability considerations may be especially important in trials with placebo and/or blinding because these factors are never present in clinical practice (Mallinckrodt 2013; Mallinckrodt et al. 2016).

2.3.2 Rescue Medication Considerations

Whether or not data should be collected after discontinuation of initially randomized study medication or initiation or rescue medication, and whether that data should be included in an analysis are critically important considerations.

Use of rescue medications for patients not adequately responding to the initially randomized medications has been suggested because this provides an assessment of pragmatic effectiveness and can reduce dropout (NRC 2010; Fleming 2011; Permutt 2015a). The need for rescue therapy is also partly motivated by arguments for ethical patient care, especially in placebo-controlled trials. However, rescue medications can mask or exaggerate the efficacy and safety effects of the initially assigned treatments, thereby biasing estimates of the effects of the originally assigned medication (Buncher and Tsay 2005; Holubkov et al. 2009; Henning 2011; Mallinckrodt et al. 2012, 2014; Leuchs et al. 2015). In placebo-controlled trials, if rescue therapy is beneficial and post-rescue data are included in the analysis, the treatment effect is likely to be substantially diminished compared to the effect if post-rescue data are not included (Mallinckrodt et al. 2016).

Another consideration is that readily available rescue medications may reduce study discontinuation, but could increase discontinuation from the initially randomized medication, which would of course be counter to the primary goal of maximizing retention on the initial medications (Mallinckrodt 2013). This issue may be particularly important in placebo-controlled trials where patients are aware that they may be randomized to an ineffective treatment but switching to rescue guarantees use of an effective treatment (Mallinckrodt et al. 2016).

With estimand 1 (de facto, treatment regimens), data after discontinuation of the initially randomized medication and/or addition of rescue medication are included in the analyses. The study protocol should specify the rescue treatment(s) and how they are administered, or specify that rescue treatment is at the discretion of the investigator. The protocol should also specify if rescue treatment is provided by the sponsor or if marketed product is to be used.

As noted above, estimand 1 is with regard to treatment policies or regimens (NRC 2010; Mallinckrodt et al. 2012; Leuchs et al. 2015). Estimand 1 is often seen as an assessment of pragmatic effectiveness (Permutt 2015a). As with estimand 2, generalizability must be considered. For estimand 1, a design comparing an experimental drug plus rescue versus a standard of care plus rescue may be appropriate. However, designs with placebo control (e.g., experimental drug plus rescue versus placebo plus rescue) may be less appropriate in some settings. Decisions regarding adherence and need for rescue in double-blind, placebo-controlled settings may not be as applicable to general clinical practice as the decisions made when all patients receive active medication. Simply put, placebo is never used in general clinical settings; therefore, when assessing pragmatic effectiveness, placebo control may not be ideal (Mallinckrodt et al. 2016). Moreover, the most relevant questions in early research and initial regulatory reviews, especially for placebo-controlled trials, are often about the effects of the investigational drugs, not treatment policies (Mallinckrodt et al. 2012; Mallinckrodt 2013).

The ICH E9 guidance is often cited when justifying choice of a primary analytic approach (http://www.ich.org/fileadmin/Public_Web_Site/ICH_Products/Guidelines/Efficacy/E9/Step4/E9_Guideline.pdf). This guidance emphasizes the ITT principle, which is defined as "the principle that asserts that the effect of a treatment policy can be best assessed by evaluating on the basis of the intention to treat a subject (i.e., the planned treatment regimen) rather than the actual treatment given. It has the consequence that subjects allocated to a treatment group should be followed up, assessed and analyzed as members of that group irrespective of their compliance to the planned course of treatment."

Thus, ITT has two parts, the patients to include and the data for each patient to include (Permutt 2015a; Mallinckrodt et al. 2016). Some deviations from one or both aspects of the intent-to-treat principles are routinely accepted (Permutt 2015a). The guidance is clear on the need to include all randomized patients and that all data should be included, but it does not specifically address data after initiation of rescue treatment.

Rescue therapy is specifically addressed in ICH E10, Section 2.1.5.2.2 (http://www.ich.org/fileadmin/Public_Web_Site/ICH_Products/Guidelines/Efficacy/E10/Step4/E10_Guideline.pdf). In referring to trials with rescue, E10 states: "In such cases, the need to change treatment becomes a study endpoint." Thus, according to E10, post-rescue data need not be included in the primary analysis.

It is important to recognize that the ICH guidance was developed before the NRC report (NRC 2010) that focused on the need for clarity on estimands. The E9 guidance refers to ITT as the best way to assess treatment policies/regimens. It does not address inference for the initially randomized medications. Considerations of estimands today are often more nuanced than anticipated by the 1998 ICH guidance. An addendum to the E9 guidance specific to choices of estimands is anticipated in 2016 or soon thereafter.

A reasonable approach is to maintain the principles of ITT, but employ a slight modification to address the need for greater specificity (Mallinckrodt et al. 2016). In this modified approach to ITT, all randomized patients are again included, thereby maintaining consistency with the first tenant of ITT. The second tenant of ITT is modified to mean that all data—*relevant to the estimand*—are included. For example, when evaluating estimand 2 (de facto, initially randomized treatments) and estimand 3 (de jure, initially randomized treatments), post-rescue data are not relevant and are therefore not included in the analysis, thereby avoiding the confounding effects of rescue medication.

O'Neill and Temple (2012) noted that estimand 1 may be a more common choice for the primary estimand in outcomes trials where the presence/absence of a major health event is the endpoint and/or the intervention is intended to modify the disease process. Symptomatic trials (symptom severity is the endpoint) often use a primary estimand where the inferential target is the initially randomized treatments. In these scenarios the confounding from rescue medications is avoided by excluding data after discontinuation of study medication/initiation of rescue from the primary analysis.

2.4 Analysis Considerations

To understand the analytic implications in choice of estimand, first consider estimand 3, the de jure effects of the initially randomized medication. The intent of estimand 3 is to assess drug effects if all randomized patients were adherent, even though in any realistically sized trial there will be some patients who do not adhere. Although failure to adhere can be manifest in many ways, the most common scenario is that of missing data. Patients may discontinue the study and all study-related procedures prior to the planned time of the primary assessment. Patients may also discontinue the randomized study medication but remain in the study for follow-up assessments.

For estimand 3, data after discontinuation of the initially randomized study medication are not needed. That is, post-rescue/post-discontinuation data are not included, thereby avoiding the potentially confounding effects of rescue medication. However, some data intended to be collected are not available. Moreover, the reason(s) data are not available are usually related to outcome. That is, patients with poor outcomes are more likely to be missing than patients with good outcomes. This selection process means that the observed data are not a random sample of the data intended to be collected. Therefore, analysis of estimand 3 requires estimates of what would have happened if all patients were adherent, but this cannot be based on only those patients who *were* adherent.

Common analytic approaches for estimand 3 involve the assumption that data are missing at random (MAR). This assumption and other missing data considerations are covered in detail in Section III. Missing at random essentially means that conditional on the observed data, the statistical behavior (means, variances, etc.) of the unobserved data is the same as the observed data. Put another way, the unobserved data can be predicted in an unbiased manner from the observed data. Analytic approaches valid under MAR include likelihood-based analyses, multiple imputation of missing values followed by an analysis that would have been appropriate had the data been complete, and weighted generalized estimating equations. These analyses are covered in detail in Section III.

Given the reliance of these methods on assumptions about the missing data, which of course cannot be verified since the data are missing, sensitivity analyses are required to assess the degree to which inferences are dependent on the assumptions (Verbeke and Molenberghs 2000; NRC 2010; Mallinckrodt 2013).

Estimand 1 can be evaluated using analyses similar to estimand 3, with the exception that estimand 1 requires including post-rescue data (Permutt 2015a).

This has several important implications. First, the confounding effects of the rescue medication necessitate that inference is on the treatment regimens, not the individual treatments to which patients were randomized. In addition, including the post-rescue data means less data will be missing compared with that same scenario when not including post-rescue data.

Approaches to assessing estimand 2 often entail ascribing unfavorable outcomes to patients who discontinue the initially randomized medication or who need rescue medication, regardless of what outcomes were actually observed while the patients were adherent (Carpenter et al. 2013; Mallinckrodt 2013; Permutt 2015a). This approach has the compelling benefit of resulting in no missing data. And for symptomatic treatments that do not change the underlying disease process, it is intuitively sensible to assume that if patients can not adhere to a drug they will not benefit from it in the long run (O'Neill and Temple 2012).

However, the generalizability considerations noted in the section on design considerations are particularly important. Fully satisfactory assessments of effectiveness from clinical trials may be problematic (NRC 2010). Adherence decisions in the clinical trial setting must sufficiently match the decisions in clinical practice for the estimand to be useful. Placebo control and blinding in a clinical trial may result in adherence decisions different from what would be seen in clinical practice (Mallinckrodt et al. 2016).

Another consideration is exactly what value(s) to impute as unfavorable outcomes for nonadherent patients. Such imputations for continuous endpoints have historically been done using baseline observation carried forward (BOCF). However, single imputation approaches such as BOCF have a number of disadvantages that are discussed in Chapters 12 and 13, and more principled approaches are gaining favor (Kenward and Molenberghs 2009; Carpenter et al. 2013; Mallinckrodt 2013; Mallinckrodt et al. 2014).

Multiple imputation-based approaches to estimate parameters for and test hypotheses about de facto estimands have come into the literature recently. These methods have been referred to as controlled imputation or more specifically reference-based controlled imputation. See Chapter 18 for detailed descriptions of these approaches. However, the general approach is to use multiple imputation in a manner that accounts for the change in/discontinuation of treatment. In so doing, patients that discontinue from an experimental arm have values imputed as if they were in the reference (e.g., placebo arm). Depending on the exact implementation, imputed values can either reflect no pharmacologic benefit from the drug immediately upon discontinuation/rescue, a decaying benefit after discontinuation/rescue, or a constant benefit after discontinuation/rescue (Carpenter et al. 2013; Mallinckrodt et al. 2014).

For categorical endpoints, nonresponder imputation (NRI) has often been used, wherein all patients that discontinue initially randomized medication and/or initiate rescue medication are considered nonresponders, regardless of the observed outcome. The term NRI is somewhat of a misnomer.

The name implies explicit imputation of repeated (binary) measurements. In this context, NRI would have the same disadvantages as BOCF. However, NRI as commonly used does not involve imputation of repeated measures. Rather, there is a single endpoint per patient, reflecting treatment success or failure. Patients that remain adherent to the protocol-specified intervention and achieve the predefined level of response are considered a treatment success (responder) and patients that either fail to achieve the needed level of response or who deviate from the protocol-specified intervention are considered treatment failures.

As with continuous endpoints, the advantage of the treatment success/failure approach is that it yields complete data; and, the important caveat is that adherence decisions in the trial must be similar to the decisions that would be made in clinical practice if results are to be generalizable.

2.5 Multiple Estimands in the Same Study

The multifaceted nature of clinical trials is important to appreciate when considering estimands (Leuchs et al. 2015; Mallinckrodt et al. 2016). Within a trial, diverse objectives are often needed to inform the decisions of the diverse stakeholders (multiple regulatory agencies, dozens of health technology assessors/payers, prescribers, patients, caregivers, sponsors, other researchers, etc.). Even for a single stakeholder in a single trial it is often important to know what happens when a drug is taken as directed (de jure estimand) and to know what happens when the drug is taken as in actual practice (de facto estimand). Therefore, no single estimand is likely to best serve the interests of all stakeholders and de jure and de facto estimands will both be of interest (Mallinckrodt et al. 2012; Leuchs et al. 2015; Mallinckrodt et al. 2016).

The following example first described in Mallinckrodt et al. (2012) illustrates the benefits of assessing both de jure and de facto estimands in the same trial. Drug A and Drug B (or Dose A and Dose B of a drug) have equal effectiveness, but drug A has superior efficacy and Drug B has greater adherence. Even if effectiveness is the primary estimand, de jure estimands are needed to understand the differences in clinical profiles.

Dose/Drug A might be the best choice for patients with more severe illness because it has greater efficacy. Dose/Drug B might be best for patients with less severe illness and/or safety and tolerability concerns because it has greater adherence resulting from fewer side effects. A more nuanced understanding of efficacy and adherence could lead to additional investigation that could lead to more optimized patient outcomes. For example, subgroups of patients who especially benefit from or tolerate the high dose might be identified from the existing data or from a new trial (nonresponders to low dose).

Or, alternate dosing regimens that might improve the safety/tolerability of the high dose, such as titration, flexible, or split dosing (40 mg every 2 weeks rather than 80 mg every 4 weeks), could be investigated in subsequent trials (Mallinckrodt et al. 2016).

One approach to evaluating multiple estimands in the same study is to have some outcomes geared toward assessing a certain estimand(s) while other outcomes address other estimand(s). However, study designs and the data generated from them are often such that multiple estimands can be evaluated from the same outcome measure.

For example, estimand 1 could be assessed by including post-rescue data in the analysis in order to provide an evaluation of pragmatic effectiveness. Estimand 2 could be evaluated in the same trial by not including post-rescue data and defining discontinuation of the initial study medication or the need for rescue medication as treatment failure. Estimand 3 could also be evaluated from the same trial by not including post-rescue data and applying an appropriate analysis.

The ability to assess multiple estimands from the same outcome variable reinforces the need for clarity as to which estimand is addressed by each analysis. This in turn highlights the need for clarity on the assumptions, strengths, and limitations of analyses, which can vary from one estimand to another.

Even though multiple estimands can be assessed from the same outcome, the internal validity and external generalizability of those results will vary. Some designs are better suited to certain estimands than others. Therefore, choice of the primary estimand has a particularly important influence on choice of design.

2.6 Choosing the Primary Estimand

Historical precedent, especially for trials submitted to regulatory authorities in support of marketing authorizations, can influence choice of the primary estimand. However, fundamental understanding of key considerations should be the primary driver in choice of primary estimands.

In the iterative study development process outlined in Section 2.1, design and analysis considerations can influence objectives and estimands. For example, consider a short-term, acute phase clinical trial where extensive efforts to maximize adherence are expected to yield 95% of patients remaining on the initially assigned study medication. Given this highly controlled setting and strong adherence, a de jure primary estimand may be most relevant. However, in a long-term trial in an otherwise similar setting, the design may need to be more similar to clinical practice, with open-label treatment, rescue therapy, etc., in order to enroll patients willing to participate in a long-term study. The more pragmatic intent and design of the long-term study, along with the inevitable loss of adherence over time, are more consistent with a de facto primary estimand than a de jure primary estimand (Mallinckrodt et al. 2016).

Mallinckrodt et al. (2016) detailed another example of how other factors can influence choice of primary estimand. Consider a trial where focus is on effectiveness, but interest is in both estimand 1 and estimand 2; that is, results with and without post-rescue data are relevant. Also consider that in this scenario it is important to keep the sample size as small as possible either because patients are hard to recruit, or for ethical reasons it is important to limit exposure to placebo. Use of estimand 2 as the primary estimand is likely to result in greater power, which translates into smaller sample sizes and reduced exposure to placebo. If estimand 2 was chosen as the primary estimand, estimand 1 with post-rescue data may still be collected and used secondarily.

2.7 Summary

An iterative process should be used to choose estimands, beginning with the objectives required to address the needs of diverse stakeholders. No single estimand is likely to meet the needs of all stakeholders. De jure (efficacy) and de facto (effectiveness) estimands each have strengths and limitations, and fully understanding a drug's effects requires understanding results from both families of estimands.

Whether or not data after initiation of rescue medication should be included in the primary analysis depends on the estimand to be tested and the clinical setting. Including versus not including post-rescue data can have an important impact on results, and therefore sample size implications and total exposure to placebo must be carefully considered.

There are many important nuances to understand about various analyses as they are applied to different estimands. These nuances are the focus of Sections II, III, and IV. However, one factor is common to all analyses for all estimands: the analysis must either entail modeling assumptions about missing data or use the fact that data are missing to ascribe an outcome. Therefore, minimizing missing data reduces sensitivity to missing data assumptions for de jure estimands, but it is also important to consider generalizability of results for de facto estimands if efforts to maximize adherence in the trial are not feasible in clinical practice. The next chapter discusses trial design and conduct for limiting missing data.

3

Study Design—Collecting the Intended Data

3.1 Introduction

The trial design element of the study development process depicted in Figure 2.1 can be parsed into two distinct components: (1) determining what data is to be collected and (2) ensuring the intended data is collected. The intent of this chapter is not to provide a broad discussion of both components. This chapter addresses the second component of ensuring that the intended data is collected. The focus is on practical aspects of preventing missing data, which is important regardless of the specific design—regardless of what data was intended to be collected. For general texts on clinical trial design, see Piantadosi (2005).

The consequences of even moderate amounts of missing data can be noteworthy and the impact of higher rates of missing data can be profound (Mallinckrodt 2013). Therefore, maximizing the number of participants who are maintained on the protocol-specified interventions until the outcome data are collected is the single most important thing that can be done to mitigate the impact of missing data (NRC 2010). That is, the best way to handle missing data is to prevent it.

Studies with more missing data than expected are suspect for poor conduct in general (LaVange and Permutt 2015). These authors noted that from a regulatory perspective, aberrantly high rates of missing data raise questions about what else may have gone awry. If a surprising number of patients miss their scheduled visits, then other aspects of patient compliance or study conduct in general may be questioned. Similarly, if a surprising number of patients are lost to follow-up with little attempt at finding out why or encouraging those still willing to participate to reconsider a decision to drop out, the study objectives may not have been adequately explained to the patients at the time of their consent, or the enrollment criteria may have been applied inconsistently, with some patients enrolled that should not have been and vice versa. A key component of study planning is to anticipate the eventualities of missed visits and attrition during the treatment and follow-up periods (LaVange and Permutt 2015).

However, minimizing missing data is not easy. Strategies for maximizing retention are difficult to study directly and what evidence there is comes from between study comparisons that are subject to confounding factors that can mask or exaggerate differences in retention due to a design feature or trial conduct strategy (Mallinckrodt 2013).

Mindful of these limitations, recent guidance on preventing and treating missing data (NRC 2010; Hughes et al. 2012; LaVange and Permutt 2015) provided a number of suggestions on ways to minimize missing data. An overview of these suggestions is provided in the following sections. Additional details on these approaches can be found elsewhere (Mallinckrodt 2013).

3.2 Trial Design

Some of the trial design options to limit missing data considered by the NRC expert panel (NRC 2010) include:

- Run-in periods and enrichment designs
- Randomized withdrawal studies
- Choice of target population
- Titration and flexible dosing
- Add-on studies
- Shorter follow-up
- Rescue medications
- Definition of ascertainable outcomes

One of the complicating aspects of lowering rates of missing data is that design options to maximize retention often entail trade-offs. A design feature that reduces the probability of dropout is likely to have consequences in other aspects of the trial. Understanding and managing the trade-offs is key to picking appropriate options for a particular scenario. The following discussion focuses on general aspects of these trade-offs. Given the idiosyncratic nature of missing data and its impacts, it is important to assess the pros and cons of the various options in the specific situation at hand.

Treatments typically do not work equally well in all patients. If there is a systematic trend for some groups of patients to have better outcomes, this knowledge can be used to reduce dropout by testing the treatment in the subpopulation with the most favorable outcome or greatest likelihood of adherence/compliance.

Selecting participants prior to randomization that are thought to have more favorable responses or other attributes is termed "enrichment" (NRC 2010). Run-in designs have an initial (run-in) period in which a subset of patients is selected based on initial response. The key difference between run-in and enrichment designs is that the active treatment is used to identify the subset of participants in a run-in design whereas prior knowledge is used in enrichment designs (NRC 2010). The trade-off with enrichment and run-in designs is that inference is restricted to the subset of patients meeting randomization criteria. Inferences do not apply to the general population because the patients available for randomization are expected to have more favorable responses than the population as a whole. For additional information on and descriptions of run-in periods and enrichment designs, see Fedorov and Liu (2007) and Temple (2005).

A randomized withdrawal design is a specific form of run-in design, typically having a longer run-in phase because the goal is to identify patients that sustain an adequate efficacy response and to then test whether or not continued treatment is needed. However, many of the same design considerations and trade-offs apply to both randomized withdrawal and run-in designs (Mallinckrodt 2013).

Protocols that allow flexible dosing to accommodate individual differences in response may reduce the frequency of dropout due of adverse events or inadequate efficacy (NRC 2010). Dose titration is when patients initially take a drug at a dose lower than the target or posited optimal dose in order to reduce adverse events and improve initial tolerability, which can reduce dropout. Flexible dosing may include dose titration, but also allows subsequent dosing adjustments. The basic idea is to set a target dose that patients may titrate to or begin initially. Dose increases above the target dose are allowed for patients with inadequate initial response, and decreases below the target dose are allowed if safety or tolerability concerns emerge (Mallinckrodt 2013).

In titration and flexible dose trials, inference is on the dosing regimen(s), not on specific doses. Hence, flexible dosing is most applicable to those situations in which inferences on dose response or specific doses are not required. However, flexible dosing may more accurately reflect actual clinical practice in many scenarios (Mallinckrodt 2013).

Add-on studies include designs for which in addition to receiving a standard of care, patients are randomized to an experimental drug versus control (usually placebo). Add-on designs may reduce dropout due to lack of efficacy and in many instances may reflect actual clinical practice (NRC 2010). However, inference is on the dosing regimen, not on the experimental drug as mono-therapy. In addition, add-on designs generally target a subset of the population with inadequate response to the standard of care because patients doing well on the background treatment are not good candidates to assess the benefits of the experimental drug (NRC 2010).

Shorter follow-up periods may lead to lower dropout rates compared with longer follow-up periods, because patients have less opportunity to experience those events that lead to dropout. In addition, shorter follow-up reduces the overall burden on patients because the number of clinical visits may be reduced, thereby fostering greater compliance with the planned assessments (Mallinckrodt 2013).

However, shorter follow-up may not be feasible because trials of specific duration are often required. In addition, shorter follow-up periods may be less efficient in those instances where the treatment benefits increase over time and are therefore larger as the duration of assessment increases (Mallinckrodt 2013). Use of shorter follow-up is essentially trading off participants who respond more slowly to study treatment with participants who drop out early. Past experience from similar trials can guide evaluation of this trade-off (NRC 2010). A potential compromise is to have the primary assessment based on shorter follow-up, but patients continue in the trial and assessments at subsequent times are secondary (NRC 2010).

Use of rescue medication was cited by the NRC expert panel (NRC 2010) as a potential means to reduce missing data. However, this approach has important implications for what estimands can be evaluated. For a complete discussion on the considerations for use of rescue medications, see Chapter 2. Importantly, if rescue medication is provided as part of the protocol, care must be taken so that availability of rescue medication does not increase discontinuation of randomized study medication (Mallinckrodt et al. 2016).

Another highlighted recommendation from the NRC guidance (NRC 2010), closely linked to use of rescue medications, was collecting follow-up data. Specifically, the panel recommended that: "Trial sponsors should continue to collect information on key outcomes on participants who discontinue their protocol-specified intervention in the course of the study, except in those cases for which compelling cost-benefit analysis argues otherwise, and this information should be recorded and used in the analysis."

The NRC guidance goes on to state that benefits of collecting follow-up data include being able to assess the impact of subsequent treatments on outcomes, to assess adverse events after discontinuation of the trial, and to help verify assumptions made about what outcomes would have been had treatment continued. If the primary estimand is to test treatment regimens that include the experimental medication and rescue medication, follow-up data is part of the primary estimand.

Given the idiosyncratic nature of missing data and its consequences, it is important to consider the specific circumstances of a trial. Following patients to monitor resolution of adverse effects is clearly necessary for ethical and scientific reasons, and is already done routinely. Sponsors should consider whether patients who discontinue due to adverse effects should be given a full assessment battery, only safety assessments, or some reduced assessment battery including safety and some efficacy outcomes (Mallinckrodt 2013). For assessing the effects of rescue treatments on outcomes, the follow-up data will often be of an observational nature—not arising from randomized comparisons. Therefore, constructing meaningful statistical comparisons may not be straightforward (Mallinckrodt 2013).

It is important to recognize that collecting follow-up data does not reduce the amount of missing data for some estimands. Therefore, collecting follow-up data should not be seen as a substitute for the most important objective of retaining as many patients as possible on the initially randomized medications (Mallinckrodt 2013).

Primary outcome measures that require invasive procedures (e.g., liver biopsies, endoscopies) are likely to result in significant missing data, and such outcome measures should be avoided whenever possible (NRC 2010). Missing data can also arise from the use of outcomes that are undefined for some patients. Therefore, primary outcomes that are ascertainable for all randomized participants should be used (NRC 2010).

One approach that may be useful in a variety of settings is to define a composite outcome that includes adherence as part of the outcome; for example, outcomes that incorporate death, or study drug discontinuation or the need for rescue medication as part of the outcome (NRC 2010; LaVange and Permutt 2015). The composite outcome may have as one component an ordinal or continuous outcome. The death and adherence components of the composite can be incorporated by ranking a continuous outcome score in a manner that assigns bad outcomes to applicable patients, regardless of the outcomes that were observed (LaVange and Permutt 2015).

Another common approach is to dichotomize the continuous outcome based on criteria for a clinically meaningful response. Patients that meet the response criteria and are adherent to study medication are considered a treatment success. Patients that did not meet response criteria, or who discontinue study medication, are considered treatment failures (LaVange and Permutt 2015).

These approaches are appealing in that they result in no missing data. However, composite outcomes should not be used to avoid the missing data if it compromises the clinical relevance of the outcome (Fleming 2011).

As detailed in Chapter 2, when including adherence as part of an outcome, it is important that the generalizability of the results is justified. For example, in a double-blind and placebo-controlled study, the decisions patients and doctors make about adhering to randomized medication may not reflect the effectiveness of the medication that will be seen in actual clinical practice. Hence, the estimator may be a biased estimate of the intended effectiveness estimand.

3.3 Trial Conduct

Trial conduct approaches to limit missing data include:

- Limiting trial burden on participants
- Providing incentives to patients and investigative sites for trial completion

- Train and educate sites and patients on the importance of complete data
- Monitoring and reporting completion rates during the trial
- Do not discontinue non-compliant patients

Trials should limit participants' burden and inconvenience in data collection. However, collecting less data means getting less information. Therefore study teams need to balance the conflicting goals of getting the most information possible from a trial and reducing patient burden in order to increase retention (NRC 2010).

Some ways to reduce patient burden include: (1) minimize the number of visits and assessments; (2) avoid redundant data collection and collect the minimum amount of information needed to address study objectives; (3) gather data efficiently using user-friendly case report forms and direct data capture (that does not require a clinic visit) whenever feasible; and, (4) allow sufficiently large time windows for assessments (NRC 2010; Mallinckrodt 2013).

Clinic visits can be made less burdensome by making the overall experience more pleasant via a welcoming environment, friendly staff that respects participant's time, provisions for transportation and availability of on-site diversions for children and/or provisions for child care. Sending visit reminders, as is routinely done in clinical practice, can also help avoid missed visits (NRC 2010).

Retention may also be increased by providing incentives for completing treatment. Some possible incentives include providing effective treatments or extension phases to participants that complete the trial (NRC 2010).

Other trial conduct features to consider include basing site/investigator selection on rates of complete data while patients are in the trial and in rates of patients who complete the trial (NRC 2010). Training provided to sites and patients on the study procedures should emphasize the importance of complete data. In those instances when follow-up data are collected, also emphasize the difference between discontinuing the study treatment and discontinuing data collection (NRC 2010).

Data completeness can be improved by monitoring and reporting it during the course of the trial. The NRC guidance (NRC 2010) suggested that the information from these assessments be available at investigator meetings and on study websites in order to create a climate that encourages study completion. Monitoring can also identify poorly performing sites and the need for remediation or site closure (Mallinckrodt 2013).

Patient education should include how their data is important to overall scientific knowledge. This information could be included in a patient video that also covers key study procedures. Participant engagement and retention can be enhanced through newsletters, regularly updated websites, study-branded gifts, regular expressions of thanks, and solicitation of input regarding relevant issues of study conduct (NRC 2010; Mallinckrodt 2013).

Investigator payments can be structured to reward completions. The NRC guidance (NRC 2010) notes that it is acceptable and generally advisable to link a final payment to completion of forms at a study closeout visit. However, the guidance goes on to caution that it is unethical for patients to continue a study if it exposes them to undue risk. But if there are minimal risks to the participant associated with data collection, it may be acceptable to provide financial incentives to continue to collect data, whether or not the participant continues treatment.

The NRC guidance (NRC 2010) also summarized what investigators and site personnel can do to reduce the amount of missing data. Suggestions included emphasizing the importance of completion (and follow-up data, if relevant) during informed consent and informed withdrawal of consent, and providing appropriate incentives for participants. The Code of Federal Regulations requires that study participant compensation is neither coercive nor at the level that would present undue influence (21CFR 50.20). Most institutional review boards allow cash payments that are slightly back-loaded, retaining a small proportion as an incentive for completion (NRC 2010).

Often, trial sponsors discontinue patients who are not compliant, justifying this practice on grounds that non-compliant patients are not useful in evaluating the effects of the drug (LaVange and Permutt 2015). However, this can unnecessarily increase the amount of missing data. Alternatively, a variable can be created in the database to note compliance status. Data can be analyzed for all patients and for compliant patients only. Whatever the reason for the protocol violation, if the patient's safety is not at risk, then encouraging discontinuation should not be necessary (LaVange and Permutt 2015)

Again, the most important aspect is to prevent missing data. Replacing language encouraging discontinuation of protocol violators with strategies for encouraging compliance and minimizing attrition would go a long way to improving study conduct and optimizing data analysis (LaVange and Permutt 2015).

3.4 Summary

Objective evidence on how trial design and trial conduct alternatives influence rates of missing data is scarce. Nevertheless, recent literature provides general recommendations that are practical to implement and consistent with good science, even if their impact on missing data rates is not certain. Although minimizing missing data is important, trials cannot be designed with this lone goal in mind. Design features to maximize retention often involve trade-offs, and these trade-offs must be considered carefully.

After choosing a design that is appropriate for the study objectives and primary estimands, appropriate investigators and patients can be chosen and trained. Trial conduct can proceed mindful of conditions and strategies to maximize retention. Progress is monitored toward study-specific goals. Reasons for dropout other than adverse events and lack of efficacy can include patient decision, physician decision, protocol violation, and loss to follow-up. These reasons leave doubt about treatment-related causality and the impact the missing data may have on treatment comparisons. The ideal trial may be one in which the only reasons for discontinuing the initially randomized study drug are lack of efficacy, adverse events, and withdrawal of consent. Depending on the goals of the study, follow-up data after discontinuation of the initial study drug and/or initiation of rescue medications might be collected.

To achieve such disposition results, proper processes, case report forms, informed consents, data capture procedures, minimal patient burden, patient accommodations, etc., need to be in place. However, trial sponsors, sites, and patients also need to believe in the importance of complete data. Rigorous selection of sites and patients, combined with education, monitoring, and incentives can help in this regard. As LaVange and Permutt (2015) noted, a key in minimizing missing data is creating a culture wherein the importance of complete data is recognized.

Importantly, changing attitudes and behaviors regarding missing data will likely help increase retention in drug groups and control groups, whereas enrichment designs, flexible dosing and other design features may have greater impact on drug groups than on the placebo groups.

4

Example Data

4.1 Introduction

Throughout this book, analyses are illustrated using various example data sets. Data sets are chosen for particular scenarios to match data characteristics with the points and principles to be illustrated. A "hand-sized" data set of four subjects is used primarily in Chapter 5 to illustrate the mixed model equations to be solved for various longitudinal models. "Small" data sets of 50 subjects (25 per arm) with three post-baseline assessments are used to illustrate the actual implementations of those analyses. Two "large" data sets are used to illustrate the analyses in real settings, one where the rate of missing data was low and one where it was high. The following sections provide more details on each data set and how they were created.

4.2 Large Data Sets

The two large data sets were based on actual clinical trial data but were somewhat contrived to avoid implications for marketed drugs tested in those studies. Nevertheless, the key features of the original data were preserved. The original data were from two nearly identically designed antidepressant clinical trials that were originally reported by Goldstein et al. (2004) and Detke et al. (2004). Each trial had four treatment arms with approximately 90 subjects per arm. The treatment arms included two doses of an experimental medication (subsequently granted marketing authorizations in most major jurisdictions), an approved medication, and placebo.

Assessments on the HAMD17 (Hamilton 17-item rating scale for depression; Hamilton 1960) were taken at baseline and Weeks 1, 2, 4, 6, and 8 in each trial. The Patient Global Impression of Improvement (PGI; Guy 1976) was taken at Weeks 1, 2, 4, 6, and 8 in each trial. The HAMD is a continuous variable. The PGI has 7 ordered categories from very much improved = 1, to very much worse = 7, with not improved = 4.

All subjects from the original placebo arm were included along with a contrived drug arm that was created by randomly selecting 100 subjects from the non-placebo arms. In addition to including all the original placebo-treated subjects, additional placebo-treated subjects were randomly re-selected so that there were also 100 subjects in the contrived placebo arms. A new identification number was assigned to the re-selected placebo-treated subjects and outcomes were adjusted to create new observations by adding a randomly generated value to each original observation.

These trials are referred to as the low and high dropout large data sets. In the high dropout data set, completion rates were 70% for drug and 60% for placebo (see Table 4.1). In the low dropout data set, completion rates were 92% in both the drug and placebo arms. The dropout rates in the contrived data sets closely mirrored those in the corresponding original studies. The design difference that may explain the difference in dropout rates between these two otherwise similar trials was that the low dropout data set came from a study conducted in Eastern Europe that included a 6-month extension treatment period after the 8-week acute treatment phase, and used titration dosing. The high dropout data set came from a study conducted in the US that did not have the extension treatment period and used fixed dosing.

Visit-wise mean changes for subjects that completed the trials versus those who discontinued early are summarized in Figures 4.1 and 4.2 for the low and high dropout data sets, respectively. In the high dropout data set, subjects who discontinued early had less favorable outcomes than completers. With only a few dropouts at each visit in the low dropout data set, trends were not readily identifiable.

4.3 Small Data Sets

Two versions of the small data set were created. The first version (complete data) had complete data where all subjects adhered to the originally assigned study medication. The second version (missing data) was identical to the first except some data were missing data such as would arise

TABLE 4.1

Number of Observations by Week in Large Data Sets

	High Dropout					Low Dropout				
Week	**1**	**2**	**4**	**6**	**8**	**1**	**2**	**4**	**6**	**8**
Placebo	100	92	85	73	60	100	98	98	95	92
Drug	100	91	85	75	70	100	98	95	93	92

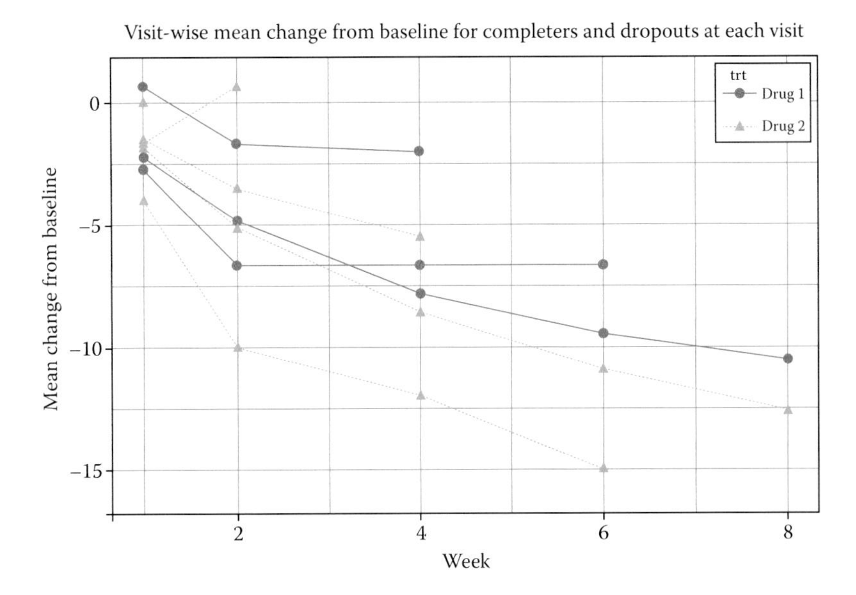

FIGURE 4.1
Visit-wise mean changes from baseline by treatment group and time of last observation in the low dropout large data set.

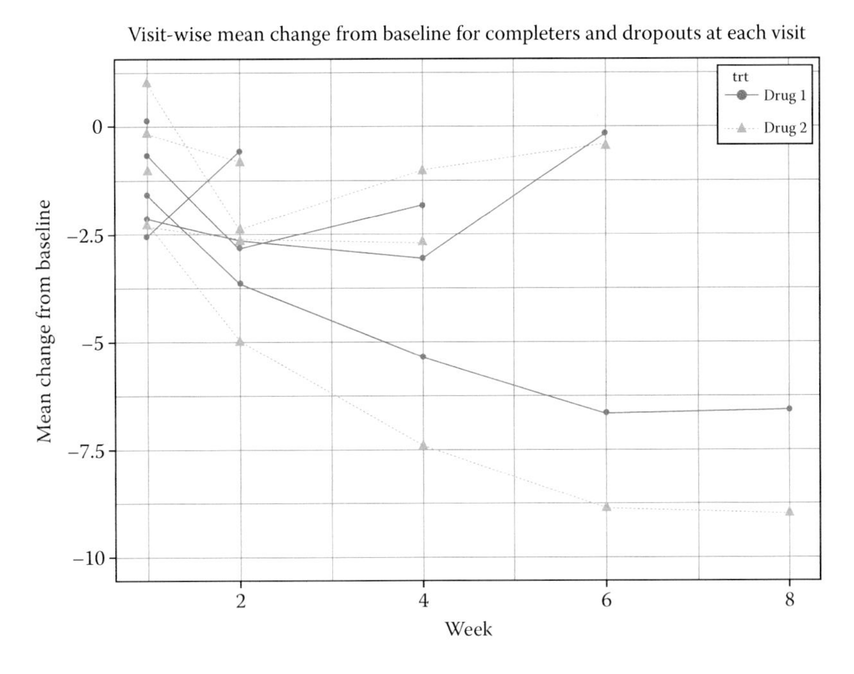

FIGURE 4.2
Visit-wise mean changes from baseline by treatment group and time of last observation in the high dropout large data set.

from subject dropout. Each data set had 50 subjects, 25 per arm, and 3 post-baseline assessments. A complete listing of these data sets is provided at the end of this chapter.

The complete data set was created from the large, low dropout data set. All subjects that completed the trial and were from the investigational site with the largest enrollment were selected. Additional subjects were selected to provide 25 subjects per arm. These additional subjects were chosen based on gender and outcome in order to yield a data set that had a significant treatment effect at endpoint and was not balanced by gender across treatments. Only data from Weeks 2, 4, and 8 were included, and then renamed as Time 1, Time 2, and Time 3. The number of observations by treatment and gender are summarized in Table 4.2. The most notable feature of the data is that the percentage of males was greater in Treatment 1 than in Treatment 2.

Baseline and visit-wise means by treatment are summarized for the complete data set in Table 4.3, and correlations between the baseline and post-baseline assessments are summarized in Table 4.4. Mean baseline values were similar across treatments. Post-baseline changes increased over time in both treatments (negative changes indicate improvement), with greater changes in Treatment 2. Baseline values had moderate to weak negative

TABLE 4.2

Number of Subjects by Treatment and Gender in Small Example Data Set

Treatment	n (%) Female	n (%) Male	Total
1	10(40)	15(60)	25
2	19(76)	6(24)	25
Total	29(58)	21(42)	50

TABLE 4.3

Baseline Means by Treatment and Visit-Wise Means by Treatment in Complete Data

Treatment	Time	N	Mean	Median	Standard Deviation
1	Baseline	25	19.80	20	3.06
1	1	25	–4.20	–4	3.66
1	2	25	–6.80	–6	4.25
1	3	25	–9.88	–10	4.85
2	Baseline	25	19.32	20	4.89
2	1	25	–5.24	–6	5.49
2	2	25	–8.60	–8	5.39
2	3	25	–13.24	–13	5.54

TABLE 4.4

Simple Correlations between Baseline Values and Post-Baseline Changes in Small Example Data Set

	Baseline	Time 1	Time 2	Time 3
Baseline	1.00	−0.26	−0.32	− 0.03
Time 1		1.00	0.76	0.52
Time 2			1.00	0.71
Time 3				1.00

TABLE 4.5

Number of Subjects by Treatment and Time in Small Data Set with Dropout

	Time		
Treatment	**1**	**2**	**3**
1	25	20	18
2	25	22	19
Total	50	42	37

correlations with post-baseline changes, such that subjects with greater symptom severity at baseline tended to have greater post-baseline improvement. Post-baseline values had strong positive correlations across time.

The small data set with (monotone) dropout had 18 completers for Treatment 1, the "placebo" group, and 19 completers for Treatment 2, the "experimental" group. Observations were deleted from the complete data set as follows: For Treatment 1, if change from baseline on the HAMD17 total score at Time 1 was less than an 8-point improvement, the probability of dropout was 30%; and, if the improvement at Time 2 was less than 10 points, the probability of dropout was 40%. For Treatment 2, if change at Time 1 was less than a 12-point improvement, the probability of dropout was 20%; and, if the improvement at Time 2 was less than 12 points, the probability of dropout was 25%. In all instances, the value that triggered the dropout was included in the data. The number of subjects by treatment and time is summarized in Table 4.5.

Visit-wise means by treatment are summarized for the data set with dropout in Table 4.6.

In contrast to the complete data set, the difference between treatments in mean change at Time 3 based on the observed data was somewhat smaller in the data with dropout. To further investigate the potential impact of incomplete data, the visit-wise mean changes from baseline for completers versus dropouts are summarized in Figure 4.3. Subjects that discontinued early tended to have worse outcomes than those that completed the trial,

TABLE 4.6

Visit-Wise Raw Means in Data with Dropout

Treatment	Time	N	Mean	Median	Standard Deviation
1	1	25	–4.20	–4.0	3.66
1	2	20	–6.80	–5.5	4.63
1	3	18	–10.17	–9.0	4.88
2	1	25	–5.24	–6.0	5.49
2	2	22	–8.14	–8.0	5.27
2	3	19	–13.11	–13.0	5.44

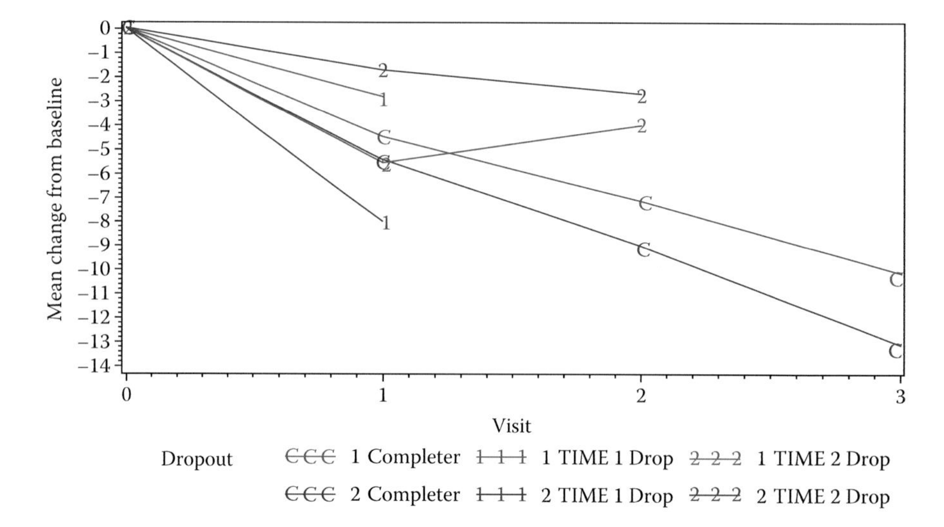

FIGURE 4.3
Visit-wise mean changes from baseline by treatment group and time of last observation in the small example data set with dropout.

mimicking dropout for lack of efficacy. However, Treatment 2 (drug-treated) subjects that discontinued at Time 1 tended to have better outcomes than those that completed the trial, thereby potentially mimicking dropout for adverse events.

Data from the small example data sets are listed in Tables 4.7 and 4.8.

TABLE 4.7

Listing of HAMD17 Data from Small Example Data Set

	Treatment			Changes from Baseline					
				Complete Data			Data with Dropout		
Subject		Gender	Baseline Value	Time 1	Time 2	Time 3	Time 1	Time 2	Time 3
1	2	F	24	–11	–16	–24	–11	.	.
2	1	F	20	–6	–8	–5	–6	.	.
3	2	F	18	–1	–1	–9	–1	–1	.
4	2	M	10	–9	–6	–9	–9	–6	–9
5	1	F	12	–6	–3	–9	–6	–3	–9
6	1	F	14	–6	–10	–10	–6	–10	–10
7	2	F	17	–7	–7	–14	–7	–7	–14
8	1	F	21	–2	–9	–9	–2	–9	–9
9	1	F	19	–9	–6	–10	–9	–6	.
10	2	F	19	–13	–12	–14	–13	–12	–14
11	2	F	20	–11	–15	–20	–11	–15	–20
12	2	F	19	–7	–15	–19	–7	.	.
13	1	M	20	–9	–12	–13	–9	–12	–13
14	1	F	19	–6	–12	–16	–6	–12	–16
15	2	F	19	–12	–15	–18	–12	–15	–18
16	1	M	19	–3	–11	–17	–3	–11	–17
17	2	F	20	–9	–13	–19	–9	–13	–19
18	1	F	23	–7	–10	–15	–7	–10	–15
19	1	M	26	–5	–5	–11	–5	–5	–11
20	2	F	19	0	–1	–8	0	–1	–8
21	2	F	24	–12	–15	–19	–12	–15	–19
22	2	M	19	0	–2	–10	0	–2	–10
23	2	F	20	–7	–8	–13	–7	–8	–13
24	1	M	20	1	–1	–6	1	–1	–6
25	1	F	22	0	–4	–9	0	–4	–9
26	2	F	23	–12	–17	–22	–12	–17	–22
27	1	M	21	–1	–2	–3	–1	–2	–3
28	1	M	21	–2	–2	–2	–2	–2	–2
29	2	F	20	–3	–8	–13	–3	–8	–13
30	1	F	19	–2	–2	0	–2	–2	.
31	2	F	13	–1	–4	–11	–1	–4	–11
32	1	M	24	–10	–14	–20	–10	–14	–20
33	2	M	18	–4	–10	–15	–4	–10	–15
34	1	M	21	–2	–1	–6	–2	–1	–6
35	2	F	20	–5	–10	–15	–5	–10	–15
36	1	M	20	–4	–4	–10	–4	.	.

(Continued)

TABLE 4.7 ***(Continued)***

Listing of HAMD17 Data from Small Example Data Set

			Changes from Baseline					
Treatment			Complete Data			Data with Dropout		
Subject	Gender	Baseline Value	Time 1	Time 2	Time 3	Time 1	Time 2	Time 3
37 2	F	20	−3	−6	−12	−3	−6	.
38 1	F	22	−3	−5	−6	−3	−5	−6
39 2	M	20	−6	−9	−13	−6	−9	−13
40 1	M	18	−5	−9	−15	−5	.	.
41 2	M	20	5	−2	−10	5	−2	−10
42 1	M	15	0	−2	−8	0	−2	−8
43 1	M	19	−3	−9	−11	−3	.	.
44 2	F	8	−6	−3	−7	−6	−3	−7
45 1	M	20	−9	−11	−9	−9	−11	−9
46 2	M	20	−6	−5	−9	−6	.	.
47 2	F	35	−8	−14	1	−8	−14	1
48 1	M	17	−10	−14	−14	−10	−14	−14
49 1	M	23	4	−4	−13	4	.	.
50 2	F	18	−1	−1	−9	−1	−1	.

TABLE 4.8

Listing of PGI Improvement from the Small Example Data Set

Subject	Treatment	Time 1	Time 2	Time 3
1	2	3	2	2
2	1	4	4	5
3	2	4	4	4
4	2	6	2	1
5	1	2	5	4
6	1	2	2	2
7	2	2	2	2
8	1	4	2	2
9	1	2	3	2
10	2	2	2	1
11	2	3	2	2
12	2	2	2	1
13	1	3	3	2
14	1	3	1	1
15	2	3	3	2

(Continued)

TABLE 4.8 ***(Continued)***

Listing of PGI Improvement from the Small Example Data Set

Subject	Treatment	Time 1	Time 2	Time 3
16	1	3	2	2
17	2	3	2	2
18	1	3	3	2
19	1	4	4	3
20	2	4	4	3
21	2	3	3	1
22	2	4	3	2
23	2	3	3	2
24	1	4	4	2
25	1	4	3	2
26	2	2	2	1
27	1	4	4	4
28	1	4	4	4
29	2	4	3	2
30	1	4	4	4
31	2	2	2	1
32	1	2	2	1
33	2	4	3	2
34	1	4	4	3
35	2	3	2	2
36	1	3	3	2
37	2	3	3	2
38	1	3	3	4
39	2	2	2	2
40	1	2	1	1
41	2	4	3	2
42	1	4	3	2
43	1	4	4	3
44	2	1	2	1
45	1	5	3	4
46	2	3	5	3
47	2	5	7	.
48	1	3	3	3
49	1	4	3	3
50	2	4	4	4

5

Mixed-Effects Models Review

5.1 Introduction

Some readers will find the material in this chapter most useful before proceeding to subsequent chapters. Other readers may benefit more from referring to this chapter during or after digesting the contents of subsequent chapters. The intent is to provide a general review of mixed-effect models and let readers refer to it as best suited to their individual needs. As such, readers are not obligated to digest this chapter before proceeding.

Mixed-effects models provide a flexible analytic framework for clinical trial data. The term mixed model refers to the use of both fixed and random effects in the same analysis. Fixed effects have levels that are of primary interest and would be used again if the experiment were repeated. Random effects have levels that are not of primary interest, at least usually not of primary interest in clinical trials, but rather are a random selection from a larger set of levels. In the clinical trial context, subject effects are usually random effects, while treatment levels are usually fixed effects.

The use of both fixed and random effects in the same model can be thought of hierarchically, and there is a close relationship between mixed models and the class of models referred to as hierarchical linear models. The hierarchy often includes one level for subjects and another level for measurements within subjects. There can be more than two levels of the hierarchy, such as investigative sites, subjects within sites, and measurements within subjects.

Although the following example is simplistic, it provides conceptual and practical motivation for the use of mixed models for analyses of longitudinal clinical trial data. Consider a typical clinical trial scenario where the fixed effect parameters explain the average difference between treatments and the random effect parameters represent the variability among subjects (and/or sites). It is possible to fit a model with subject as a fixed effect, with for example, a unique intercept (and possibly slope) for each subject. In addition to mistreating the conceptually random subject effect as fixed, the analysis estimates one intercept parameter for each subject. Alternatively, fitting a random subject intercept requires estimating only one variance parameter that represents the spread of the random intercepts around the common intercept. Therefore, conceptual and practical motivations support use of mixed-effect models for analyses of clinical trial data.

5.2 Notation and Definitions

Laird and Ware (1982) introduced the general linear mixed-effects model to be any model that satisfies

$$Y_i = X_i\beta + Z_i b_i + \varepsilon_i \tag{5.1}$$

$$b_i \sim N(0, D)$$

$$\varepsilon_i \sim N(0, \Sigma_i)$$

$$b_1 \ldots b_N, \varepsilon_1 \ldots \varepsilon_N \text{ independent}$$

where Y_i is the n_i-dimensional response (column) vector for patient i; β is the p-dimensional vector of fixed effects; b_i is the q-dimensional vector of random (patient-specific) effects; X_i and Z_i are $(n_i \times p)$- and $(n_i \times q)$-dimensional matrices relating the observations to the fixed and random effects, respectively; ε_i is the n_i-dimensional vector of residuals; D is a general $(q \times q)$-dimensional covariance matrix with (i,j) element $d_{ij} = d_{ji}$; and Σ_i is a general $(n_i \times n_i)$-dimensional covariance matrix (usually the same for all *i*). It follows from this model that, marginally,

$$Y_i \sim N(X_i\beta, V)$$

$$\text{and } V = Z_i D Z_i' + \Sigma_i$$

In other words, mixed-effects models include fixed and random effects, with overall variability (V in the above equation) that can be partitioned into a part due to the random effects $(Z_i D Z_i')$ and a part due to the errors (Σ_i). In contrast, analysis of variance models include only fixed effects (apart from the residuals).

In clinical trials, the subject-specific (random) effects are seldom the focus. Rather, the trials are typically designed to assess differences in fixed effects, most notably treatment effects. However, accounting for the random effects is needed in order to properly assess the precision of estimates and to make the most appropriate inferences regarding the fixed effects. Specifically, the difference between subjects and/or the similarity within subjects must be taken into account in order to have standard errors and confidence intervals that reflect the true uncertainty in parameter estimates.

5.3 Building and Solving Mixed Model Equations

Data from four subjects (1, 7, 9, and 14) in the small complete data set are used to illustrate the formulation of the mixed model equations. These data are listed below

			Change from Baseline on HAMD17		
Subject	**Treatment**	**Baseline**	**Time1**	**Time2**	**Time3**
1	2	24	–11	–16	–24
7	2	17	–7	–7	–14
9	1	19	–9	–6	–10
14	1	19	–6	–12	–16

Mechanically, mixed model equations are constructed by matrix manipulations. However, concepts underlying the manipulations are covered before illustrating the actual mechanics. The first step, whether mechanical or conceptual, is to define the linear model. Illustrations begin with a simple fixed effects model for which ordinary least squares can be applied. Subsequently, more detailed generalized least squares and mixed-effects approaches are illustrated.

5.3.1 Ordinary Least Squares

For the hand-sized example data listed above, consider a fixed effects model where only Time 3 data are used as the dependent variable, with treatment and intercept as the only fixed effects. In scalar notation

$$Y_{ij} = \mu + \beta_i + \varepsilon_{ij}$$

where μ is the population mean (intercept), β_i is the fixed effect of treatment i, and ε_{ij} is the error (residual) for subject j in treatment i.

The equations that solve for the unknown parameters (μ, β_1, and β_2) in this model can be constructed so as to minimize the error sums of squares. The sum of squared residuals for linear models is minimized by equating the means of the observed data to the associated expected values under the model.

As the simplest case, the squared sum of deviations from the mean $\Sigma(y_i - \overline{y})^2$ is smaller than the sum of squared deviations around any other provisional value, c, $\Sigma(y_i - c)^2$; hence, the least square estimate of the grand mean μ is the sample mean, $\overline{y}$. Equivalently, the estimate of grand mean can be obtained by equating the sum of observed values with the sum of expected values under the assumed model: $\Sigma\, y_i = \Sigma\, \hat{E}(Y_i) = N\hat{\mu}$.

Thus, for each effect in the model (except residual error), compute a sum such that each observation that contains the effect is included in the sum. These sums form a vector of "observations" (observed data summaries), Y. In this model, equations are needed for μ and for each treatment group, three equations total. All observations contain the effect of μ; hence, the sum for the μ effect is the sum of all observations. Likewise, the sum for each treatment group equation is the sum of all observations for the subjects in that group. The transpose of the Y vector of sums is (–64, –26, –38).

The next step is to construct the ordinary least squares equations by writing the model associated with each sum in Y and equating each sum to the associated sum of the model-based predictions. The sum for the μ equation contains all four observations; therefore, the μ equation contains four μ and two β_i of one kind or another. The model and the associated equations can be written in matrix form as follows:

$$X\beta = Y$$

$$= \begin{pmatrix} 4 & 2 & 2 \\ 2 & 2 & 0 \\ 2 & 0 & 2 \end{pmatrix} \begin{pmatrix} \mu \\ \beta_1 \\ \beta_2 \end{pmatrix} = \begin{pmatrix} -64 \\ -38 \\ -26 \end{pmatrix}$$

While it is important to bear in mind the concept of equating sums to effects, the task of building the equations (coefficient matrix and right-hand side) is made much easier via the use of design (aka incidence) matrices. Incidence matrices are matrices of 0s and 1s that relate observations to the various effects. These matrices have a row for each observation and a column for each effect in the model. Whenever an observation contains an effect, a 1 is placed in the cell corresponding to the appropriate row and column, otherwise place a 0. In the example above, the X incidence matrix is

$$\begin{pmatrix} 1 & 1 & 0 \\ 1 & 1 & 0 \\ 1 & 0 & 1 \\ 1 & 0 & 1 \end{pmatrix}$$

Pre-multiplying X by its transpose (X′) creates the coefficient matrix (X′X):

$$\begin{pmatrix} 1 & 1 & 1 & 1 \\ 1 & 1 & 0 & 0 \\ 0 & 0 & 1 & 1 \end{pmatrix}\begin{pmatrix} 1 & 1 & 0 \\ 1 & 1 & 0 \\ 1 & 0 & 1 \\ 1 & 0 & 1 \end{pmatrix} = \begin{pmatrix} 4 & 2 & 2 \\ 2 & 2 & 0 \\ 2 & 0 & 2 \end{pmatrix}$$

Pre-multiplying the vector of observations Y by X′ creates the appropriate sums:

$$\begin{pmatrix} 1 & 1 & 1 & 1 \\ 1 & 1 & 0 & 0 \\ 0 & 0 & 1 & 0 \end{pmatrix}\begin{pmatrix} -24 \\ -14 \\ -10 \\ -16 \end{pmatrix} = \begin{pmatrix} -64 \\ -38 \\ -26 \end{pmatrix}$$

Hence, the matrix equations are now

$$(X'X)\beta = X'Y$$

And the solutions to the ordinary least square equations are

$$\beta = (X'X)^{-1} X'Y$$

Therefore, solving the equations requires an inverse of the coefficient matrix X′X. Unfortunately, the equations as written cannot be solved due to dependencies. That is, the two equations for the two treatments sum to the equation for μ. Therefore, the equations are not independent. The coefficient matrix is said to be singular and it cannot be inverted, nor can the equations be solved using iterative techniques.

The solution to this dilemma is to create a generalized inverse by first imposing constraints on the coefficient matrix that eliminate the dependency. For example, the coefficients for one row of the equations, which corresponds to one of the effects in β, can be set equal to zero, which eliminates the dependency of the two treatment equations summing to the μ equation. When a dependency is eliminated by using coefficients of zero for a row, zeros must also replace the original coefficients in the corresponding column for that effect.

The effects of imposing constraints, in addition to facilitating inversion of the coefficient matrix, include:

1. The expected values of solutions for fixed effects do not equal the actual fixed effect, but rather equal estimable functions of the fixed effects.

2. Solutions depend on the specific constraint(s) imposed. Different constraints for the same set of equations yield different solutions that reflect different estimable functions of the fixed effects.
3. Typically, regardless of specific constraints, the expected value of the difference in solutions reflects the difference in fixed effects. That is, the differences are estimable even if the actual effects are not.
4. Random effects solutions are unaffected by the constraints imposed on the fixed effects equations, and are said to be "translation invariant."

For the present simple example, one constraint that can be imposed is set the μ equation equal to 0, or simpler still, not include μ in the model. With this constraint the equations are:

$$\begin{pmatrix} 2 & 0 \\ 0 & 2 \end{pmatrix}\begin{pmatrix} \beta_1 \\ \beta_2 \end{pmatrix} = \begin{pmatrix} -26 \\ -38 \end{pmatrix}$$

The solutions vector β' is (–13, –19), which in this simplistic example is also the simple averages for each treatment. With this constraint, the first solution represents $\mu + \beta_1$ and the second solution is $\mu + \beta_2$. The solutions in this unique example are conveniently the least square means (lsmeans) for the treatments. Typically, the estimable functions will be more complex and less convenient.

An lsmean is an estimate from a linear model, whereas a raw (arithmetic) mean is the simple average. In this simple model, the lsmeans for treatment are also the simple averages. As illustrated in later sections, the lsmeans seldom equal the raw means because the lsmeans are adjusted for other terms (covariates) in the model, thereby reflecting the independent effect of the fixed effects.

Another interesting aspect of this simple model is that changing the data for a subject in one treatment only influences the solution for that effect and the other solution is unaffected. For example, if the outcome for Subject 1 was 0 instead of 24 then $\beta' = (-13, -7)$. Later examples with more complex models will illustrate that such independence is usually not the case as estimates of fixed effects are typically correlated. That is, changing the data for a subject in treatment 1 can change the estimates of not just treatment 1 but also other effects in the model.

Another possible constraint would be to "zero out" the equation for β_2. The resulting equations with this constraint are

$$\begin{pmatrix} 4 & 2 & 0 \\ 2 & 2 & 0 \\ 0 & 0 & 0 \end{pmatrix} \begin{pmatrix} \mu \\ \beta_1 \\ \beta_2 \end{pmatrix} = \begin{pmatrix} -64 \\ -26 \\ 0 \end{pmatrix}$$

The solution vector $\beta' = 19, 6, 0$. The estimable functions with these solutions are that the first element $= \mu + \beta_2$ and the second element is $\beta_1 - \beta_2$.

A slightly more complex model that includes in addition to treatment the fixed covariate of baseline severity can be fit by including the actual covariate values in X. The appropriate X matrix is:

$$\begin{matrix} & \mu & \beta_1 & \beta_2 & \beta_3 \end{matrix}$$
$$X = \begin{pmatrix} 1 & 1 & 0 & 19 \\ 1 & 1 & 0 & 19 \\ 1 & 0 & 1 & 24 \\ 1 & 0 & 1 & 17 \end{pmatrix}$$

The resulting coefficient matrix (X′X) has four effects, μ, two treatment effects, and the covariate.

$$\begin{pmatrix} 4 & 2 & 2 & 79 \\ 2 & 2 & 0 & 38 \\ 2 & 0 & 2 & 41 \\ 79 & 38 & 41 & 1587 \end{pmatrix} \begin{pmatrix} \mu \\ \beta_1 \\ \beta_2 \\ \beta_3 \end{pmatrix} = \begin{pmatrix} -64 \\ -26 \\ -38 \\ -1308 \end{pmatrix}$$

The equation for the covariate is in the fourth row (and fourth column). The value in the first position of row 4 (79) is the sum of all baseline values, the second and third positions are sums of the baseline values in the respective treatment groups (38, 41), and the last entry (1587) is the sum of the squared baseline values. The last entry in the Y vector (–1308) is the sum of cross products. Adding this continuous covariate does not add a dependency, and (as before) only one constraint is needed to yield a coefficient matrix that can be inverted.

To fit more complex models with multiple fixed effects, the same process is used as with simple models, but the design (incidence) matrices and coefficient matrices are more extensive. Recall that the example data from four subjects includes three assessments per subject taken at 3 time points. To include time in the model, the X matrix now has 12 rows and 6 columns to associate the 12 observations with the 6 fixed effects (μ, 2 treatments, and 3 time points).

$$
X = \begin{pmatrix}
1 & 1 & 0 & 1 & 0 & 0 \\
1 & 1 & 0 & 1 & 0 & 0 \\
1 & 1 & 0 & 0 & 1 & 0 \\
1 & 1 & 0 & 0 & 1 & 0 \\
1 & 1 & 0 & 0 & 0 & 1 \\
1 & 1 & 0 & 0 & 0 & 1 \\
1 & 0 & 1 & 1 & 0 & 0 \\
1 & 0 & 1 & 1 & 0 & 0 \\
1 & 0 & 1 & 0 & 1 & 0 \\
1 & 0 & 1 & 0 & 1 & 0 \\
1 & 0 & 1 & 0 & 0 & 1 \\
1 & 0 & 1 & 0 & 0 & 1
\end{pmatrix}
\quad \text{(columns: } \mu, \beta_1, \beta_2, \tau_1, \tau_2, \tau_3\text{)}
$$

And the coefficient matrix and right-hand sides are

$$
\begin{pmatrix}
12 & 6 & 6 & 4 & 4 & 4 \\
6 & 6 & 0 & 2 & 2 & 2 \\
6 & 0 & 6 & 2 & 2 & 2 \\
4 & 2 & 2 & 4 & 0 & 0 \\
4 & 2 & 2 & 0 & 4 & 0 \\
4 & 2 & 2 & 0 & 0 & 4
\end{pmatrix}
\begin{pmatrix} \mu \\ \beta_1 \\ \beta_2 \\ \tau_1 \\ \tau_2 \\ \tau_3 \end{pmatrix}
=
\begin{pmatrix} -138 \\ -59 \\ -79 \\ -33 \\ -41 \\ -64 \end{pmatrix}
$$

To solve these equations, two constraints are needed; for example, the last treatment equation and the last time equation can be set to zero.

$$
\begin{pmatrix}
12 & 6 & 0 & 4 & 4 & 0 \\
6 & 6 & 0 & 2 & 2 & 0 \\
0 & 0 & 0 & 0 & 0 & 0 \\
4 & 2 & 0 & 4 & 0 & 0 \\
4 & 2 & 0 & 0 & 4 & 0 \\
0 & 0 & 0 & 0 & 0 & 0
\end{pmatrix}
\begin{pmatrix} \mu \\ \beta_1 \\ \beta_2 \\ \tau_1 \\ \tau_2 \\ \tau_3 \end{pmatrix}
=
\begin{pmatrix} -138 \\ -59 \\ 0 \\ -33 \\ -41 \\ 0 \end{pmatrix}
$$

The solution vector $\beta' = 17.67, 3.33, 0, 7.75, 5.75, 0$. And the lsmeans derived from these solutions are

trt	1	−9.83
trt	2	−13.16
Time	1	−8.25
Time	2	−10.25
Time	3	−16.00

While it is easy to see that the differences in solutions for the treatment effects and the time effects match the differences in lsmeans, the estimable functions represented by each solution are more complex when more constraints are imposed.

It is often of interest to model the effects of interactions between main effects. For example, the effect of treatment may not be constant over time. The X matrix for the example data with a model that includes the effects of treatment (β_i), time (τ_j) and the treatment-by-time interaction ($\beta\tau_{ij}$) is given below.

$$\begin{array}{cccccccccccc} \mu & \beta_1 & \beta_2 & \tau_1 & \tau_2 & \tau_3 & \beta\tau_{11} & \beta\tau_{12} & \beta\tau_{13} & \beta\tau_{21} & \beta\tau_{22} & \beta\tau_{23} \end{array}$$

$$X = \begin{pmatrix} 1 & 1 & 0 & 1 & 0 & 0 & 1 & 0 & 0 & 0 & 0 & 0 \\ 1 & 1 & 0 & 1 & 0 & 0 & 1 & 0 & 0 & 0 & 0 & 0 \\ 1 & 1 & 0 & 0 & 1 & 0 & 0 & 1 & 0 & 0 & 0 & 0 \\ 1 & 1 & 0 & 0 & 1 & 0 & 0 & 1 & 0 & 0 & 0 & 0 \\ 1 & 1 & 0 & 0 & 0 & 1 & 0 & 0 & 1 & 0 & 0 & 0 \\ 1 & 1 & 0 & 0 & 0 & 1 & 0 & 0 & 1 & 0 & 0 & 0 \\ 1 & 0 & 1 & 1 & 0 & 0 & 1 & 0 & 0 & 1 & 0 & 0 \\ 1 & 0 & 1 & 1 & 0 & 0 & 1 & 0 & 0 & 1 & 0 & 0 \\ 1 & 0 & 1 & 0 & 1 & 0 & 0 & 0 & 0 & 0 & 1 & 0 \\ 1 & 0 & 1 & 0 & 1 & 0 & 0 & 0 & 0 & 0 & 1 & 0 \\ 1 & 0 & 1 & 0 & 0 & 1 & 0 & 0 & 0 & 0 & 0 & 1 \\ 1 & 0 & 1 & 0 & 0 & 1 & 0 & 0 & 0 & 0 & 0 & 1 \end{pmatrix}$$

Nested effects are similar to interaction effects except that one factor of the interaction effect does not appear as a main effect. Consider again the X matrix described earlier for the model with treatment and baseline severity as fixed effects:

$$\begin{array}{cccc} \mu & \beta_1 & \beta_2 & \gamma \end{array}$$

$$\begin{pmatrix} 1 & 1 & 0 & 19 \\ 1 & 1 & 0 & 19 \\ 1 & 0 & 1 & 24 \\ 1 & 0 & 1 & 17 \end{pmatrix}$$

The X matrix for a model with categorical treatment, baseline severity as a covariate, and the treatment-by-baseline severity interaction is:

$$\begin{matrix} \mu & \beta_1 & \beta_2 & \gamma & (\beta\gamma)_1 & (\beta\gamma)_2 \end{matrix}$$
$$\begin{pmatrix} 1 & 1 & 0 & 19 & 19 & 0 \\ 1 & 1 & 0 & 19 & 19 & 0 \\ 1 & 0 & 1 & 24 & 0 & 24 \\ 1 & 0 & 1 & 17 & 0 & 17 \end{pmatrix}$$

The X matrix for a model that included treatment and baseline severity nested within treatment is:

$$\begin{matrix} \mu & \beta_1 & \beta_2 & (\beta\gamma)_1 & (\beta\gamma)_2 \end{matrix}$$
$$\begin{pmatrix} 1 & 1 & 0 & 19 & 0 \\ 1 & 1 & 0 & 19 & 0 \\ 1 & 0 & 1 & 0 & 24 \\ 1 & 0 & 1 & 0 & 17 \end{pmatrix}$$

As an artifact of the small example, both subjects in treatment 1 have a value of 19 for baseline severity, which creates an additional dependency making the equations unsolvable. However, in realistic scenarios where not all baseline values within a treatment were the same, the equations would be solvable and the interaction model and the nested model would yield identical fits to the data and identical treatment contrasts.

5.3.2 Generalized Least Squares

Ordinary least squares assume that observations are independent, an assumption that is not justifiable when subjects are measured repeatedly over time. Therefore, now assume that errors have a general covariance matrix, $\text{Var}[\varepsilon] = \Sigma$, such that the model becomes

$$Y = X\beta + \varepsilon \qquad \varepsilon \sim (0, \Sigma)$$

Generalized least squares minimizes the generalized error sum of squares

$$SSE_g = (Y - X\beta)'\Sigma^{-1}(Y - X\beta)$$

This leads to the generalized normal equations

$$(X'\Sigma^{-1}X)\beta = X'\Sigma^{-1}Y$$

and the GLS estimator

$$\hat{\beta}_g = (X'\Sigma^{-1}X)^{-}X'\Sigma^{-1}Y$$

5.3.3 Mixed-Effects Models

As noted earlier, the mixed model is written as

$$Y = X\beta + Zb + \varepsilon$$

where terms are the same as in the general linear model described above except for the addition of the known design matrix, Z, and the vector b of unknown random-effects parameters. The Z matrix can contain either continuous or dummy variables, just like X. The model assumes that b and ε are normally distributed with

$$E\begin{bmatrix} b \\ \varepsilon \end{bmatrix} = \begin{bmatrix} 0 \\ 0 \end{bmatrix}$$

$$Var\begin{bmatrix} b \\ \varepsilon \end{bmatrix} = \begin{bmatrix} G & 0 \\ 0 & R \end{bmatrix}$$

The variance of Y is $V = ZGZ' + R$, and is modeled via the random-effects design matrix Z and covariance structures G and R.

Building the coefficient matrix and right-hand side proceeds as before, albeit with more steps to incorporate both the X and Z design matrices. For simplicity, consider the example data and a model that includes only treatment and a random intercept for each subject, ignoring the correlation between the repeated observations (G and R) for now. Because the fixed effects in this model are the same as previously described, the X matrix will be the same. The Z matrix for this example is as follows:

$$\begin{pmatrix} 1 & 0 & 0 & 0 \\ 1 & 0 & 0 & 0 \\ 1 & 0 & 0 & 0 \\ 0 & 1 & 0 & 0 \\ 0 & 1 & 0 & 0 \\ 0 & 1 & 0 & 0 \\ 0 & 0 & 1 & 0 \\ 0 & 0 & 1 & 0 \\ 0 & 0 & 1 & 0 \\ 0 & 0 & 0 & 1 \\ 0 & 0 & 0 & 1 \\ 0 & 0 & 0 & 1 \end{pmatrix}$$

The mixed model equations are

$$\begin{pmatrix} X'X & X'Z \\ Z'X & Z'Z \end{pmatrix}\begin{pmatrix} \beta \\ b \end{pmatrix} = \begin{pmatrix} X'Y \\ Z'Y \end{pmatrix}$$

which for the example data yields:

$$\begin{pmatrix} 12 & 6 & 6 & 3 & 3 & 3 & 3 \\ 6 & 6 & 0 & 0 & 0 & 3 & 3 \\ 6 & 0 & 6 & 3 & 3 & 0 & 0 \\ 3 & 0 & 3 & 0 & 3 & 0 & 0 \\ 3 & 0 & 3 & 0 & 3 & 0 & 0 \\ 3 & 3 & 0 & 0 & 0 & 3 & 0 \\ 3 & 3 & 0 & 0 & 0 & 0 & 3 \end{pmatrix}\begin{pmatrix} \mu \\ \beta_1 \\ \beta_2 \\ b_1 \\ b_2 \\ b_3 \\ b_4 \end{pmatrix} = \begin{pmatrix} -138 \\ -59 \\ -79 \\ -51 \\ -28 \\ -25 \\ -34 \end{pmatrix}$$

The mixed model equations that take into account the within-subject correlations include the G and R matrices. In practice estimates of G and R, which are denoted $\hat{G}$ and $\hat{R}$, respectively, are usually needed since the true values are not known. Estimates of β and b can be obtained from solving the following equations (Henderson 1984):

$$\begin{bmatrix} X'\hat{R}^{-1}X & X'\hat{R}^{-1}Z \\ Z'\hat{R}^{-1}X & Z'\hat{R}^{-1}Z+\hat{G}^{-1} \end{bmatrix}\begin{bmatrix} \hat{\beta} \\ \hat{b} \end{bmatrix} = \begin{bmatrix} X'\hat{R}^{-1}Y \\ Z'\hat{R}^{-1}Y \end{bmatrix}$$

The solutions can obtained as

$$\hat{\beta} = (X'\hat{V}^{-1}X)^{-}X'\hat{V}^{-1}Y$$

$$\hat{b} = \hat{G}Z'\hat{V}^{-1}(Y - X\hat{\beta})$$

If G and R are known, $\hat{\beta}$ is the best linear unbiased estimator (BLUE) of β, and $\hat{b}$ is the best linear unbiased predictor (BLUP) of b (Searle 1971; Harville 1988, 1990). In this context, "best" means minimum mean squared error.

The covariance matrix of $(\hat{\beta}-\beta, \hat{b}-b)$ is

$$C = \begin{bmatrix} X'R^{-1}X & X'R^{-1}Z \\ Z'R^{-1}X & Z'R^{-1}Z + G^{-1} \end{bmatrix}^{-}$$

Again, in practice $\hat{G}$ and $\hat{R}$ are substituted into the preceding expression to obtain

$$\hat{C} = \begin{bmatrix} X'\hat{R}^{-1}X & X'\hat{R}^{-1}Z \\ Z'\hat{R}^{-1}X & Z'\hat{R}^{-1}Z + \hat{G}^{-1} \end{bmatrix}^{-}$$

as the approximate variance-covariance matrix of $(\hat{\beta}-\beta, \hat{b}-b)$. The matrix C has as diagonal elements error variances and off-diagonals are error covariances. With estimated G and R ($\hat{G}$ and $\hat{R}$), the solutions are approximate BLUE and BLUP, which are often referred to as empirical BLUE and BLUP (EBLUE and EBLUP).

True sampling variability is underestimated by $\hat{C}$ because the uncertainty in estimating G and R is not taken into account. Inflation factors have been proposed (Prasad and Rao 1990), but they tend to be small for data sets that are fairly balanced. Another approach to accounting for the underestimation of uncertainty is approximate *t* and *F* statistics that are based on Kenward-Roger or Satterthwaite-based degrees of freedom (SAS 2013).

Returning to the example data introduced at the beginning of Section 5.3 and a model with treatment and a random intercept, now incorporating G and R, assuming values of 1 for both the random intercept and residual variances, the mixed model equations become

$$\begin{pmatrix} 12 & 6 & 6 & 3 & 3 & 3 & 3 \\ 6 & 6 & 0 & 0 & 0 & 3 & 3 \\ 6 & 0 & 6 & 3 & 3 & 0 & 0 \\ 3 & 0 & 3 & 4 & 0 & 0 & 0 \\ 3 & 0 & 3 & 0 & 4 & 0 & 0 \\ 3 & 3 & 0 & 0 & 0 & 4 & 0 \\ 3 & 3 & 0 & 0 & 0 & 0 & 4 \end{pmatrix} \begin{pmatrix} \mu \\ \beta_1 \\ \beta_2 \\ b_1 \\ b_2 \\ b_3 \\ b_4 \end{pmatrix} = \begin{pmatrix} -138 \\ -59 \\ -79 \\ -51 \\ -28 \\ -25 \\ -34 \end{pmatrix}$$

A residual variance of 1 results in no change to the X′X, X′Z, and Z′X parts of C. However, the Z′Z part of C now has 4s as non-zero values rather than 3s due to the addition of G^{-1} to that part of the coefficient matrix. If the residual variance again = 1 and the random intercept variance = 9, then the coefficient matrix and right-hand side become

$$\begin{pmatrix} 12 & 6 & 6 & 3 & 3 & 3 & 3 \\ 6 & 6 & 0 & 0 & 0 & 3 & 3 \\ 6 & 0 & 6 & 3 & 3 & 0 & 0 \\ 3 & 0 & 3 & 3.11 & 0 & 0 & 0 \\ 3 & 0 & 3 & 0 & 3.11 & 0 & 0 \\ 3 & 3 & 0 & 0 & 0 & 3.11 & 0 \\ 3 & 3 & 0 & 0 & 0 & 0 & 3.11 \end{pmatrix} \begin{pmatrix} \mu \\ \beta_1 \\ \beta_2 \\ b_1 \\ b_2 \\ b_3 \\ b_4 \end{pmatrix} = \begin{pmatrix} -138 \\ -59 \\ -79 \\ -51 \\ -28 \\ -25 \\ -34 \end{pmatrix}$$

Note that with a larger value for intercept variance, the Z′Z part of C is augmented with smaller values.

If the residual variance = 9 and the random intercept variance = 1 then the coefficient matrix and right-hand side become

$$\begin{pmatrix} 1.33 & 0.66 & 0.66 & 0.33 & 0.33 & 0.33 & 0.33 \\ 0.66 & 0.66 & 0 & 0 & 0 & 0.33 & 0.33 \\ 0.66 & 0 & 0.66 & 0.33 & 0.33 & 0 & 0 \\ 0.33 & 0 & 0.33 & 1.33 & 0 & 0 & 0 \\ 0.33 & 0 & 0.33 & 0 & 1.33 & 0 & 0 \\ 0.33 & 0.33 & 0 & 0 & 0 & 1.33 & 0 \\ 0.33 & 0.33 & 0 & 0 & 0 & 0 & 1.33 \end{pmatrix} \begin{pmatrix} \mu \\ \beta_1 \\ \beta_2 \\ b_1 \\ b_2 \\ b_3 \\ b_4 \end{pmatrix} = \begin{pmatrix} -15.33 \\ -6.55 \\ -8.77 \\ -5.66 \\ -3.11 \\ -2.77 \\ -3.77 \end{pmatrix}$$

Note that with a larger residual variance the values in R^{-1} are smaller; therefore, the $X'R^{-1}X$, $X'R^{-1}Z$, and $Z'R^{-1}X$ parts of C and the right-hand side $Z'R^{-1}Y$ are also smaller.

5.3.4 Inference Tests

Inferences regarding fixed- and random-effects parameters in the mixed model are obtained by testing the hypothesis

$$H : L\begin{bmatrix} \beta \\ b \end{bmatrix} = 0$$

where L is a contrast vector or matrix with coefficients that pull the needed elements from β and b. When L consists of a single row, a general ***t*** statistic is constructed as illustrated below by again using L to pull the appropriate solutions for the numerator and the appropriate variances and covariances from the coefficient matrix C for the denominator. For example, the variance of the difference between Treatment 1 and Treatment 2 is equal to the variance of Treatment 1 + the variance of Treatment 2 – 2 times the covariance between Treatments 1 and 2 (McLean and Sanders 1988; Stroup 1989). The L vector is set up to extract these elements from the coefficient matrix.

$$t = \frac{L\begin{bmatrix} \hat{\beta} \\ \hat{b} \end{bmatrix}}{\sqrt{L\hat{C}L'}}$$

Under the assumed normality of b and ε, t is in general only approximately t-distributed, and its degrees of freedom must be estimated. With $\hat{v}$ being the approximate degrees of freedom, the associated confidence interval is

$$L\begin{bmatrix} \hat{\beta} \\ \hat{b} \end{bmatrix} \pm t_{\hat{v},\alpha/2}\sqrt{L\hat{C}L'}$$

where $t_{\hat{v},\alpha/2}$ is the (1–α/2)100th percentile of the $t_{\hat{v}}$ distribution. If the rank of L is greater than 1, the following general F statistic can be constructed:

$$F = \frac{\begin{bmatrix} \hat{\beta} \\ \hat{b} \end{bmatrix}' L'(L\hat{C}L')^{-1}L\begin{bmatrix} \hat{\beta} \\ \hat{b} \end{bmatrix}}{r}$$

where $r = \text{rank}(L\hat{C}L')$. Analogous to t, F in general has an approximate F distribution with r numerator degrees of freedom and $\hat{v}$ denominator degrees of freedom (SAS 2013).

5.4 Impact of Variance, Correlation, and Missing Data on Mixed Model Estimates

5.4.1 Impact of Variance and Correlation in Complete and Balanced Data

Important properties of mixed models can be illustrated by examples. For that purpose, consider the hand-sized complete data set of four subjects introduced at the beginning of Section 5.3. To these data fit a model that includes treatment, time, treatment-by-time interaction, and a random intercept for each subject. Further assume the following four combinations of values for the intercept (between subject) (σ_b^2) and residual (σ_e^2) variances:

Random Intercept Variance	Residual Variance	Total Variance
1	1	2
1	9	10
5	5	10
9	1	10

Lsmeans and standard errors for these scenarios are summarized in Table 5.1.

With complete data, the values of variance components do not influence estimates of fixed effect means. The Time 3 and treatment main effect contrast lsmeans are the same across the four combinations of variance components. However, the variance components do influence the standard errors. As expected, increasing the total variance from 2 to 10 increased the standard error of Time 3 and treatment main effect lsmeans (not shown) and of the standard error of the contrast between these lsmeans. Among the three

TABLE 5.1

Least Squares Means and Standard Errors from Mixed Model Analyses of Complete Data from the Hand-Sized Data Set

Scenario	Treatment	LSMEANS	Contrast	Contrast SE
Treatment main effect results				
$\sigma_b^2 = 1, \sigma_e^2 = 1$	1	−9.83	3.33	1.15
	2	−13.16		
$\sigma_b^2 = 9, \sigma_e^2 = 1$	1	−9.83	3.33	3.06
	2	−13.16		
$\sigma_b^2 = 5, \sigma_e^2 = 5$	1	−9.83	3.33	2.58
	2	−13.16		
$\sigma_b^2 = 1, \sigma_e^2 = 9$	1	−9.83	3.33	2.00
	2	−13.16		
Time 3 results				
$\sigma_b^2 = 1, \sigma_e^2 = 1$	1	−13.00	6.00	1.41
	2	−19.00		
$\sigma_b^2 = 9, \sigma_e^2 = 1$	1	−13.00	6.00	3.16
	2	−19.00		
$\sigma_b^2 = 5, \sigma_e^2 = 5$	1	−13.00	6.00	3.16
	2	−19.0		
$\sigma_b^2 = 1, \sigma_e^2 = 9$	1	−13.00	6.00	3.16
	2	−19.00		

scenarios where total variance = 10, that is total variance is equal, standard errors for the treatment main effect contrast increased as between-subject variance increased and residual variance decreased. In contrast, variance components did not influence standard errors of the Time 3 contrast.

The results in Table 5.1 can be explained as follows. As the between-subject variance increases, the covariance within subjects increases. That is, as the variance between subjects increases, correlation between the repeated observations on the same subjects increase and the amount of information gained from additional assessments on the same subject is decreased. Hence, standard errors for the treatment main effect are larger when the between-subject variance (and within-subject covariance) is greater. For the Time 3 contrast, a single point in time, the treatment contrast standard error is not influenced by the ratio of the variance components, only total variance. If data were unbalanced, (e.g., due to missing values) variance ratios would influence treatment contrasts at specific time points.

Generally, as the eigenvalues of G increase, G^{-1} contributes less to the equations and $\hat{b}$ is closer to what it would be if b contained fixed-effects parameters. When the eigenvalues of G decrease, G^{-1}dominates the equations and $\hat{b}$ is close to 0. For intermediate cases, G^{-1} can be viewed as shrinking the estimates of b toward 0 (Robinson 1991). This shrinkage can be seen in the estimates of the random intercepts across the varying levels of G and R. These results are summarized in Table 5.2.

The observation for Subject 1 at Time 3 (–24) was an improvement of 5 points more than the group mean. When $\sigma_b^2 = 9$ and $\sigma_e^2 = 1$ this 5-point advantage yielded an estimate for the random intercept of –3.70; that is, a result better than group average. However, when $\sigma_b^2 = 5$ and $\sigma_e^2 = 5$, the same observation yielded a random intercept estimate of –2.88, and when $\sigma_b^2 = 1$ and $\sigma_e^2 = 9$, the estimate was further shrunk to –0.96. The estimate of the intercept when $\sigma_b^2 = 5$ and $\sigma_e^2 = 5$ was the same as when $\sigma_b^2 = 1$ and $\sigma_e^2 = 1$ because the shrinkage is determined by variance ratios. A similar effect is seen in subjects who were doing worse than group mean, but of course the sign of the intercept is opposite, reflecting below-average intercepts for subjects with observations

TABLE 5.2

Estimated Intercepts and Residuals at Time 3 for Subject 1 from Mixed Model Analyses of Complete Data across Varying Values of G and R

Scenario	Observed Value	Group Mean	Estimated Intercept	Predicted Value	Residual
$\sigma_b^2 = 1, \sigma_e^2 = 1$	–24	–19	–2.88	–21.88	–2.12
$\sigma_b^2 = 9, \sigma_e^2 = 1$	–24	–19	–3.70	–22.70	–1.30
$\sigma_b^2 = 5, \sigma_e^2 = 5$	–24	–19	–2.88	–21.88	–2.12
$\sigma_b^2 = 1, \sigma_e^2 = 9$	–24	–19	–0.96	–19.96	–4.04

below average. Estimates of the intercept are again regressed toward the mean in accordance with the ratio of the variance components.

5.4.2 Impact of Variance and Correlation in Incomplete (Unbalanced) Data

Next, consider the impact of variance components in unbalanced (incomplete) data by re-examining the example data, but delete the Time 2 and Time 3 values for Subject 1 and the Time 3 value for Subject 9. Lsmeans, contrasts, and standard errors are summarized in Table 5.3. In contrast to the scenario with complete and therefore balanced data, with missing and therefore unbalanced data, variance components influenced both lsmeans and standard errors.

For the treatment main effect, increasing total variance again increased standard errors, and when σ_b^2 was a greater fraction of total variance, standard errors were larger. Changes in the lsmeans due to incomplete data were greater for the Treatment 2 main effect than the Treatment 1 main effect because more data were deleted for Treatment 2. The Time 3 contrast standard errors changed with variance components but in the opposite direction

TABLE 5.3

Least Squares Means and Standard Errors from Mixed Model Analyses of Incomplete Data from the Hand-Sized Data Set

Scenario	Treatment	LSMEANS	Contrast	Contrast SE
Treatment main effect results				
$\sigma_b^2 = 1, \sigma_e^2 = 1$	1	–10.70	0.00	1.30
	2	–10.70		
$\sigma_b^2 = 9, \sigma_e^2 = 1$	1	–10.60	0.60	3.12
	2	–11.20		
$\sigma_b^2 = 5, \sigma_e^2 = 5$	1	–10.70	0.00	2.87
	2	–10.70		
$\sigma_b^2 = 9, \sigma_e^2 = 1$	1	–10.78	–0.65	2.40
	2	–10.13		
Time 3 results				
$\sigma_b^2 = 1, \sigma_e^2 = 1$	1	–15.50	–0.50	1.91
	2	–15.00		
$\sigma_b^2 = 9, \sigma_e^2 = 1$	1	–15.29	0.51	3.42
	2	–15.80		
$\sigma_b^2 = 5, \sigma_e^2 = 5$	1	–15.50	–0.50	4.17
	2	–15.00		
$\sigma_b^2 = 1, \sigma_e^2 = 9$	1	–15.86	–1.66	4.47
	1	–14.20		

as for the treatment main effect. With a fixed total variance, as σ_b^2 increases, σ_e^2 decreases and the within-subject correlation increases. As with complete data, larger within-subject correlation resulted in smaller gain in precision from repeated observations. However, with fixed total variance, for a contrast at a single time point, as σ_b^2 increases, σ_e^2 decreases, which decreases error variance and reduces the standard error.

The shrinkage of random effect estimates can again be seen in the estimates of the random intercepts across the varying levels of σ_b^2 and σ_e^2. These results are summarized in Table 5.4 for Subject 1. The observation for Subject 1 was missing at Time 2 and Time 3. At Time 1, Subject 1's observation was 2 points better than the group mean. In contrast to the complete data, this is the only evidence about Subject 1 and it is easier to see how σ_b^2 and σ_e^2 influence estimates.

In this simple situation, the estimate of the random intercept for Subject 1 is calculated as that subject's deviation from the mean multiplied by the shrinkage factor determined by the variance components. With Subject 1, the two-point superiority in improvement resulted in an estimated intercept of –1.8 when $\sigma_b^2 = 9$, $\sigma_e^2 = 1$. The estimated intercept is 90% of the magnitude of the deviation from the group mean when the ratio of σ_b^2 to total variance (9/(9 + 1)) is 90%.

With $\sigma_b^2 = 5$, $\sigma_e^2 = 5$ and $\sigma_b^2 = 1$, $\sigma_e^2 = 1$, the estimated intercept was –1.0, 50% of the observed deviation from the group mean, and the ratio of σ_b^2 to total variance = 0.5. With $\sigma_b^2 = 1$, $\sigma_e^2 = 9$, the estimated intercept was –0.2, 1/10 the observed deviation, and the ratio of σ_b^2 to total variance = 0.1. If Subject 1's observation had been 2 points below the group mean, the estimated intercept would have been the same magnitude but opposite in sign (–2 × the shrinkage factor). If the observed deviation had been 4 points above average, the estimated intercept would have been calculated as four × the shrinkage factor.

These results illustrate that σ_b^2 and σ_e^2 define the regression of estimated intercept on deviation from the group mean. In this simple setting,

TABLE 5.4

Estimated Intercepts and Group Means at Time 3 for Subject 1 from Mixed Model Analyses of Incomplete Data across Varying Values of G and R

Scenario	Group Mean	Estimated Intercept	Predicted Value
$\sigma_b^2 = 1, \sigma_e^2 = 1$	–15.00	–1.00	–16.00
$\sigma_b^2 = 9, \sigma_e^2 = 1$	–15.80	–1.80	–17.60
$\sigma_b^2 = 5, \sigma_e^2 = 5$	–15.00	–1.00	–16.00
$\sigma_b^2 = 1, \sigma_e^2 = 9$	–14.20	–0.20	–14.40

when $\sigma_b^2/(\sigma_b^2 + \sigma_e^2) = 0.9$, the regression = 0.9, when $\sigma_b^2/(\sigma_b^2 + \sigma_e^2) = 0.5$, the regression = 0.5, etc. This makes intuitive sense because σ_b^2 and σ_e^2 define the intra-class correlation (a.k.a. repeatability) of the multiple observations on the same subjects. As error variance (σ_e^2) decreases, the reliability or repeatability of observations increases and the observations more closely reflect the true value; hence, a smaller shrinkage factor is applied.

The same general relationships were present in the complete data, but they were less obvious because, with three observations on each subject, the setting was that of multiple regression. With only one observation on Subject 1, the setting is simple regression and relationships are easier to see.

Although specific results are idiosyncratic to specific combinations of variance components and deviations from group means, the general idea of ratios in variance components defining the magnitude of shrinkage to estimates of random effects is common to all mixed-effect analyses. Importantly, change to random effect estimates due to changes in variance components in unbalanced data also influence estimates of fixed effects.

5.5 Methods of Estimation

5.5.1 Inferential Frameworks

Three general frameworks for inference are frequentist, Bayesian, and likelihood-based. With frequentist inference conclusions are drawn from significance tests, or results are expressed in terms of sample-derived confidence intervals. With Bayesian inference results are expressed in terms of probability distributions for the parameters being estimated. Likelihood-based inference arises from the assertion that all the information in samples is contained in probability distributions—called likelihood functions. The extent to which the evidence supports one parameter value or hypothesis against another is therefore equal to the ratio of their likelihoods. From these likelihoods (probabilities), confidence intervals and hypothesis tests can be constructed.

Obviously, method of inference and method of estimation are linked. Subsequent sections in this chapter briefly review common methods of estimation: least squares and generalized estimating equations (GEE), and takes a more in-depth look at maximum likelihood-based estimation.

5.5.2 Least Squares

A standard reference for least squares estimation is Snedecor and Cochran (1980). Least squares minimizes $(Y–X\beta)'(Y–X\beta)$, that is, minimizes squared deviations. The mechanics of least squares estimation for fixed effects was illustrated in Section 5.3.1. The following section provides additional detail.

Fisher (1925) introduced the method for estimating variance components by equating sum of squares to their expected values. Possibly the most important paper in least squares estimation for unbalanced data is Henderson (1953). The three methods presented in that paper, later known as Henderson's methods, were the standard estimation methods for linear mixed-effect models until fast computers became available.

In simple regression, the method of least squares determines the best fit line to the data by minimizing the error sums of squares. The degree to which the data points are scattered around the line determines how well the model "fits" the data. The more tightly clustered the points are around the line, the better the fit to the data. Best fit can be determined for any finite linear combination of specified functions and is not limited to regression settings. That is, any number of categorical and continuous independent variables can be fit via least squares.

Least squares has been used broadly across many fields of research because it is a flexible method that can be applied to simple data structures using simple models, or can be adapted to complex situations with complex models. A simple data structure could have, for example, one observation on the outcome variable per subject. More complex data structures arise when the outcome variable is measured repeatedly on each subject (or experimental unit). Least squares can be adapted to these more complex data structures. As illustrated in Sections 5.3.1 and 5.3.2, least squares can be subdivided into two categories: ordinary least squares for simple data structures and generalized least squares to accommodate correlated data.

An important attribute of least squares estimation and the associated frequentist inference is that missing data are only ignorable if arising from a missing completely at random (MCAR) mechanism. Important missing data concepts are covered in Section III, including the benefits of ignorability. See in particular Chapters 12 and 13. For now, it is sufficient to know that methods such as least squares that require MCAR for ignorability are less well-suited to longitudinal clinical trial data than methods that require the less restrictive assumption of missing at random (MAR).

5.5.3 Generalized Estimating Equations

A standard reference for generalized estimating equations (GEE) is Liang and Zeger (1986). Intuitively, GEE allows for correlation between repeated measurements on the same subjects without explicitly defining a model for the origin of the dependency. As a consequence, GEE is less sensitive to parametric assumptions than maximum likelihood, and is computationally more efficient. Some connections can be drawn between the origins of GEE and maximum likelihood. However, GEE is a non-likelihood based method, and hence frequentist, and similar to least squares. The very restrictive assumption of an MCAR missing data mechanism is required for ignorabily of missing data in GEE.

In GEE, estimates arise as generalizations of both quasi-likelihood and generalized linear models from univariate to multivariate outcomes. It is a viable approach for conducting inference on parameters that can be expressed via the first moments of some underlying multivariate distributions (e.g., treatment contrast in repeated measures analysis), especially in situations when specification of the entire multivariate distribution may be challenging. For example, GEE can be useful for analysis of non-normally distributed (e.g., binary) correlated data when maximum likelihood methods either do not exist or are hard to implement. See Chapter 10 for additional details on analyses of categorical data.

The attractiveness of GEE is in that it does not require modeling within-subject correlation structures. Even if the structure is incorrectly specified (e.g., assumed to be independent), the point estimates of parameters are consistent and the correct standard errors can be computed by using the robust sandwich estimator that is based on residuals from the fitted model. However, the relaxed distributional assumptions and non-reliance on correlation structure comes at the price of generally decreased statistical efficiency. That is, all else equal, parameter estimates from GEE will have greater standard errors than corresponding maximum likelihood estimates.

GEE obtains estimates as solutions of estimating equations that have the following form.

$$s(\beta) = \sum_{i=1}^{N} D_i^T V_i^{-1} \left(Y_i - \mu_i(\beta) \right) = 0$$

Here, the summation is over N patients, μ_i is a vector of expected marginal means for the ith subject (i.e., the set of n_i visit-wise marginal means μ_{ij} for the ith subject with evaluations at visits $j=1,...,n_i$) that are expressed in terms of linear combination $X_{ij}^T\beta$ through an appropriate link function. For example, when modeling binary data using the logit link, the marginal means are probabilities of the event of interest that are related to a linear predictor $l_{ij} = X_{ij}^T\beta$ via an inverse logit transformation $Pr(Y_{ij}=1) = \mu_{ij}=1/(1+\exp(-l_{ij}))$. The linear combination l_{ij} is the product of row-vector X_{ij}^T in the $N \times p$ design matrix X_j and the p-dimensional vector of parameters β (e.g., associated with treatment variable, baseline severity score).

The $n_i \times p$ matrix D_i contains partial derivatives of μ_i with respect to parameters β and the $n_i \times n_i$ matrix V_i is essentially a "working model" for the covariance of Y_i that is decomposed into a so-called working correlation matrix R(α) (where α is the vector of estimated parameters) that is pre- and post-multiplied by the square root of diagonal matrix A_i with marginal variances.

$$V_i = \phi A_i^{\frac{1}{2}} R(\alpha) A_i^{\frac{1}{2}}$$

Note that the GEE actually contains p equations. In the simplest case of a univariate normal regression, these specialize to p "normal equations" that are obtained by differentiating the log-likelihood (or least squares) with respect to p parameters in β.

5.5.4 Maximum Likelihood

Maximum likelihood (ML) estimation for normal distribution variance component models was considered by Crump (1947). The landmark papers on ML estimation include Hartley and Rao (1967), in which the first asymptotic results for the maximum likelihood estimators (MLE) were established. Restricted maximum likelihood was introduced by Thompson (1962) and later extended by Patterson and Thompson (1971). Harville (1977) presented a comprehensive review of maximum likelihood and restricted maximum likelihood estimation in linear mixed-effects models and is a standard reference, along with papers by Laird and Ware (1982), and Jennrich and Schluchter (1986).

Loosely speaking, a likelihood function is the probability distribution function associated with the parameter(s) being estimated from the observed data sample. Parameter values are set such that the observed data sample is most likely to be generated from the underlying probability distribution. In maximum likelihood estimation, the value of a parameter that maximizes the likelihood function is chosen as the estimate for that parameter. For example, the appropriate likelihood function for a continuous variable may be the normal probability distribution, which includes parameters for the mean and variance. A key implication is that parameters for the mean and variance need to be estimated. When extending this to repeated measures taken in a longitudinal clinical trial, parameters for mean, variance, and covariance (correlation) need to be estimated.

With likelihood-based estimation and inference (as well as with Bayesian inference), missing data can be ignored if it arises from either an MCAR or MAR mechanism. This is an extremely important advantage for longitudinal clinical trial data analyses over least squares and GEE that require the more restrictive assumption of MCAR for ignorability. (See Section III, especially Chapter 12 and 13, for additional details.)

Use of least squares does not mean the errors (residuals from the model) will be small, only that no other estimates will yield smaller errors.

And ML does not guarantee the parameter estimates have a high likelihood of being the true value, only that there is no other value of the parameter that has a greater likelihood, given the data. Under certain conditions, ML and least squares yield the same results.

Restricted maximum likelihood estimates (RMLE) of the variance-covariance components are usually preferred to MLE in linear mixed-effects models because RMLEs take into account the estimation of the fixed effects when calculating the degrees of freedom associated with the variance-components estimates, while MLEs do not.

Maximum likelihood and restricted maximum likelihood estimates of G and R can be obtained by constructing appropriate objective functions and maximizing that function over the unknown parameters. The corresponding log-likelihood functions are as follows:

$$\text{ML:}\quad l(\mathrm{G},\mathrm{R}) = -\frac{1}{2}\log|\mathrm{V}| - \frac{1}{2}\mathrm{r}'\mathrm{V}^{-1}\mathrm{r} - \frac{n}{2}\log(2\pi)$$

$$\text{REML:}\quad l_R(\mathrm{G},\mathrm{R}) = -\frac{1}{2}\log|\mathrm{V}| - \frac{1}{2}\log|\mathrm{X}'\mathrm{V}^{-1}\mathrm{X}| - \frac{1}{2}\mathrm{r}'\mathrm{V}^{-1}\mathrm{r} - \frac{n-p}{2}\log(2\pi)\}$$

where $\mathrm{r} = \mathrm{Y} - \mathrm{X}(\mathrm{X}'\mathrm{V}^{-1}\mathrm{X})^{-}\mathrm{X}'\mathrm{V}^{-1}\mathrm{Y}$ and p is the rank of X.

In practice, commercial software packages minimize –2 times these functions by using a ridge-stabilized Newton–Raphson algorithm, which is generally preferred over the expectation-maximum algorithm (Lindstrom and Bates 1988). One advantage of using the Newton–Raphson algorithm is that the second derivative matrix of the objective function evaluated at the optima (H) is available upon completion.

The asymptotic theory of maximum likelihood shows that H^{-1} is an estimate of the asymptotic variance-covariance matrix of the estimated parameters of G and R. Therefore, tests and confidence intervals based on asymptotic normality can be obtained. However, these tests can be unreliable in small samples, especially for parameters such as variance components that have sampling distributions that tend to be skewed to the right (SAS 2013). See Verbeke and Molenberghs (2000) for additional details on estimation and testing of variance components in likelihood-based models.

5.6 Marginal, Conditional, and Joint Inference

Within each inferential framework/method of estimation, it is also important to consider whether marginal, conditional, or joint inference is most relevant for the clinical question at hand.

To illustrate the conceptual distinctions between marginal, conditional, and joint inference, consider the following example regarding the probability of developing a certain disease. Assume that D is a discrete random variable with a value of 1 for subjects with the disease and 0 for those who do not have the disease. Further assume that R is a discrete random variable with a value of 1 for subjects with known risk factors for the disease and 0 for those who do not have risk factors. Further assume that the probabilities of D depend on R. That is, P(D = 1) and P(D = 0) vary depending on whether R is 0 or 1. With R = 1, P(D = 1) is greater than if R = 0. Hypothetical probabilities for the example are listed below.

	R = 0	R = 1	Marginal Probability
D = 0 (healthy)	0.70	0.10	0.80
D = 1 (disease)	0.10	0.10	0.20
Total	0.80	0.20	1.0

Finding the probability for specific pairs of outcomes, D and R, requires knowledge of the joint probability distribution. An example would be the probability of a subject having D = 1 and R = 0. That is, what is the probability of having the disease and no risk factors, which in this example is 0.10 (10%).

An example of marginal inference from these data would be questions about the probability of D without regard for R. That is, what is the probability of having the disease without regard for whether or not risk factors are present? The marginal P(D = 1) can be found by summing the joint probabilities for D = 1 across levels of R. In the example, the marginal P(D = 1) = 0.10 + 0.10 = 0.20. The marginal P(D = 0) can be found similarly by summing across levels of R where D = 0 (0.80 in the example). Thus the marginal probability of having the disease = 20% and the marginal probability of not having the disease = 80%.

An example of conditional inference from these data would be questions about the probability of having the disease conditional on having (or not having) risk factors. The conditional probability of having disease in subjects with risk factors is based on only those subjects with R = 1. Hence, the probability D = 1 given R = 1 (which can be denoted as $P(D = 1 | R = 1) = 0.10/(0.10 + 0.10) = 50\%$. Similarly, the probability of having the disease in subjects with no risk factors is $P(D = 1 | R = 0)$, which is calculated as $0.10/(0.70 + 0.10) = 12.5\%$.

None of these three inferential frameworks (joint, marginal, and conditional) is inherently more relevant than the others; each can be the most relevant or not relevant depending on the question being addressed. The distinction between marginal and conditional inference is relevant in longitudinal trials of medical interventions, but perhaps not as straightforward as in the previous simplistic example.

This topic is most often considered with regard to random effects, such as subject.

The marginal and conditional means in the linear mixed model are $E[Y] = X\beta$ and $E[Y|b] = X\beta + Zb$, respectively. Therefore, the marginal and conditional residuals are $Y - X\beta$ and $Y - X\beta - Zb$, respectively. Recall that random effects are constrained to have mean = 0. Therefore, in normally distributed data with a linear model $X\beta = X\beta + Zb$. That is, with regard to fixed effects contrasts, there is no difference between the marginal and the conditional result. However, for data that are not normally distributed, this will not be the case.

Another way to conceptualize the distinction is that marginal inference involves the estimate of the average response in the population of subjects whereas conditional inference involves the estimates of response for the average subject (the subject for which $b = 0$). In normally distributed data, the average response and the response of the average subject are identical. In nonnormal data, they are not identical. However, the important issues are not so much numeric equality or inequality, but rather which estimate is best to address the question at hand.

Section II

Modeling the Observed Data

Given the variety of scenarios that may be encountered in longitudinal clinical trials, no universally best model or modeling approach exists. This implies that the analysis must be tailored to the situation at hand. To an extent, characteristics of the data are driven by the design of the study. And, an appropriate analysis therefore follows logically from the design—and the estimand. The analyst must therefore understand how data characteristics and estimands influence choice of analysis. In Section II, each chapter addresses a common modeling consideration for the analysis of longitudinal clinical trial data. Chapter 6 discusses various choices for the dependent variable. Chapter 7 covers approaches to modeling mean trends over time. Chapter 8 covers common methods to account for correlation between repeated measurements. Chapter 9 covers considerations for whether covariates should be included and, if so, how best to include them. Chapter 10 covers categorical data. Chapter 11 covers model checking and validation.

6

Choice of Dependent Variable and Statistical Test

6.1 Introduction

A logical place to begin in developing analyses for longitudinal clinical trial data is to determine the dependent (i.e., response or outcome) variable and upon what basis it will be evaluated. These may seem like obvious decisions dictated by the design of the trial and historical precedent. However, a number of subtleties apply and these factors reinforce the need for the iterative study development process detailed in Chapter 2. Specifically, the trial design informs the analysis, but analytic consequences also need to inform the design.

Of course, the distribution of the outcome variable influences the method of analysis. Statistical methods for a wide array of distributions are well known. In many longitudinal clinical trials the primary analysis is based on a continuously distributed variable. Continuous outcome variables can be analyzed as: the actual outcomes collected, change from baseline, percent change from baseline, or a dichotomized version of the outcome indicating whether or not some relevant threshold in the actual score, change, or percent change is achieved.

In addition, the statistical test used to evaluate these various versions of the outcome variable could be based on a contrast at a single, landmark time point, or based on multiple time points, such as a slopes analysis, treatment main effect or treatment-by-time interaction. Convention may guide the analyst to choices for the primary analysis. Nevertheless, consequences of the conventional choice should be understood. Secondary analyses of alternative choices or an alternative choice may be needed as the primary analysis.

6.2 Statistical Test—Cross-Sectional and Longitudinal Contrasts

In clinical trials, it is common to base the primary analysis on a contrast at a landmark time point. Such contrasts are often referred to as cross-sectional contrasts because the focus is on a "cross section in time." However, other "longitudinal contrasts" that involve multiple time points, for example, the entire longitudinal profile, are often worth considering for the primary analysis or secondary analysis.

An important distinction must be made for cross-sectional contrasts. Historically, cross-sectional contrasts have often been based upon just the data at the landmark time point. However, it is possible to construct the same cross-sectional contrast from the longitudinal sequence of data. Single-point-in-time analyses were likely motivated by simplicity and ease of computation in an era when computational efficiency was a legitimate concern. However, with advancements in hardware and software, such compromises are no longer needed.

Incorporating all repeated measures from a subject into an analysis rather than including just a single outcome per subject opens many possibilities for analyses. Perhaps the most important benefit from longitudinal analyses, regardless of whether or not focus is on a landmark time point, is in accounting for missing data. With repeated measurements, the correlation between outcomes within subjects can be exploited under certain conditions to provide safeguards against potential bias from missing data. Missing data is a nuanced and detailed discussion that is covered in detail in Section III of this book. The important point here is that longitudinal data require a longitudinal analysis, even when focus is on a single point in time. Therefore, the emphasis throughout this book is on longitudinal analysis, with illustrations of how contrasts can be constructed if focus is on a single point in time.

The following examples in Figures 6.1 through 6.3 illustrate some of the key considerations in choosing between test statistics that involve a single landmark time point versus test statistics that include data from all time points.

Figure 6.1 illustrates a significant treatment-by-time interaction wherein the difference between treatments varies over time. The two groups are equal at endpoint, but the effect evolved more slowly in one group. Such a scenario reinforces the need to understand the longitudinal profiles that lead to the endpoint results.

Figure 6.2 illustrates a significant treatment main effect, with a rapidly evolving treatment effect that is sustained until endpoint. The consistency of the time trends suggests the treatment main effect, which includes data from all time points, could be a useful primary analysis. The treatment main effect is in essence an average effect over all visits and can be interpreted similarly to an area under the curve analysis.

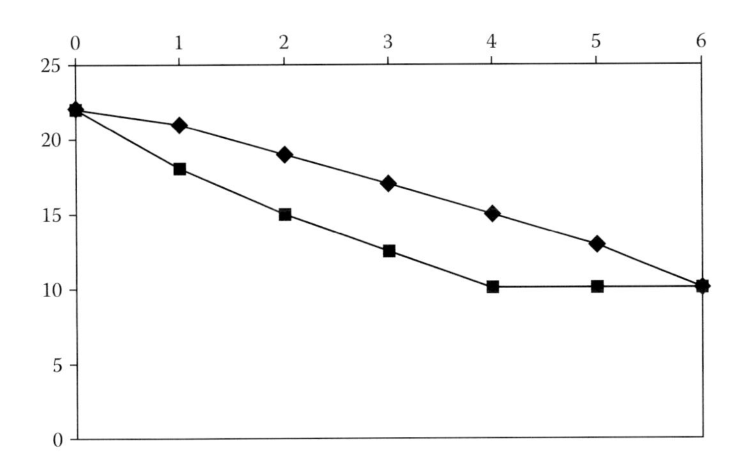

FIGURE 6.1
Illustration of a significant treatment-by-time interaction with a transitory benefit in one arm.

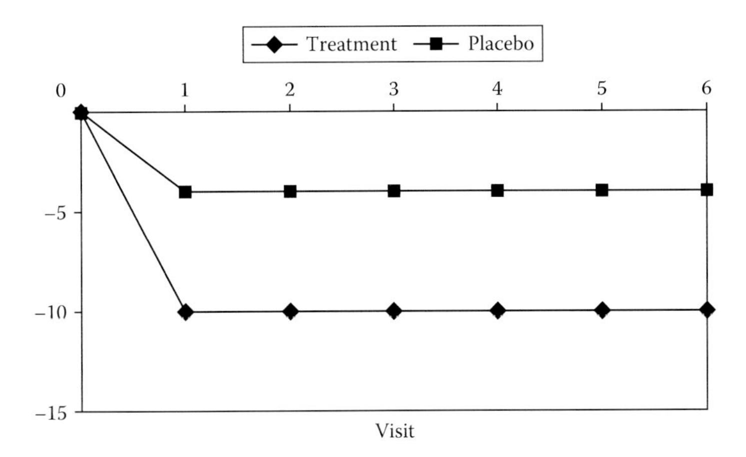

FIGURE 6.2
Illustration of a significant treatment main effect.

Figure 6.3 illustrates a significant treatment-by-time interaction where the treatment effect increases over time. The treatment contrast at endpoint is usually of particular interest in such scenarios. However, in certain situations similar to this example, focus may be on the rate of change over time, that is, time is fit as a continuous effect (see Chapter 8 for further examples).

In situations with more than two treatment arms, additional options for primary test statistics exist. For example, a global F test might be used at a landmark time point to assess if any differences exist between treatments at that visit. Or, if treatment main effects are relevant, a global F test for the treatment main effect can be used that includes data from all visits in all arms.

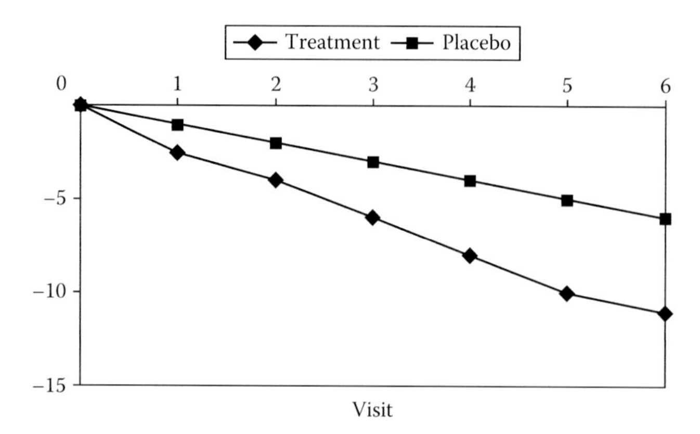

FIGURE 6.3
Illustration of a significant treatment-by-time interaction with an increasing treatment difference over time.

6.3 Form of Dependent Variable (Actual Value, Change, or Percent Change)

Clinical relevance is an important factor in the choice of how a continuous outcome is expressed. In some scenarios, the outcomes are well-understood at face value and the actual values may be favored for the dependent variable. Consider blood pressure, a well-understood, objective measure for which the actual outcomes are meaningful and could be used in the primary analysis. However, medical interventions are hoped to elicit change in a condition. Therefore, even if the actual outcome is meaningful and well-understood, change from baseline may be the more intuitive and preferred outcome.

For other outcomes, the actual values may not be readily meaningful or widely understood. Take, for example, the psoriasis area and severity index (PASI) (Langley et al. 2004). The PASI combines the amount of skin covered by the psoriatic plaques (area) and the severity (thickness, redness, etc.) of the plaques into a single number that can range from 0 to 72. Experienced researchers understand PASI scores, but the broader dermatology community may lack context and find such values difficult to interpret. Similarly, if the actual values have limited meaning, then change scores may also be difficult to interpret. Therefore, psoriasis clinical trials typically use percent change from baseline because relative changes are easier for broader audiences to appreciate.

However, the analytic consequences of the choices need to be considered. Perhaps foremost among these analytic consequences is the distribution of the dependent variable. To illustrate key points, consider the histograms of all post-baseline values for actual HAMD17 total scores, change from baseline, and percent change from baseline obtained from the small complete data set that are depicted in Figures 6.4 through 6.6.

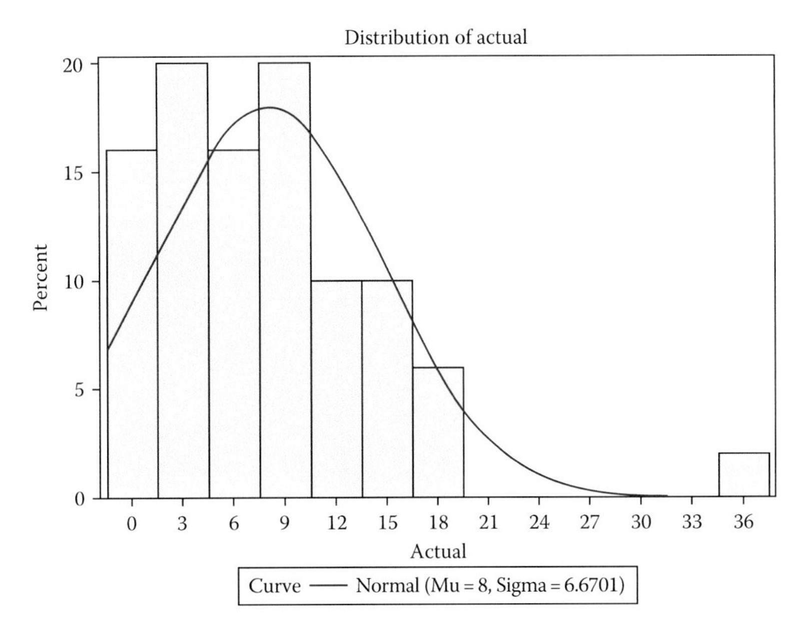

FIGURE 6.4
Distribution of actual scores in the small complete data set.

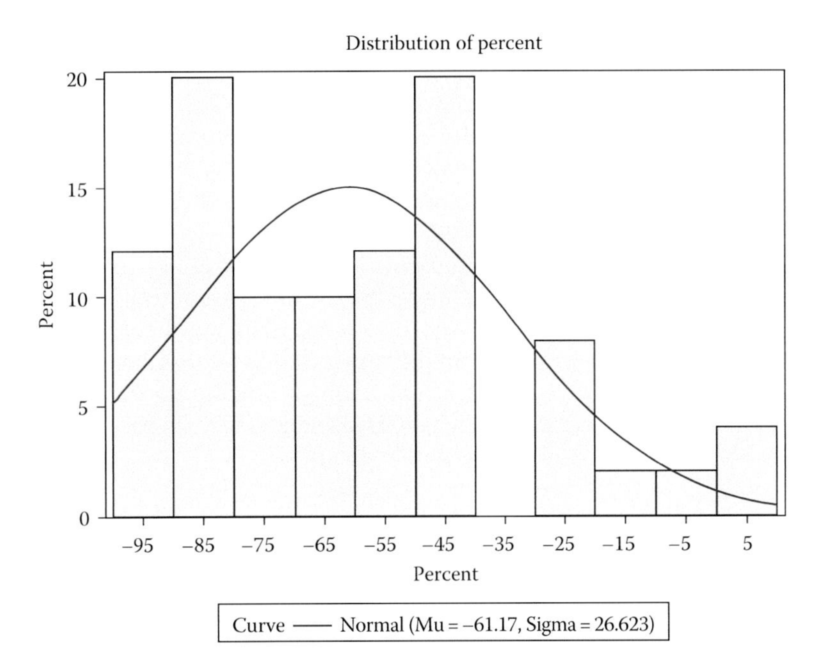

FIGURE 6.5
Distribution of percent changes from baseline in the small complete data set.

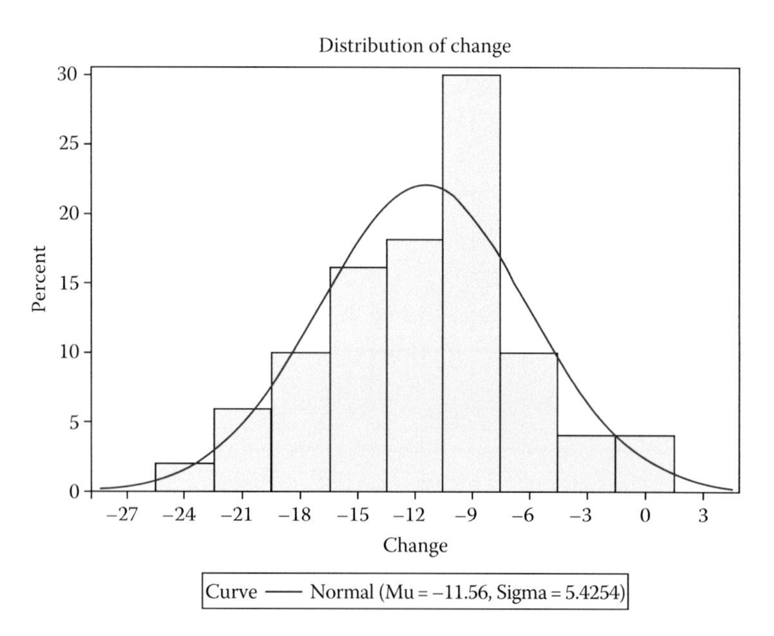

FIGURE 6.6
Distribution of changes from baseline in the small complete data set.

The actual values and the percent changes have truncated distributions, bounded by 0 for actual values and –100% for percent change. Actual scores and percent changes also have skewed distributions, with actual scores having an extreme outlier value. In contrast, changes from baseline are not truncated and are more symmetrically distributed. Of course, this is only one example and situations vary. However, whenever an appreciable portion of subjects have a score of 0, and accordingly –100 percent change, truncation and its impact should be considered.

To that end, nonnormality of the outcome variable is not the key issue. Normality of the residuals is the key distributional assumption. However, residuals are more likely to be nonnormal as the distribution of the outcome variable departs further from normality. As will be seen in Chapter 9, under certain formulations of a longitudinal analysis (including baseline score for the outcome variable as a covariate) treatment contrasts based on actual change and change from baseline will be identical.

Considerations for percent change are particularly important when there is no minimum requirement for baseline severity, as would be the case for many secondary outcomes. To illustrate, consider the hypothetical data in Table 6.1 for a 100 mm visual analog scale for pain. Subjects rate pain by marking a spot in the line describing their pain (current pain, pain during the assessment interval, etc.). Zero denotes no pain and 100 denotes the worst possible pain.

TABLE 6.1

Hypothetical Data Illustrating Actual Outcomes, Change from Baseline, and Percent Change from Baseline

Subject	Treatment	Baseline	Endpoint	Change	Percent Change
1	1	60	30	–30	–50%
2	1	1	10	9	900%
3	2	20	10	–10	–50%
4	2	80	30	–50	–62%
Mean	1		20	–10.5	425%
Mean	2		20	–30	–56%

TABLE 6.2

Hypothetical Data Illustrating Dichotomization of a Continuous Endpoint

Subject	Treatment	Percent Change	Response Status
1	1	–70%	Yes
2	1	+20%	No
3	2	–49%	No
4	2	–50%	Yes

Based on the unadjusted (raw) means, mean endpoint scores are equal for Treatments 1 and 2 (20 for each treatment). The mean change from baseline is nearly threefold greater for Treatment 2 (30 versus –10.5). The mean percent change from baseline for Treatment 1 is strongly influenced by Subject 2, who had minimal pain at baseline and a small increase at endpoint. The low baseline severity results in an extreme outlier value for percent change. While this hypothetical example is purposefully extreme, it illustrates how percent change can create outlier values and nonnormal distributions, especially when analyzing a variable with no minimum requirement for baseline severity.

In situations where percent change is customary, an alternative may be to conduct the analyses based on changes from baseline and then convert the mean changes into *percent mean change*, rather than using percent change as the dependent variable to assess *mean percent change*. In the example above, the percent mean changes for Treatments 1 and 2 are approximately –34% (mean change of –10.5 divided by baseline mean of 30.5) and –60% (mean change of –30 divided by baseline mean of 50), respectively.

Dichotomization of continuous outcomes into binary outcomes of whether or not a certain threshold of response was met causes a loss of information. To illustrate, consider the hypothetical data in Table 6.2. Assume that a 50% improvement from baseline is used as the cut off to define responder status.

The percent changes for Subjects 2 and 3 are very different (20% worsening vs. 49% improvement), but both are classified as nonresponders. The percent changes for Subjects 3 and 4 are essentially identical, but Subject 3 is a nonresponder and Subject 4 is a responder. Both treatment groups have a 50% responder rate, whereas the mean percent change is approximately twofold greater for Treatment 2.

In situations where responder rate is a common outcome, it may be useful to consider some form of mean change analysis to assess if a treatment signal exists and then use the dichotomized responder status to describe the clinical relevance of a signal, if one is found based on the mean change analysis.

6.4 Summary

Cross-sectional contrasts have often been based upon just the data at the landmark time point. However, it is possible to construct the same cross-sectional contrast from the longitudinal sequence of data. Using longitudinal analyses rather than cross-sectional analyses opens many possibilities for tailoring the analysis to the situation at hand. Actual change from baseline will usually have better distributional properties than percent changes, especially when there is no baseline minimum requirement for the dependent variable.

7

Modeling Covariance (Correlation)

7.1 Introduction

Clinical trials often assess subjects repeatedly over time. Correlations between repeated measurements *within* the same subjects often arise from between-subject variability and adjacency in time or location of evaluations. Therefore, independence of observations cannot be assumed in longitudinal trials. Failure to properly account for the association between observations can result in biased point estimates and standard errors that do not properly reflect the uncertainty in the data.

Between-subject variability (i.e., heterogeneity between individual profiles) may arise from inherent, subject-specific factors, such as genotype. Additional association may arise from unaccounted for fixed effects, such as age or gender, which like genotype influence every observation and therefore create association between repeated observations. Further association may arise due to time course (i.e., serial) correlation, which exists when observations closer to each other in time (or location) are more similar than observations further apart in time (or location).

Correlation *between* subjects is generally less of a concern in longitudinal clinical trials than correlations within subjects. Sources of correlation between subjects may include genetic or environmental factors. Generally, the frequency of relatives in a clinical trial is so low that genetic correlation can be ignored. The most common environmental source of correlation is that observations on subjects at the same investigative site (location) may be more similar to each other than to the sample as a whole.

Random measurement errors contribute to variability. In the longitudinal setting it is particularly important to consider the potential for error variance to increase or decrease over time (Mallinckrodt et al. 2003). Measurement errors tend to weaken the association between the measurements.

Longitudinal analyses can account for the correlation between observations as functions of the random effects, the residual effects, or both. Appropriate means of accounting for correlations between observations begins with considering the sources of covariation. The relative importance of the various sources of (co)variance can be useful in guiding modeling choices for specific circumstances.

For example, in analyses of objective physical measures such as blood pressure or laboratory values, subject-specific factors may have the greatest contribution to within-subject correlations. Fixed effects that are not included in the analysis (e.g., subject's age or gender) may also give rise to a compound symmetric error structure because, like random effects, these fixed effects may have the same effect on each observation. Detailed descriptions for a wide array of correlation structures are available (SAS 2013).

In analyses of subjective ratings, such as the Hamilton Depression Rating Scale (Hamilton 1960), serial correlation that decays with increasing distance in time (such as in an autoregressive structure) may also be important.

In clinical trials where the focus is primarily on the fixed effects, it may be equally appropriate, and more straightforward, to omit explicit modeling of the subject-specific effects and model them as part of the within-subject error (residual) correlation structure. In such cases, the subject-specific effects and serial correlations combine, with or without changes in error variance over time, to yield what is often an unstructured correlation pattern for the within-subject (residual) errors.

In certain settings the number of parameters that must be estimated for an unstructured covariance matrix can be prohibitive. However, many clinical trials have observations taken on the primary outcome measure at a relatively small number of time points. These measurement times are typically fixed, with narrow intervals. Thus measurements may be taken perhaps once per week, with the Week 1 observation mandated to take place between days 5 and 9, the Week 2 observation between days 12 and 16, and so on.

Therefore, unstructured modeling of residual correlation is a popular approach in clinical trials, especially confirmatory trials, because fewer restrictions/assumptions are imposed on the pattern of correlations over time. However, this should not be confused with an assumption-free approach. For example, unstructured modeling of within-subject correlation may still require assumptions, such as the same correlation structure applies to each treatment group. Of course, this restriction can be relaxed by specifying separate structures for each treatment group. However, separate structures for each group may trigger the issue of having to estimate a prohibitively large number of parameters relative to the number of subjects.

7.2 Assessing Model Fit

Given the importance of appropriately modeling the covariance between repeated measures, and the variety of approaches that can be used, it is important to assess the fit of a prespecified model and to compare the fit of alternative models.

With likelihood-based estimation the objective function can be used to assess model fit and to compare the fit of candidate models. If one model is a submodel of another, likelihood ratio tests can be used to assess if the more general model provides superior fit. The likelihood ratio test is constructed by computing –2 times the difference between the log likelihoods of the candidate models. This statistic is then compared to the χ^2 distribution with degrees of freedom equal to the difference in the number of parameters for the two models.

For models that are not submodels of each other, various information criteria can be used to determine which model provides the best fit. The Akaike (AIC) and Bayesian (BIC) information criteria are two common approaches (Hurvich and Tsai 1989). These criteria are essentially log likelihood values adjusted (penalized) for the number of parameters estimated, and can thus be used to compare different models. The criteria are set up such that the model with the smaller value is preferred.

7.3 Modeling Covariance as a Function of Random Effects

Two common means of modeling within-subject correlation include fitting a random intercept or the random coefficient regression approach that fits a random intercept and random effect(s) for time. Random coefficient regression is covered in Section 8.3. Code fragments for fitting a random intercept model in SAS and R for the small complete data set are listed in Section 7.8 (Code Fragment 7.1). Results from fitting a random intercept model are summarized in Table 7.1.

The between-subject variance (random intercept) was 15.08 and the residual variance was 8.11, resulting in within-subject correlations of approximately 0.65 [15.08/(15.08 + 8.11)]. This formulation of the mixed model assumes constant variance over time. Therefore, the within-treatment standard errors and the standard errors of the contrasts between treatments do not change over time. At Time 3 the between-treatment contrast was 3.39 and the SE was 1.36.

The correlation between observations on different subjects at the same investigative site could be modeled by adding a random intercept for site to the model above.

TABLE 7.1

Results from Fitting a Random Intercept Model to the Small Complete Data Set

Visit-wise Least Square Means			
Treatment	**Time**	**LSMEAN**	**Standard Error**
1	1	−4.120	0.9641
1	2	−6.70	0.9641
1	3	−9.86	0.9641
2	1	−5.31	0.9641
2	2	−8.69	0.9641
2	3	−13.25	0.9641

Visit-wise Contrasts			
Time	**Difference LSMEAN**	**Standard Error**	**P**
1	1.19	1.36	0.3860
2	1.99	1.36	0.1487
3	3.39	1.36	0.0151

Random intercept variance = 15.08

Residual variance = 8.11

−2 res log likelihood = 823.2

AIC = 827.2

7.4 Modeling Covariance as a Function of Residual Effects

Subject-specific effects and serial correlation or other sources of correlation can be modeled simultaneously. However, if the subject-specific effects are not of direct interest, a simpler formulation of the model can be implemented in which the random effects are not explicitly modeled, but rather are included as part of the error correlation matrix, leading to what could be described as a multivariate normal model. Under certain model specifications discussed in Section 7.5, fitting versus not fitting a random intercept in addition to fitting a residual correlation structure has no effect on treatment contrasts.

Modeling the random effects as part of the within-subject error correlation structure is the feature that distinguishes the so-called MMRM (mixed model for repeated measures) analysis from other implementations of mixed-effects models (Mallinckrodt 2013).

Many residual covariance structures can be implemented for analyses. Some example structures are described below and subsequently used in analyses of the small example data set. The compound symmetric (CS) structure has constant variance and constant covariance across all assessments. The heterogeneous compound symmetric (CSH) structure has a different variance for each assessment time and it uses the square roots of these parameters in the off-diagonal entries. The heterogeneous Toeplitz (TOEPH) structure has a different variance for each assessment time and uses the same correlation value whenever the degree of adjacency is the same (correlation between Time 1 and 2 is the same as between Times 2 and 3). An unstructured covariance matrix is completely unstructured, with different variances at each visit and different covariances for each combination of visits.

Each of the selected structures is described in further detail in Figure 7.1. Those descriptions use four assessment times even though the example data set has only three assessment times. Adding a fourth assessment time makes it easier to appreciate how the structures differ.

Code fragments for fitting the selected residual covariance structures in SAS and R for the small complete data set are listed in Section 7.8 (Code Fragment 7.2). Estimated covariance matrices from fitting these structures are summarized in Table 7.2.

With a compound symmetric structure the within-subject covariance is equal to the between-subject variance when fitting a random intercept model and the total variance is equal for the two models. When adding heterogeneous variance over time to the compound symmetric structure variance estimates increase over time, especially at Time 3. Compound symmetric models fit a single correlation parameter for all combinations of visits. Therefore, when variance increases over time the covariance must increase for observations further apart in time to maintain equal correlation.

Covariance estimates from the unstructured model and the TOEPH model were similar, with variances increasing over time and covariance decreasing for observations further apart in time. Given only three assessment times, the number of parameters estimated for the various structures did not differ

$$\begin{bmatrix} \sigma^2+\sigma_1 & \sigma_1 & \sigma_1 & \sigma_1 \\ \sigma_1 & \sigma^2+\sigma_1 & \sigma_1 & \sigma_1 \\ \sigma_1 & \sigma_1 & \sigma^2+\sigma_1 & \sigma_1 \\ \sigma_1 & \sigma_1 & \sigma_1 & \sigma^2+\sigma_1 \end{bmatrix} \quad \begin{bmatrix} \sigma_1^2 & \sigma_1\sigma_2\rho & \sigma_1\sigma_3\rho & \sigma_1\sigma_4\rho \\ \sigma_2\sigma_1\rho & \sigma_2^2 & \sigma_2\sigma_3\rho & \sigma_2\sigma_4\rho \\ \sigma_3\sigma_1\rho & \sigma_3\sigma_2\rho & \sigma_3^2 & \sigma_3\sigma_4\rho \\ \sigma_4\sigma_1\rho & \sigma_4\sigma_2\rho & \sigma_4\sigma_3\rho & \sigma_4^2 \end{bmatrix}$$

(a) (b)

$$\begin{bmatrix} \sigma_1^2 & \sigma_1\sigma_2\rho_1 & \sigma_1\sigma_3\rho_2 & \sigma_1\sigma_4\rho_3 \\ \sigma_2\sigma_1\rho_1 & \sigma_2^2 & \sigma_2\sigma_3\rho_1 & \sigma_2\sigma_4\rho_2 \\ \sigma_3\sigma_1\rho_2 & \sigma_3\sigma_2\rho_1 & \sigma_3^2 & \sigma_3\sigma_4\rho_1 \\ \sigma_4\sigma_1\rho_3 & \sigma_4\sigma_2\rho_2 & \sigma_4\sigma_3\rho_1 & \sigma_4^2 \end{bmatrix} \quad \begin{bmatrix} \sigma_1^2 & \sigma_{21} & \sigma_{31} & \sigma_{41} \\ \sigma_{21} & \sigma_2^2 & \sigma_{32} & \sigma_{42} \\ \sigma_{31} & \sigma_{32} & \sigma_3^2 & \sigma_{43} \\ \sigma_{41} & \sigma_{42} & \sigma_{43} & \sigma_4^2 \end{bmatrix}$$

(c) (d)

FIGURE 7.1
Description of selected covariance structures for data with four assessment times: (a) compound symmetry, (b) heterogeneous CS, (c) heterogeneous Toeplitz, and (d) unstructured.

TABLE 7.2

Residual (Co)variances and Correlations from Selected Models

	Covariances					
Time	**1**	**2**	**3**	**1**	**2**	**3**
	Compound Symmetric (CS)			*CS with Heterogeneous Variance*		
1	23.19	15.08	15.08	21.28	13.62	16.24
2	15.08	23.19	15.08	13.62	20.08	15.77
3	15.08	15.08	23.19	16.24	15.77	28.54
	Unstructured			*Toeplitz with Heterogeneous Variance*		
1	20.61	15.30	12.28	20.59	15.28	12.28
2	15.30	21.36	17.67	15.28	21.36	17.70
3	12.28	17.67	27.61	12.28	17.70	27.64
	Correlations					
Time	**1**	**2**	**3**	**1**	**2**	**3**
	Compound Symmetric (CS)			*CS with Heterogeneous Variance*		
1	1.00	0.65	0.65	1.00	0.66	0.66
2	0.65	1.00	0.65	0.66	1.00	0.66
3	0.65	0.65	1.00	0.66	0.66	1.00
	Unstructured			*Toeplitz with Heterogeneous Variance*		
1	1.00	0.73	0.51	1.00	0.73	0.51
2	0.73	1.00	0.72	0.73	1.00	0.73
3	0.51	0.72	1.00	0.51	0.73	1.00

TABLE 7.3

Treatment Contrasts, Standard Errors, P Values, and Model Fit Criteria from Selected Residual Correlations Structures

Structure	**AIC**	**Time 3 Contrast**	**Standard Error**	**P**
CSH	828	3.391	1.514	0.0299
TOEPH	820	3.391	1.490	0.0272
UN	823	3.391	1.489	0.0274
UN GROUP = TRT	831	3.381	1.490	0.0279

Note: CSH = compound symmetric with heterogeneous variance, TOEPH = toeplitz with heterogeneous variance, UN = unstructured, GROUP = TRT indicates separate structures were fit for each treatment group.

as much as would be the case with more assessment times. Therefore, results from the different covariance structures were more similar than would be the case with more assessment times.

Treatment contrasts, standard errors, P values and model fit criteria for fitting selected residual correlation structures are summarized in Table 7.3.

The treatment contrasts from models that fit a single covariance structure for all subjects were identical. This would not be expected to happen if some data were missing or the data were otherwise unbalanced. Fitting separate structures by treatment had a small effect on the contrast. Standard errors and P values varied slightly across the various models. The best fit came from the TOEPH model. Although the unstructured covariance model yielded nearly identical results to the TOEPH model, the TOEPH yielded the best fit based on Akaike's information criteria because it estimated fewer parameters.

A banded correlation structure may be useful in scenarios where fitting an unstructured correlation matrix is desired but problematic due to the number of parameters to be estimated. In a banded unstructured covariance matrix, not all covariance parameters are estimated. Instead, only those covariance terms within the specified degree of adjacency (number of bands) are fit and all other covariance terms are set to zero. For example, in a study with 10 post-baseline visits, if an unstructured matrix with 3 bands is fit, then for any time point only those assessments within 3 visits of the reference visit are fit, with all other covariances assumed to = 0. With 10 post-baseline assessments, a fully unstructured approach requires estimation of $10(10 + 1)/2 = 55$ variance and covariance parameters. Banding can therefore dramatically reduce the number of parameters to be fit, but imposes restrictions on how rapidly the correlations decay.

A vast array of residual correlation structures may be fit, far too many to fully consider here. See, for example, the SAS PROC Mixed documentation (SAS 2013) for full descriptions of the structures that can be fit within that software. While choice of covariance structure is in general an important issue, for clinical trials an unstructured approach, either overall or separate structures for each treatment, is generally preferred and almost always feasible given the number of observations relative to the number of parameters to be estimated.

7.5 Modeling Covariance as a Function of Random and Residual Effects

Code fragments for fitting a random intercept and residual correlations in SAS and R for the small complete data set are listed in Section 7.8 (Code Fragment 7.3).

Results from fitting a random intercept and an unstructured residual covariance structure is summarized below. Standard errors, treatment contrasts, and P values were identical for models with unstructured residual covariance structures that fit and did not fit a random intercept for subject.

In actual practice, a model with unstructured covariance and random effects should not be fit because this results in overspecified models. Specifically, if an unstructured covariance is fit, there is nothing left for random effects to explain about the within-subject correlations.

An unstructured covariance was used here in conjunction with a random intercept to illustrate the very point that random effects can be accounted for via residual within-subject correlations and that there is nothing left in addition to be explained by the random intercept. Note that the model fit in SAS as specified in code fragment 7.3 yields the following warning: "NOTE: Convergence criteria met but final hessian is not positive definite." Results from fitting versus not fitting a random intercept will not be identical if a residual structure other than unstructured is fit, but usually results are similar.

Even when interest centers on the fixed effects, it is still useful to understand the random effects. Variance and covariance parameters from the model fitting a random intercept and an unstructured residual covariance structure are summarized in Table 7.4. Adding the random intercept variance to each element of the residual covariance matrix in Table 7.4 reproduces the unstructured covariance matrix in Table 7.3 that was estimated from the model that did not fit the random intercept. The random intercept accounts for most of the total variance at Time 1 and Time 2, and over half the total variance at Time 3. The random intercept accounts for virtually all of the within-subject covariance.

As further noted in Chapter 8, a variety of means can be used to model correlations as a function of the random effects, and as noted above, many possibilities exist for modeling correlations as a function of the residual effects. In principle, most of the approaches can be combined in order to model correlations as functions of random and residual effects. However, model complexity should be considered and it is seldom necessary to fit both a complex random effects and residual effects modeling of correlation; usually, at least one of the two will involve a simple structure and require only one or a few parameters to be estimated.

TABLE 7.4

Variance and Covariance Parameters from the Model Fitting a Random Intercept and an Unstructured Residual Covariance Structure

Intercept Variance 16.06

	Residual Covariance		
Time	**1**	**2**	**3**
1	4.56	−0.75	−3.77
2	−0.75	5.30	1.61
3	−3.78	1.61	11.56

7.6 Modeling Separate Covariance Structures for Groups

In Section 7.3, results from separate residual correlation structures by treatment group were included. In this example, there was little difference in results from fitting separate structures by treatment versus a single, common structure for both treatments. However, in many realistic scenarios it is necessary to at least consider the possibility that correlation structures differ for certain groups of patients. In principle, this is an extension of a *t*-test with heterogeneous variance to the repeated measures setting.

Code fragments for fitting separate random intercepts (Code Fragment 7.4) and separate residual correlations (Code Fragment 7.5) by treatment group in SAS and R for the small complete data set are listed in Section 7.8. Results in Table 7.3 showed that in these examples, fitting separate residual correlation structures by treatment had little effect on results. However, in other scenarios, especially those with unbalanced data and/or missing data, choice of correlation structure is likely to have a greater impact. Therefore, consideration of separate structures for groups is important. Separate correlation structures based on demographic or illness characteristics can also be considered.

7.7 Study Design Considerations

Although understanding the relative magnitude of, for example, a random intercept variance and residual (co)variances is not necessary to interpret fixed effects results, the variance components have implications for study design and power. Refer to the examples in Section 5.4 where given a fixed total variance, the ratio of between-subject variance to within-subject variance influenced standard errors, with the direction (increase or decrease) of effect varying depending on what parameter was being estimated.

Therefore, in powering and designing studies, it is not sufficient to consider only the total variance, rather the between-subject variance and within-subject variance both need to be considered. Historical data can be mined to determine plausible variances for the study under development. Simulations can be used to assess how differing combinations of between- and within-subject variance influence power for specific parameters.

7.8 Code Fragments

CODE FRAGMENT 7.1 SAS and R Code for Fitting a Random Intercept Model

SAS code

```
PROC MIXED DATA=ONE;
 CLASS SUBJECT TRT TIME;
 MODEL CHANGE = BASVAL TRT TIME BASVAL*TIME TRT*TIME /
   DDFM=KR;
 RANDOM INT / SUBJECT=SUBJECT*;
 LSMEANS TRT*TIME/DIFFS;
RUN;
```

R code[†]

```
# using lme function from nlme package
require(nlme)

# setting the time and treatment variables as factors
# (corresponds to the use of CLASS statement in SAS
  procedures
# Note: unlike SAS, R is case-sensitive and variable names
# should be written exactly
# as they are imported in R data frame from a csv file
complete$TIME <-as.factor(complete$TIME)
complete$trt <-as.factor(complete$trt)

# specifying random intercept model in nlme
fitmle<-lme(change ~ basval +trt+ TIME + basval*TIME+
  trt*TIME, data = complete, random = ~ 1 |subject)

# displaying model fit summary
summary(fitmle)

#displaying variance components
VarCorr(fitmle)

# evaluating treatment least square means and contrast at
  specific visit
require(contrast)
```

* In the data set, the patient identification variable is named "subject." If that variable were named ID, then the statement would read RANDOM INT / SUBJECT=ID;

† Obtaining P-values using the Kenward–Roger approximation in R to match results from SAS requires first fitting a random effects model using the lme4 package and then computing KR degrees of freedom using another package (pbkrtest).

```
# least squares means
contrast(fitmle ,a = list(trt = "1", basval=
  mean(complete$basval), TIME = "3"),
     type = "individual")
contrast(fitmle ,a = list(trt = "2", basval=
  mean(complete$basval), TIME = "3"),
     type = "individual")

contrast(fitmle ,a = list(trt = "1", basval=
  mean(complete$basval), TIME = "3"),
                  b = list(trt = "2", basval=
                    mean(complete$basval), TIME = "3"),
     type = "individual")

# Computing p-value based on KR df can be done using lme4
    and pbkrtest packages.
require(lme4)
require(pbkrtest)

# setting the reference (base) level for time and treatment
  variables as the last level
contrasts(complete$TIME) <- contr.treatment(3, base = 3)
contrasts(complete$trt) <- contr.treatment(2, base = 2)

# runs a random effect model using lmer procedure from lme4
  package
lmerfit<-lmer(change ~ basval +trt+ TIME + basval*TIME+
  trt*TIME+(1|subject), data = complete, REML = TRUE)
sumlmer<-summary(lmerfit)

# displays estimated variance components
sumlmer$varcor

# displays estimated coefficients; since we set reference
  levels for trt and time at the last visit the coefficient
  for variable trt estimates treatment effect at the last
  visit.
coefs<-data.frame(coef(sumlmer))
coefs

# obtaining Kenward-Roger degrees of freedom for treatment
  contrast at time 3 using pbkrtest package
trt.df.KR <-get_Lb_ddf(lmerfit, c(0,0,1,0,0,0,0,0,0))
trt.df.KR

# computing p-value from t-distribution with KR degrees of
  freedom
trt.p.KR <- round(2 * (1 - pt(abs(coefs["trt1","t.value"]),
  trt.df.KR)),5)
trt.p.KR.
```

CODE FRAGMENT 7.2 SAS and R Code for Fitting Residual Correlations

SAS code

```
PROC MIXED DATA=ONE;
 CLASS SUBJECT TRT TIME;
 MODEL CHANGE = BASVAL TRT TIME BASVAL*TIME TRT*TIME /
   DDFM=KR;
 REPEATED TIME / SUBJECT=SUBJECT TYPE =XX;*
 LSMEANS TRT*TIME/DIFFS;
RUN;
```

R code

```
require(nlme)

fitmodel <- gls(change ~ basval +trt+ TIME + basval*TIME+
  trt*TIME, data = complete,
      weights = varFunc(form= ~ 1 | TIME),
      correlation= corStruct(form=~ 1| subject))
```

Notes

corStruct is specific error correlation structure, e.g. corAR1, corCompSymm, corSymm (see R help for *corClasses*{nlme}), specifying weights via *varFunc* allows for various error covariance structures, for example, combining varFunc =varIdent with correlation = corCompSymm fits a model with heterogeneous compound symmetry (see help for varFunc{nlme}

To evaluate treatment contrasts at time x, one can use the contrast function from the contrast package as shown in code fragment 7.3.

CODE FRAGMENT 7.3 SAS and R Code for Fitting a Random Intercept and Residual Correlations

SAS code

```
PROC MIXED DATA=ONE;
 CLASS SUBJECT TRT TIME;
 MODEL CHANGE = BASVAL TRT TIME BASVAL*TIME TRT*TIME /
   DDFM=KR;
```

* TYPE = XX indicates entries for this option determine the correlation structure that is fit, e.g., UN, AR(1), ARH(1)

```
 RANDOM INT / SUBJECT=SUBJECT;
 REPEATED TIME / SUBJECT=SUBJECT TYPE =XX;
 LSMEANS TRT*TIME/DIFFS;
 ODS OUTPUT DIFFS=_DIFFS (where=(TIME= _TIME))
 LSMEANS=_LSMEANS;
RUN;

Type = XX indicates entries for this
```

R code

```
fitLME.erun.rint <- lme(change ~ basval +trt+ TIME +
  basval*TIME+ trt*TIME, data = complete, random = ~ 1
  |subject, weights = varIdent(form= ~ 1 | TIME),
correlation=corSymm(form=~ 1| subject))

summary(fitLME.erun.rint)

# treatment contrasts can be evaluated using the contrast
  package (see Code Fragment 7.5)
```

CODE FRAGMENT 7.4 SAS Code for Fitting Separate Random Intercepts by Treatment

```
ODS LISTING CLOSE;
PROC MIXED DATA=ONE;
 CLASS SUBJECT TRT TIME;
 MODEL CHANGE=BASVAL TRT TIME BASVAL*TIME TRT*TIME /
   DDFM=KR;
 RANDOM INT / SUBJECT=SUBJECT GROUP=TRT G GCORR;
 LSMEANS TRT*TIME/DIFFS;
 ODS OUTPUT DIFFS=_DIFFS LSMEANS=_LSMEANS G=_G;
RUN;
```

CODE FRAGMENT 7.5 SAS Code for Fitting Separate Residual Correlation Structures by Treatment

```
PROC MIXED DATA=ONE
 CLASS SUBJECT TRT TIME;
 MODEL CHANGE =BASVAL TRT TIME BASVAL*TIME TRT*TIME /
   DDFM=KR;
 REPEATED TIME / SUBJECT=SUBJECT TYPE=UN Group=TRT;
 LSMEANS TRT*TIME/DIFFS;
 ODS OUTPUT DIFFS=_DIFFS LSMEANS=_LSMEANS R=_R
   RCORR=_RCORR;
RUN;
```

7.9 Summary

The association between repeated measurements on the same subjects can be modeled as a function of the random effects, the residual effects, or both. No approach is universally better than another. The analysis must be tailored to the situation at hand.

In clinical trials, the random effects are seldom of direct interest and the number of assessment times relative to the number of subjects is often fairly small. Such situations are amenable to unstructured modeling of within-subject covariance (residual errors). Unstructured modeling places few restrictions (assumptions) on the model and is often a preferred modeling approach, especially in large, confirmatory trials.

The number of parameters for unstructured modeling of correlations is equal to $n(n + 1)/2$, where n is the number of assessment times. However, it is unlikely that the number of covariance parameters to be estimated is prohibitively large in clinical trial settings unless separate unstructured matrices are fit for multiple groups (e.g., treatment arms) within the same data set.

Model fitting criteria can be used to pick the best fitting model after data become available. Alternatively, an unstructured (or other appropriate) approach can be prespecified and alternative structures tested for better fit.

8

Modeling Means Over Time

8.1 Introduction

In longitudinal clinical trials, means can vary over time due to, among other things, study effects and the natural evolution of the disease. Even when focus is on a single landmark time point (e.g., endpoint visit), properly understanding and modeling the time trends is important.

In mixed-effects models, time can be modeled in either a structured or unstructured manner. In unstructured modeling of time, the time variable is considered a categorical (i.e., class) effect. The fixed effect solutions in such a mixed model represent the unique effects of each assessment time and have t-1 degrees of freedom for t time points. In structured modeling of time, the time variable is treated as a continuous independent variable (covariate) as is typically done in regression and covariate analyses. Therefore, structured models for time can use fewer degrees of freedom and be more powerful than unstructured approaches, provided that the functional form of the time trend is correctly specified. In structured approaches the time variable can be considered strictly a fixed effect, strictly a random effect or have both fixed and random components. Models with time as a random effect are commonly referred to as random coefficients regression models (SAS 2013).

Although the longitudinal pattern of treatment effects is usually of interest, the functional form of the mean responses over time may be difficult to anticipate. In particular, linear time trends may not adequately describe the mean responses. Nonlinear trends may arise from inherent characteristics of the particular disease and the drug under study, and/or from trial design features. For example, if titration dosing is used with initial dosing at a subtherapeutic level to reduce adverse events, there may be a lag period with little or no improvement. Conversely, if a drug has rapid onset of a fully therapeutic effect, the beneficial effects may increase rapidly across early assessments and then level off thereafter. In such cases, parsimonious approaches to modeling means over time may lead to inaccurate results and more general unstructured models may be preferred (Mallinckrodt et al. 2003). Therefore, in many scenarios, an unstructured modeling of means over assessment times requires fewer assumptions, does not require estimation of an inordinate number of parameters, and can be depended upon to yield a useful result (Mallinckrodt et al. 2003).

Figure 8.1 illustrates linear time trends for means superimposed on top of unstructured time trends. In this example, the treatment group differences at the endpoint (Time 8) visit appear relatively equal for the unstructured and linear approaches. However, the linear model underestimates within-group changes at early visits and overestimates within-group changes at later visits.

Figure 8.2 illustrates the same unstructured time trends for treatment means with linear plus quadratic trends for means by treatment superimposed. The two models yield similar within-group changes and between-group contrasts at each time point.

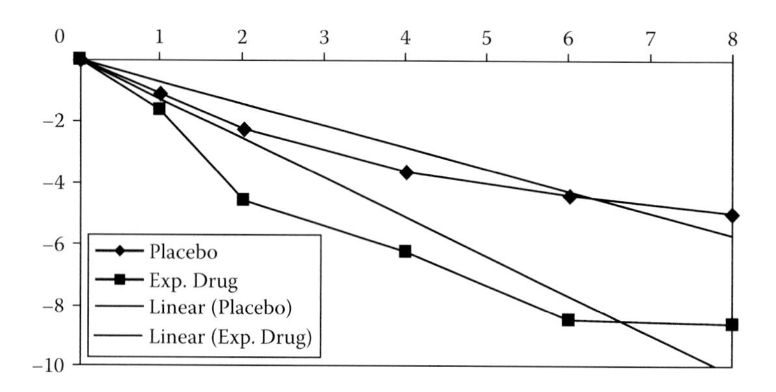

FIGURE 8.1
Unstructured modeling of time compared with linear trends.

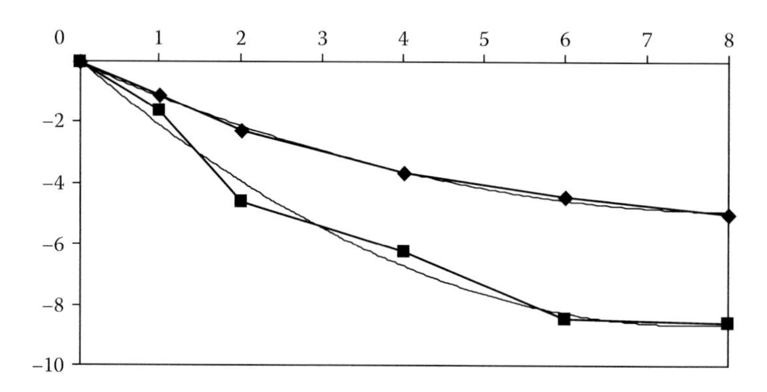

FIGURE 8.2
Unstructured modeling of time compared with linear plus quadratic trends.

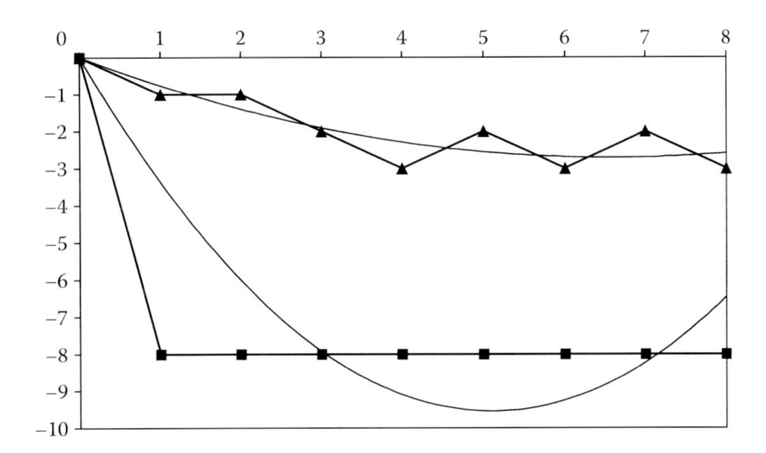

FIGURE 8.3
Unstructured modeling of time compared with linear plus quadratic trends in a scenario with a rapidly evolving treatment effect.

Figure 8.3 illustrates a scenario where one treatment has a rapid and sustained effect and the other treatment has a smaller effect that evolves more slowly over time. The linear plus quadratic model provides good fit to the treatment arm with smaller changes. Compared to the unstructured model, the linear plus quadratic model smoothed the somewhat erratic and seemingly random mean changes around the overall trend. However, the linear plus quadratic model provides poor fit to the arm with a rapid and sustained effect.

The examples are not intended to be a full exploration of modeling alternatives. Rather, the intent is merely to show that in some cases structured time models adequately describe mean trends over time and in other situations they don't.

Another aspect of mean trends over time that must be considered is with regard to the other covariates included in the analysis and their interaction with time. For example, the effect of baseline severity may be an important covariate because subjects' responses may depend on their condition at the start of the trial. It is usually preferable to allow a full interaction of covariates with time because, if not, a restriction is imposed that the dependence of response on the covariate is the same at all assessment times (Mallickrodt et al. 2008, 2014).

Alternatively, both the baseline and post-baseline measures can be treated as response variables (Liang and Zeger 2000). This topic is covered in detail in Chapter 9. For other covariates, it may be appropriate not to include interaction with time because the effects are constant; but such decisions need to be justified a priori (Mallinckrodt et al. 2008).

TABLE 8.1

Results from the Unstructured Time Model in SAS PROC MIXED

Treatment	TIME	Estimate	Standard Error	LSMEAN Difference	P
1	1	−4.12	0.91	1.19	0.360
2	1	−5.31	0.91		
1	2	−6.70	0.93	1.99	0.135
2	2	−8.69	0.93		
1	3	−9.86	1.05	3.39	0.0274
2	3	−13.25	1.05		

Residual covariance matrix

1	20.61	15.30	12.28
2	15.30	21.36	17.67
3	12.28	17.67	27.61

Note: P values for treatment main effect, the main effect of time, and treatment-by-time interaction were 0.073, 0.001, and 0.287, respectively. The values for − 2 x residual log likelihood and AIC were 810.4 and 822.4, respectively.

8.2 Unstructured Modeling of Means Over Time

Code fragments for fitting an unstructured model for means over time in SAS and R for the small complete data set are listed in Section 8.4 (Code Fragment 8.1). Key aspects of this code include specifying time as a class effect and fitting the treatment-by-time interaction along with all other two-way interactions of covariates with time. Unstructured modeling of means over time was used throughout Chapter 7 when considering approaches to model correlations between repeated measurements.

Results from the unstructured means model in SAS PROC MIXED are summarized in Table 8.1. Both the treatment (2) and control group (1) had significant mean improvement over time (P = 0.001). The mean difference between treatments increased over time, reaching statistical significance (P < 0.05) at the endpoint visit (Time 3). The treatment main effect approached significance (P < 0.10).

8.3 Structured Modeling of Means Over Time

8.3.1 Time as a Fixed Effect

Code fragments for fitting time as a linear fixed effect in SAS and R for the small complete data set are listed in Section 8.4 (Code Fragment 8.2).

Key aspects of this code include specifying time as a continuous effect (time not included in class statement), thereby using a single degree of freedom each for time and the treatment-by-time interaction. The endpoint contrast is obtained by comparing treatment lsmeans at the value of 3 for time.

Results from fitting time as a linear fixed effect are summarized in Table 8.2. Results did not differ remarkably from fitting time as unstructured in this example. However, the model fit was slightly worse for the linear fixed effect analysis.

Code fragments for fitting time as linear plus quadratic fixed effects in SAS and R for the small complete data set are listed in Section 8.4 (Code Fragment 8.3). In this approach, as in the unstructured model, time and the treatment-by-time interaction both use two degrees of freedom. In fact, the two approaches are equivalent and yield identical results. Fitting time as unstructured is equivalent to fitting a t-1 degree polynomial. Therefore, with 3 time points, a model with linear and quadratic terms for time is equivalent to the unstructured model. Of course, a linear plus quadratic model would not be equivalent to unstructured with more than 3 time points.

8.3.2 Time as a Random Effect—Random Coefficients Regression

Code fragments for SAS and R implementations of a random coefficients regression model with random terms for intercept and slope (i.e., time is a linear random effect) are listed in Section 8.4 (Code Fragment 8.4). Key aspects of this code include specifying time as a continuous fixed effect (continuous variable TIME not included in class statement) and as a random effect, along with intercept. The Type = option in the random statement allows for correlation between the random terms. As in the fixed

TABLE 8.2

Results from Fitting Time as a Linear Fixed Effect in SAS PROC MIXED

Treatment	TIME	Estimate	Standard Error	LSMEAN Difference	P
1	1	–4.07	0.92	1.14	0.389
2	1	–5.21	0.92		
1	2	–6.91	0.86	2.21	0.076
2	2	–9.13	0.86		
1	3	–9.76	1.06	3.28	0.034
2	3	–13.05	1.06		

Note: P values for treatment main effect, the main effect of time, and treatment-by-time interaction were 0.076, 0.003, and 0.133, respectively. The values for – 2 x residual log likelihood and AIC were 819.5 and 831.5, respectively.

TABLE 8.3

Results from Fitting a Random Coefficient Regression Model with Intercept and Time as Random Effects in SAS PROC MIXED

Treatment	TIME	Estimate	Standard Error	LSMEAN Difference	P
1	1	– 4.03	0.91	1.09	0.401
2	1	– 5.12	0.91		
1	2	– 6.90	0.84	2.19	0.073
2	2	– 9.09	0.8		
1	3	– 9.77	1.04	3.29	0.030
2	3	– 13.06	1.04		

Estimated G Matrix

	Intercept	Time	Residual
Intercept	24.14	– 0.528	
Time	– 0.528	3.54	
Residual			4.75

Note: P values for treatment main effect, the main effect of time, and treatment-by-time interaction were 0.073, 0.001, and 0.117, respectively. The values for –2 x residual log likelihood and AIC were 820.1 and 828.1, respectively.

effects model, the endpoint contrast is obtained by comparing treatment lsmeans at the value of 3 for time.

Results from fitting the random coefficient regression model with intercept and time as random effects are summarized in Table 8.3. Results did not differ remarkably from fitting time as unstructured or as a linear fixed effect in this example.

A quadratic term for time could be added to the random statement. However, in such models it may be useful to center the time variable (subtract the mean time from each value for time) and to use a time scale that is not overly granular. For example, fitting time in years may be preferable to fitting time in days because the latter is likely to yield smaller variance, which could cause convergence problems or result in a nonpositive definite hessian matrix. It may also be useful to transform time variables into orthogonal polynomials, especially for fitting higher-order (e.g., cubic) terms.

It is possible to capture additional correlation between repeated measurements in a random coefficients regression analysis via a residual correlation structure. However, guarding against overspecification of models is important. For example, fitting random intercepts and slopes plus an unstructured error covariance specifies too many parameters for the variance function, and a more parsimonious error covariance structure is needed.

8.4 Code Fragments

CODE FRAGMENT 8.1 SAS and R Code for Fitting an Unstructured Time Model

SAS code

```
PROC MIXED DATA=ONE;
 CLASS SUBJECT TRT TIME;
 MODEL CHANGE = BASVAL TRT TIME BASVAL*TIME TRT*TIME /
   DDFM=KR;
 REPEATED TIME / SUBJECT=SUBJECT TYPE =UN R;
 LSMEANS TRT*TIME/DIFFS;
 ODS OUTPUT DIFFS=_DIFFS (where=(TIME= _TIME)) LSMEANS=_
   LSMEANS ;RUN;
```

R code

```
fitgls.erun <- gls(change ~ basval +trt+ TIME +
            basval*TIME+ trt*TIME, data = complete,
            weights = varIdent(form= ~ 1 | TIME),
            correlation=corSymm(form=~ 1| subject))

summary(fitgls.erun)

# computing error variance-covariance matrix
getVarCov(fitgls.erun)

# evaluating least squares means at time 3
contrast(fitgls.erun ,a = list(trt = "1",
                basval= mean(complete$basval), TIME = "3"),
                type = "individual")
contrast(fitgls.erun ,a = list(trt = "2",
                basval= mean(complete$basval), TIME = "3"),
                type = "individual")

# evaluating treatment contrast at time 3
contrast(fitgls.erun ,a = list(trt = "1", basval=
                mean(complete$basval), TIME = "3"),
                b = list(trt = "2", basval=
                mean(complete$basval), TIME = "3"),
                type = "individual")
```

CODE FRAGMENT 8.2 SAS and R Code for Fitting Time as a Linear Fixed Effect

SAS code

TIME2 is continuous time variable assuming values 1, 2, 3. Variable TIME is also needed as a CLASS variable because it is used in REPEATED statement.

```
 PROC MIXED DATA=ONE;
 CLASS SUBJECT TRT TIME;
 MODEL CHANGE =BASVAL TRT TIME2 BASVAL*TIME2 TRT*TIME2 /
   DDFM=KR;
 REPEATED TIME/SUBJECT=SUBJECT TYPE=UN R RCORR;
 LSMEANS TRT / at TIME2 = 1 DIFFS;
 LSMEANS TRT / at TIME2 = 2 DIFFS;
 LSMEANS TRT / at TIME2 = 3 DIFFS;
 ODS OUTPUT DIFFS=_DIFFS (where=(TIME= _TIME))
   LSMEANS=_LSMEANS;
RUN;
```

R code

```
# using continuous time, creating timec variable
complete$timec<-as.numeric(complete$TIME)

fitgls.cont.time <- gls(change ~ basval +trt+ timec +
                 basval*timec+ trt*timec, data = complete,
                 weights = varIdent(form= ~ 1 | timec),
                 correlation=corSymm(form=~ 1| subject))

# note since timec is continuous variable, it is set at
  numerical value=3, not a character value ="3"
contrast(fitgls.cont.time ,a = list(trt = "1",
                basval= mean(complete$basval), timec = 3),
                b = list(trt = "2", basval=
                mean(complete$basval), timec = 3),
                type = "individual")
```

CODE FRAGMENT 8.3 SAS and R Code for Fitting Time as Linear + Quadratic Fixed Effects

SAS code

TIME2 is continuous time variable assuming values 1, 2, 3.

```
PROC MIXED DATA=ONE;
 CLASS SUBJECT TRT;
 MODEL CHANGE =BASVAL TRT TIME2 BASVAL*TIME2 TRT*TIME2
   TIME2*TIME2 TRT*TIME2*TIME2 BASVAL*TIME2*TIME2 /
   DDFM=KR;
 REPEATED TIME/SUBJECT=SUBJECT TYPE=UN R RCORR;
 LSMEANS TRT/ at TIME2= 1 DIFFS;
 LSMEANS TRT/ at TIME2= 2 DIFFS;
 LSMEANS TRT/ at TIME2= 3 DIFFS;
 ODS OUTPUT DIFFS=_DIFFS (where=(TIME= _TIME))
   LSMEANS=_LSMEANS;
RUN;
```

R Code

```
# creating additional variable, time squared
complete$tsq<-complete$timec^2

fitgls.cont.time2 <- gls(change ~ basval +trt+ timec +
                   basval*timec+ trt*timec+tsq+trt*tsq+
                   basval*tsq, data = complete, weights =
                   varIdent(form= ~ 1 | timec),
                   correlation=corSymm(form=~ 1| subject))

summary(fitgls.cont.time2)

# evaluating treatment contrast at time=3
# need to specify squared time tsq in the contrast at fixed
  value
contrast(fitgls.cont.time2, a = list(trt = "1",
                basval = mean(complete$basval), timec = 3,
                tsq = 9), b = list(trt = "2", basval=
                mean(complete$basval), timec = 3, tsq=9),
                type = "individual")
```

CODE FRAGMENT 8.4 SAS and R Code for Fitting a Random Coefficient Regression Model with Intercept and Time as Random Effects

SAS Code

```
PROC MIXED DATA=ONE;
 CLASS SUBJECT TRT;
 MODEL CHANGE =BASVAL TRT TIME BASVAL*TIME TRT*TIME /
   DDFM=KR;
 RANDOM INT TIME / SUBJECT=SUBJECT TYPE=UN G GCORR;
 LSMEANS TRT/ at TIME= 1 DIFFS;
 LSMEANS TRT/ at TIME= 2 DIFFS;
 LSMEANS TRT/ at TIME= 3 DIFFS;
 ODS OUTPUT DIFFS=_DIFFS LSMEANS=_LSMEANS;
RUN;
```

R Code

```
fitLME.rint.time <- lme(change ~ basval +trt+ timec +
               basval*timec+ trt*timec, data =complete,
               random = ~ 1+timec |subject)

summary(fitLME.rint.time)
getVarCov(fitLME.rint.time)

# lsmeans at timec=3
contrast(fitLME.rint.time ,a = list(trt = "1", basval=
                        mean(complete$basval), timec = 3)
                        type = "individual")
contrast(fitLME.rint.time ,a = list(trt = "2", basval=
                        mean(complete$basval), timec = 3)
                        type = "individual")

# treatment contrast at timec=3
contrast(fitLME.rint.time ,a = list(trt = "1", basval=
                        mean(complete$basval), timec = 3),
                        b = list(trt = "2", basval=
                        mean(complete$basval), timec = 3),
                        type = "individual")
```

8.5 Summary

Although the longitudinal pattern of mean treatment effects is usually of interest, the functional form of the response profiles may be difficult to anticipate. Structured (parsimonious) approaches to modeling means over time may be more powerful if appropriate, but may not fit the data adequately, leading to inaccurate results.

Clinical trials typically have a set number of assessment times that are fixed within narrow intervals. The number of assessment times relative to the number of patients is typically small. The number of parameters to describe the means over time from an unstructured model increase linearly with the number of assessment times. These attributes suggest that unstructured modeling of mean trends over time is often possible. This is important, especially in confirmatory studies, because an unstructured model for the means requires no assumption about the time trend and models with fewer assumptions are preferred.

In many situations, an unstructured model for the mean trends over time can be prespecified because the number of parameters to be estimated relative to the number of observations is small. If the anticipated data structure is not expected to be amenable to unstructured modeling, likelihood ratio tests can be used to pick the best fitting model after data become available.

9

Accounting for Covariates

9.1 Introduction

Covariates are commonly included in analyses of longitudinal clinical trials. In Section 8.1, it was noted that it is usually preferable, or at least it should be considered, to allow a full interaction of covariates with time. Fitting covariate-by-time interactions avoids imposing restrictions that the dependence of response on the covariates is the same at all assessment times. Therefore, throughout this chapter, examples will be used that include not only the covariate but also the covariate interaction with time.

Covariates are often included in longitudinal analyses to account for the variability due to these effects, thereby yielding more precise estimates of treatment effects. This can be particularly important when values of continuous covariates or levels of categorical covariates are not balanced across treatments.

Covariate-by-treatment interactions, commonly called subgroup analyses when the covariate is a categorical effect, are included in longitudinal analyses to assess the consistency of treatment effects across levels of the covariate. Consistency of treatment effect across subgroups indicates that the average treatment effect is in general applicable regardless of the specific characteristic described by the covariate. Substantial heterogeneity in treatment effect may indicate that treatment benefit pertains only to a subset of the population. However, apparent heterogeneity in the observed treatment effect across subgroups can arise due to chance as a result of partitioning the population into several subgroups. Furthermore, clinical trials are generally not powered for detecting heterogeneity in treatment effects, thus statistical tests may miss detection of existing heterogeneity due to low power (Alosh et al. 2015). This chapter emphasizes how to fit covariates and the consequences of so doing. It does not cover model building approaches to decide which covariates to include. For more details on model building, see Verbeke and Molenberghs (2000).

The impact of baseline severity on outcomes is an important consideration in longitudinal clinical trials. Baseline severity is a special case of covariate adjustment because it can be taken into account either through covariate adjustment or by including baseline as part of the response vector. Both approaches, along with their respective strengths, limitations, and considerations, will be illustrated.

This chapter begins with an illustration of including a continuous covariate for baseline severity. Other continuous covariates can be fit in the same manner as illustrated for baseline severity. Subsequent sections illustrate how baseline severity can be accounted for as a response variable, how to account for categorical covariates, and covariate-by-treatment interactions. Covariates and model development can be an important consideration in the handling of missing data. See Chapter 12 and Chapter 15 for more details on the role of covariates with regard to handling missing data.

9.2 Continuous Covariates

9.2.1 Baseline Severity as a Covariate

The small complete data set is used to illustrate key concepts in fitting covariates. Code Fragment 9.1 in Section 9.5 provides details on fitting a model with baseline severity as a covariate in SAS and R.

To illustrate covariate adjustment, consider the results in Table 9.1 from likelihood-based analyses. Two models were used. The "simple" model included only treatment, time, and the treatment-by-time interaction. The "baseline" or ANCOVA model included those same effects plus baseline and baseline-by-time interaction as specified in Code Fragment 9.1. In the simple model, because the data were completely balanced (same number of observations for each treatment-by-time combination) the lsmeans for the treatment-by-time interaction effects are equal to their

TABLE 9.1

Results from Analyses of Small Complete Data Set with and without Baseline Severity as a Covariate

		Simple Model		Model Including Baseline	
Treatment	Time	LSMEAN	SE	LSMEAN	SE
1	1	−4.20	0.94	−4.13	0.91
2	1	−5.24	0.94	−5.32	0.91
1	2	−6.80	0.97	−6.70	0.93
2	2	−8.60	0.97	−8.70	0.93
1	3	−9.88	1.04	−9.86	1.05
2	3	−13.24	1.04	−13.26	1.05
Endpoint Contrast		3.36	1.47 ($p = 0.0270$)	3.39	1.49 ($p = 0.0274$)

corresponding raw means. In the model with baseline and baseline-by-time interaction, the lsmeans do not equal the raw means, thereby reflecting the influence of correcting for differences between treatments in baseline values.

Recall from Table 4.3 that the mean baseline values were 19.80 and 19.32 for Treatments 1 and 2, respectively. Given this similarity of baseline means, differences in treatment contrasts between models fitting versus not fitting baseline severity are expected to be small. With greater imbalance between baseline means, the greater the potential for covariate adjusted results to differ from unadjusted results.

The relationship between baseline and change was such that for each 1 point increase in baseline severity, change (improvement) from baseline increased on average approximately 0.06 points. Therefore, correcting for the approximately 0.50 point greater mean baseline in Treatment 1 (by including baseline as a covariate) increased the difference between treatments in change at Time 3 by about 0.03 (0.50 mean difference in baseline × the 0.06 change in response per unit change in baseline severity).

To further clarify how including baseline as a covariate influenced results, consider the observed and predicted values for selected subjects summarized in Table 9.2. In the simple model, each subject's predicted value equals the corresponding lsmean for the treatment-by-time combination. That is, the model contained only group effects; no information unique to individual subjects was in the model. Therefore, individuals' predictions were entirely derived from the group means. Including baseline as a covariate introduced information specific to individual subjects, and the predicted values for each subject were based on a combination of group means and individual subject data (baseline values). Lower baseline values

TABLE 9.2

Predicted Values for Selected Subjects from Analyses of Complete Data with a Simple Model and a Model that Included Baseline Values as a Covariate

Subject	Model[a]	Treatment	Time	Baseline	Actual Change	Predicted Change
1	Simple	2	3	24	−24	−13.24
	Baseline					−13.54
2	Simple	1	3	20	−5	−9.88
	Baseline					−9.89
4	Simple	2	3	10	−9	−13.24
	Baseline					−12.64
5	Simple	1	3	12	−9	−9.88
	Baseline					−9.37

[a] Simple model: Change = trt time trt*time. Baseline model added basval and basval*time.

were predictive of smaller improvements and higher baseline values were predictive of greater improvements.

The mean baseline value was 19.56 (approximately 20). The baseline value for Subject 1 was 24, approximately 4 points higher than the baseline mean; the baseline values for Subjects 4 and 5 were 10 and 12, respectively, considerably below the mean. Therefore, when including baseline as a covariate, the predicted improvement for Subject 1 was greater than the corresponding treatment group mean. Similarly, when including baseline as a covariate, the predicted improvements for Subjects 4 and 5 were smaller than the corresponding group means. Subject 2 had a baseline value of 20, close to the overall mean; therefore, the predicted values from the models including versus not including baseline were nearly identical.

By default, lsmeans are typically estimated based on the mean value of continuous covariates. However, it is also useful to look at results when values other than the mean are used. [See the "AT" option in the lsmean statement of SAS PROC MIXED (SAS 2013) for implementation]. Treatment lsmeans and contrasts based on baseline severity of 15 and 25 are summarized in Table 9.3. The treatment contrasts, standard errors, and P values are the same across baseline severities of 15, 25, or the default, which is the mean value of 19.56. Within-group means, however, are influenced by the baseline value, consistent with the regression coefficient for change on baseline severity, which in this case is approximately 0.06. Therefore, conditioning on a baseline value of 15 resulted in lsmeans approximately 0.60 lower than when conditioning on a baseline value of 25.

9.2.2 Baseline Severity as a Response

Although fitting baseline severity as a covariate is a common approach, it is not the only option. Baseline severity is a special case of covariate adjustment because baseline severity can be considered a response at Time 0 and therefore may also be accounted for through including baseline outcomes as part of the response vector (Liang and Zeger 2000). This subsection details two methods that include baseline as a response, the so-called LDA (longitudinal data analysis) and the cLDA (constrained longitudinal data analysis)

TABLE 9.3

Least Squares Means and Treatment Contrasts Conditioning on Various Levels of Baseline Severity

Baseline	TRT	LSMEAN	LSMEAN Difference	Standard Error	P Value
15	1	−9.57			
	2	−12.96	3.39	1.49	0.0274
25	1	−10.21			
	2	−13.60	3.39	1.49	0.0274

(Liu et al. 2009). The constraint in cLDA is that the baseline values are equal in the intervention groups.

Code fragments are listed in Section 9.5 to implement LDA and cLDA models in SAS and R (Code Fragments 9.2 and 9.3, respectively). For these analyses, data are arranged so that there are four responses per subject, with baseline being the Time = 0 response. For the cLDA analysis, additional steps are required to create the time-specific treatment indicators tt0-tt3. These dummy variables are components of the treatment-by-time interaction: ttk=I(TIMEk*TRT) for k=1,2,3, where I(.) is the indicator function, returning 1 when the argument is TRUE and 0 if FALSE. The model is fit with time as a class variable (to estimate time-specific least squares means at Time=1, 2, 3) and the three dummy variables tt1, tt2, tt3 that capture treatment-specific least-squares means at time=1, 2, 3.

The tt0 variable and the I(Time=0)*Treatment interaction term are not fit in the model in order to implement the constraint of equal baseline means. The two treatments in essence have a common set of baselines, hence equal baselines, as would be expected on average from randomization; Table 9.4 lists data for selected subjects as prepared for LDA and cLDA.

TABLE 9.4

Data for LDA and cLDA Analyses

Subject	TRT	TIME	Y
Data for LDA			
16	1	0	19
16	1	1	16
16	1	2	8
16	1	3	2
17	2	0	20
17	2	1	9
17	2	2	5
17	2	3	1

Subject	TIME	Y	TT0	TT1	TT2	TT3
Data for cLDA						
16	0	19	0	0	0	0
16	1	16	0	0	0	0
16	2	8	0	0	0	0
16	3	2	0	0	0	0
17	0	20	1	0	0	0
17	1	9	0	1	0	0
17	2	5	0	0	1	0
17	3	1	0	0	0	1

Note: The tt0 variable is not fit in the model in order to constrain lsmean by omitting the (Time=0)*TRT interaction term.

Endpoint contrasts from the various methods of accounting for baseline severity in the small complete data set are summarized in Table 9.5 and residual variances and correlations are summarized in Table 9.6. The endpoint (Time 3) contrast from the cLDA and ANCOVA models were identical. This will only be the case in complete data. Standard errors and P values were similar across methods, as were correlations between the residuals. However, residual variances were greater for the LDA and cLDA models.

Although results from the ANCOVA, LDA, and cLDA methods tend to be similar in many situations, circumstances exist when important differences are likely. To illustrate, data from the small complete data set were

TABLE 9.5

Endpoint Contrasts from Various Methods of Accounting for Baseline Severity in the Small, Complete Data Set

Method	LSMEAN Difference	Standard Error	P
ANCOVA	3.391	1.489	0.0274
LDA	3.360	1.473	0.0270
cLDA	3.391	1.501	0.0284

TABLE 9.6

Residual Variances and Correlations from Various Methods of Accounting for Baseline Severity in the Small, Complete Data Set

Time	0	1	2	3
Baseline as Covariate (ANCOVA)				
1		20.612	0.729	0.515
2			21.358	0.724
3				27.614
LDA				
0	16.613	0.529	0.473	0.591
1		28.038	0.796	0.665
2			26.938	0.797
3				41.577
cLDA				
0	16.333	0.526	0.470	0.588
1		27.906	0.795	0.663
2			26.836	0.796
3				41.331

altered in the following ways. In alteration 1, the *baseline values* for Subjects 1 to 15 were deleted. In alteration 2, no baseline values were deleted but *all post-baseline data* for Subjects 1 to 15 were deleted. Endpoint contrasts from the three methods of handling baseline severity (ANCOVA, LDA, cLDA) are summarized in Table 9.7 for alteration 1 and in Table 9.8 for alteration 2.

For the ANCOVA method, results were identical from the two alterations, with the treatment contrast smaller than in the complete data. That is, when fitting baseline as a covariate, deleting 15 baseline values had the same impact as deleting all the post-baseline data for those 15 subjects—because observations with missing covariates are not used in the analysis. However, in the LDA and cLDA analyses where baseline is considered a response, deleting 15 baseline values left 185 of the 200 values to be used in the analysis, and all post-baseline observations are used. Therefore, missing baseline values had a smaller effect on the LDA and cLDA analyses than on the ANCOVA analyses.

For alteration 2, deleting all the post-baseline data for Subjects 1 to 15, results were similar across methods.

9.2.3 Choosing the Best Approach

In the ANCOVA model where baseline is accounted for as a covariate, baseline is considered a fixed effect. In the LDA and cLDA models where baseline

TABLE 9.7

Endpoint Contrasts from Various Methods of Accounting for Baseline Severity in the Small, Complete Data Set with 15 Baseline Values Deleted

Method	LSMEAN Difference	Standard Error	P Value	Number of Observations Used	Number of Observations Not Used
ANCOVA	2.239	1.846	0.234	155	45
LDA	3.125	1.619	0.060	185	15
cLDA	3.323	1.613	0.045	185	15

TABLE 9.8

Endpoint Contrasts from Various Methods of Accounting for Baseline Severity in the Small, Complete Data Set with All Post Baseline Values Deleted for 15 Subjects

Method	LSMEAN Difference	Standard Error	P Value	Number of Observations Used	Number of Observations Not Used
ANCOVA	2.239	1.846	0.234	155	45
LDA	2.264	1.828	0.224	155	45
cLDA	2.239	1.862	0.238	155	45

is considered a response, it is a random effect. The ANCOVA model tends to be the easier and the more common approach. In the ANCOVA model, F tests for the treatment main effect and treatment-by-time interaction are more meaningful than in the LDA or cLDA approaches. Treatment main effects in LDA and cLDA are diluted because at Time 0 (baseline) there is no difference between treatments. This zero difference at Time 0 can also inflate the treatment-by-time interaction term in LDA and cLDA.

However, when an appreciable number of baseline observations are missing, or when an appreciable number of subjects have a baseline but no postbaseline values, the LDA or cLDA approaches can have advantages, and it is important for analysts to understand the strengths and limitations of various approaches to account for baseline severity.

If baseline severity is considered a fixed effect, then the ANCOVA model is appropriate. This model addresses the conditional question of the treatment effect in subjects with the baseline values fixed as in the current clinical trial. If baseline severity is considered a random effect, then the LDA and cLDA models are appropriate. By considering baseline severity as a random effect, inference can be extended to the general population of subjects from which the sample was drawn.

9.3 Modeling Categorical Covariates

Categorical covariates are fit in longitudinal models similar to continuous covariates, except the covariate is considered a class effect. Code fragments are listed in Section 9.5 to fit gender as a categorical variable in the small complete data set using SAS and R (Code Fragment 9.4). As with continuous covariates, adding just the main effect of the covariate assumes a constant covariate effect at all assessments. Therefore, it is often useful to fit the interaction of the categorical covariate with time, and that is the approach taken in this section. However, if the categorical covariate has many levels, especially when combined with numerous assessment times, fitting the covariate-by-time interaction can require estimating too many parameters unless the sample size is large. In practice, this consideration most often comes into play for fitting investigative site and its interaction with time.

Results from fitting a model with gender and gender-by-time interaction are compared to results from the simple model that included only treatment, time, and the treatment-by-time interaction in Table 9.9. As illustrated in Section 9.2 for continuous covariates, because the data were completely balanced (same number of observations for each treatment-by-time combination), the lsmeans for the treatment-by-time interaction effects in the simple model are equal to their corresponding raw means. In the model with gender and gender-by-time interaction, the lsmeans for each treatment-by-time

TABLE 9.9

Results from Analyses of Small Complete Data Set with and without Gender as a Covariate

		Simple Model		Model Including Gender	
Treatment	**Time**	**LSMEAN**	**SE**	**LSMEAN**	**SE**
1	1	–4.20	0.94	–4.53	0.90
2	1	–5.24	0.94	–4.39	0.96
1	2	–6.80	0.97	–6.98	0.98
2	2	–8.60	0.97	–8.14	1.04
1	3	–9.88	1.04	–9.91	1.06
2	3	–13.24	1.04	–13.15	1.13
Endpoint Contrast		3.36	1.47 (p = 0.0270)	3.24	1.60 (p = 0.049)

combination do not equal the raw means, thereby reflecting covariate adjustments for gender.

Treatment 1 included 40% females and 60% males, whereas Treatment 2 had 76% females and 24% males. Females tended to have greater changes from baseline than males. Therefore, the covariate-adjusted analyses correct for the overrepresentation of females—subjects with more favorable outcomes—in Treatment 2, resulting in smaller mean changes for Treatment 2 and smaller differences between treatments than in the unadjusted analyses.

9.4 Covariate-by-Treatment Interactions

Sections 9.2 and 9.3 discussed models with continuous and categorical covariates. In longitudinal clinical trials, it can also be useful to understand if the effects of the covariate differed by treatment group; that is, to assess subgroup-by-treatment interactions. A full discussion of model development and testing is beyond our present scope. The intent here is to illustrate an implementation of such models and to consider what the results imply.

9.4.1 Continuous Covariates

Code fragments are listed in Section 9.5 to implement models with baseline severity-by-treatment interactions in SAS and R (Code Fragment 9.5). Results from models using the default approach that conditions on the mean baseline value are compared to results when conditioning on baseline values of 15 and 25 in Table 9.10. Increasing baseline from 15 to 25 increased the lsmean for Treatment 1 by 1.40, whereas the increase for Treatment 2 was only 0.35, reflecting heterogeneity in the regression of change on baseline

TABLE 9.10

Least Square Means at Time 3 Conditioning on Various Levels of Baseline Severity in Models Including Baseline-by-Treatment Interaction

Baseline	Treatment	Time 3 LSMEAN	LSMEAN Difference	Standard Error
Mean	1	−9.85		
	2	−13.25	3.40	1.50
15	1	−9.20		
	2	−13.08	3.88	2.46
25	1	−10.60		
	2	−13.43	2.83	2.69

across treatments. Therefore, the net impact of adding the various interaction terms to account for differential baseline effects across treatments was greater treatment differences at lower baseline severity.

As in simpler regression settings, moving further away from mean levels of an independent variable increased uncertainty. Therefore, the standard error of the treatment contrast was smaller when assessed at the mean level of baseline severity.

9.4.2 Categorical Covariates

Code fragments are listed in Section 9.5 to implement models with gender-by-treatment interaction in SAS and R (Code Fragment 9.6). Lsmeans for the three-way gender-by-treatment-by-time interaction and the two-way treatment-by-time interaction are summarized in Table 9.11. From the three-way interaction, the difference between treatments at Time 3 was approximately 5 in females and 0.5 in males. The two-way interaction lsmeans reflect the equal weighting given to each gender and the lsmean is the average of the corresponding gender-specific lsmeans from the three-way interaction. For example, the treatment difference at Time 3 = 2.75, which is the average of the 5 point treatment contrast in females and the 0.5 point treatment contrast in males.

Recall that in the simple model that included only treatment, time and treatment-by-time interaction, the difference between treatments was 3.36. Therefore, when correcting for the imbalance in the number of subjects by gender in each treatment via including gender and gender-by-time interactions, the treatment difference was 3.24. When including the gender-by-treatment interaction terms to further account for a differential treatment effect by gender, the treatment effect was further reduced to 2.75.

Code fragment 9.5 includes as part of the SAS code an option in the lsmeans statement "SLICE=GENDER*TIME". The slice option is a convenient way to partition interactions into component parts. Specifying slices

TABLE 9.11

Least Square Means at Time 3 by Gender and Treatment

Treatment	Gender	N	LSMEAN	LSMEAN Difference
Gender-by-Treatment lsmeans at Time 3				
1	F	10	–8.90	5.04
2	F	19	–13.94	
1	M	15	–10.53	
2	M	6	–11.00	0.47
Treatment lsmeans at Time 3				
1		25	–9.72	
2		25	–12.47	2.75

TABLE 9.12

Significance Tests Based on the Slices Option in SAS

Treatment Contrast		
Time	**Gender**	**P**
1	F	0.220
1	M	0.096
2	F	0.169
2	M	0.648
3	F	0.017
3	M	0.854

for gender by time yields significance tests for treatment contrasts for each gender-by-time combination.

Because this example has two treatment arms, the P values are essentially *t*-tests, but with three or more groups these would be *F*-tests. Similar tests could be achieved via contrast statements. However, correctly coding the series of three-way interaction contrasts is far more tedious than simply specifying the slices option. Results from the slices option are summarized in Table 9.12.

The slice option allows partitioning of a three-way interaction into its component two-way interactions and to assess a main effect for each level of the other two factors, as was done in assessing treatment differences for each gender-by-time combination. For example, the slice option could be used to assess gender differences for each treatment-by-time combination (slice=trt*time); the two-way treatment-by-time interaction for each gender (slice=gender); the gender-by-treatment interaction for each time (slice=time), or the gender-by-time interaction for each treatment (slice=treatment).

9.4.3 Observed versus Balanced Margins

Further consideration of the results in the previous section illustrates an important point for categorical subgroup-by-treatment interactions. Treatment 1 had 40% females and Treatment 2 had 76% females. By default, when the three-way gender-by-treatment-by-time interaction is fit, lsmeans for treatment-by-time reflect equal weighting by gender—the results expected if there were 50% males and 50% females in each treatment.

It is important to consider if the question being addressed by the analysis is best approached with lsmeans reflecting these so-called balanced margins (equal weightings). When subjects are randomized to treatment, gender representation in each treatment is expected to be equal. If by chance that is not the case, covariate adjustment can help restore analytically the balance that did not materialize via design. However, randomization is expected to yield equal (similar) representation of gender in each treatment, but not equal representation of gender within each group. For example, if 2/3 of the clinical trial population is female, randomization is expected to yield approximately 2/3 females in each treatment group. However, by default lsmeans are based on complete balance such that lsmeans reflect 50% females and 50% males in each treatment group.

If the population from which a clinical trial sample is drawn is not approximately 50/50 male/female, then default lsmeans assuming balance in number by gender within treatment would not be appropriate. It is possible to use software options to obtain lsmeans that reflect the margins observed in the actual sample, or user-specified margins. [See, for example, the observed margins option for the lsmean statement in SAS PROC MIXED (SAS 2013).] This feature allows an interaction to be fit without forcing the use of balanced margins.

9.5 Code Fragments

CODE FRAGMENT 9.1 SAS and R Code for Fitting Baseline Severity as a Covariate

SAS Code

```
PROC MIXED DATA=All;
 CLASS SUBJECT TRT TIME;
 MODEL Y = BASVAL TRT TIME BASVAL*TIME TRT*TIME/ DDFM=KR;
 REPEATED TIME / SUB=SUBJECT TYPE=UN R RCORR;
 LSMEANS TRT*TIME /DIFFS;
RUN;
```

R Code

```
fitgls.bas <- gls(Y ~ basval +trt+ TIME + basval*TIME,
  data = complete,
     weights = varIdent(form= ~ 1 | TIME),
     correlation= corSymm(form=~ 1| subject))
```

CODE FRAGMENT 9.2 SAS and R Code for Fitting an LDA Model

SAS Code

```
PROC MIXED DATA=RESPONSE;
 CLASS SUBJECT TRT TIME;
 MODEL Y = TRT TIME TRT*TIME / DDFM=KR;
 REPEATED TIME / SUB=SUBJECT TYPE=UN R RCORR;
 ESTIMATE' ' trt*time -1 0 0  1
                      1 0 0 -1;
 RUN;
```

R Code

```
# setting reference for TIME and trt factors at the last
level
contrasts(response$TIME) <- contr.treatment(4, base = 4)
contrasts(response$trt) <- contr.treatment(2, base = 2)

fitgls.resp <- gls(Y ~ trt+ TIME + trt*TIME,
  data = response,
     weights = varIdent(form= ~ 1 | TIME),
     correlation= corSymm(form=~ 1| subject))

# with the parameterization of factors used the difference
between treatment effects at TIME 3
# and at baseline time is the -1* [coefficient at
interaction effect trt1:TIME1]
```

CODE FRAGMENT 9.3 SAS and R Code for Fitting a cLDA Model

SAS Code

```
PROC MIXED DATA=cLDA;
Class SUBJECT TRT TIME;
MODEL Y = TIME TT1 TT2 TT3 / DDFM=KR;
REPEATED TIME / SUBJECT=SUBJECT TYPE=UN R RCORR;
ESTIMATE 'endpoint diff (trt-pbo)' TT3 -1 /cl;
ESTIMATE 'trt main effect' tt1 -1 tt2 -1 tt3 -1;
CONTRAST 'trt*time interaction' tt1 1 tt2 0 tt3 -1,
                                tt1 0 tt2 1 tt3 -1;
RUN;
```

R Code

```
fitgls.cLDA <- gls(Y ~ TIME + tt1+tt2+tt3, data = cLDA,
     weights = varIdent(form= ~ 1 | TIME),
     correlation= corSymm(form=~ 1| subject))

# evaluating treatment contrast at TIME=3
contrast(fitgls.cLDA, a = list(TIME = "3", tt1=0,tt2=0,
        tt3=-1), b = list(TIME = "3", tt1=0,tt2=0, tt3=0),
        type = "individual")

# evaluating the overall treatment effect
contrast(fitgls.cLDA, a = list(TIME = "3", tt1=-1, tt2=-1,
        tt3=-1), b = list(TIME = "3", tt1=0, tt2=0,tt3=0),
        type = "average")

Note: contrast package does not allow evaluation of
contrasts with DF>1)
```

CODE FRAGMENT 9.4 SAS and R Code for Fitting Gender as a Categorical Covariate

SAS Code

```
PROC MIXED DATA=ONE;
CLASS SUBJECT TRT TIME GENDER;
MODEL CHANGE = GENDER TRT TIME GENDER*TIME TRT*TIME/DDFM=KR
OUTP=Cov;
REPEATED TIME/SUBJECT=SUBJECT TYPE=UN R RCORR;
LSMEANS TRT*TIME/DIFFS;
ODS OUTPUT DIFFS=_DIFFS (where=(TIME= _TIME)) LSMEANS=_
  LSMEANS ;
RUN;
```

R Code

```
complete$GENDER <- as.factor(complete$GENDER)

fitgls.gender <- gls(change ~ GENDER +trt+ TIME +
  GENDER*TIME+ trt*TIME, data =complete, weights =
  varIdent(form= ~ 1 | TIME), correlation= corSymm(form=~ 1|
  subject))

# treatment effect at TIME=3 (note since gender by treatment
    interaction is not fit in the # model, GENDER can be
    fixed at any level in the call to contrast function

cont <- contrast(fitgls.gender,a = list(trt = "1",
        TIME = "3", GENDER=c("F")), b = list(trt = "2",
        TIME = "3", GENDER=c("F")), type = "individual")
```

CODE FRAGMENT 9.5 SAS and R Code for Fitting Baseline as a Covariate and its Interaction with Treatment

SAS Code

```
PROC MIXED DATA=ALL ;
 CLASS SUBJECT TRT TIME;
 MODEL CHANGE =BASVAL TRT TIME BASVAL*TIME TRT*TIME
              BASVAL*TRT
 BASVAL*TRT*TIME/DDFM=KR;
 REPEATED TIME/SUBJECT=SUBJECT TYPE=UN R RCORR;
 LSMEANS TRT*TIME/DIFFS;
 LSMEANS TRT*TIME/DIFFS at BASVAL=15;
 LSMEANS TRT*TIME/DIFFS at BASVAL=25;
 ODS OUTPUT DIFFS=_DIFFS (where=(TIME= _TIME)) LSMEANS=_
   LSMEANS ;
RUN;
```

R Code

```
fitgls.base <- gls(change ~ basval +trt+ TIME + basval*TIME+
  trt*TIME+basval*trt+basval*trt*TIME, data = complete,
  weights = varIdent(form= ~ 1 | TIME),
  correlation=corSymm(form=~ 1| subject))

# evaluating treatment contrast at TIME=3 and baseline
    value =25
cont <- contrast(fitgls.base, a = list(trt = "1",
        TIME = "3", basval=25), b = list(trt = "2",
        TIME = "3",basval=25), type = "individual")
```

CODE FRAGMENT 9.6 SAS and R Code for Fitting Gender as a Categorical Covariate and its Interaction with Treatment

SAS Code

```
PROC MIXED DATA=ALL;
 CLASS SUBJECT TRT TIME GENDER;
 MODEL CHANGE =GENDER TRT TIME GENDER*TIME TRT*TIME
              GENDER*TRT
 GENDER*TRT*TIME/DDFM=KR;
 REPEATED TIME/SUBJECT=SUBJECT TYPE=UN R RCORR;
 LSMEANS GENDER*TRT*TIME/DIFFS SLICE=GENDER*TIME;
 LSMEANS TRT*TIME/DIFFS;
 ODS OUTPUT DIFFS=_DIFFS (where=(TIME= _TIME))
   LSMEANS=_LSMEANS;
RUN;
```

R Code

```
# fitting in "gender-by-treatment" interactions
fitgls.gender <- gls(change ~ GENDER +trt+ TIME +
              GENDER*TIME+ trt*TIME+GENDER*trt+GENDER*trt*
              TIME, data = complete,
              weights = varIdent(form= ~ 1 | TIME),
              correlation=corSymm(form=~ 1| subject))

# least squares means by gender for trt=1, TIME=3
contrast(fitgls.gender, a = list(trt = "1", TIME = "3",
        GENDER=c("F","M")), type = "individual")

# treatment contrast at TIME=3, for Gender="F"
contrast(fitgls.gender, a = list(trt = "1",
TIME = "3", GENDER=c("F")), b = list(trt = "2",
TIME = "3",GENDER=c("F")), type = "individual")

# treatment contrast (averaged across gender groups)
cont <- contrast(fitgls.gender, a = list(trt = "1",
        TIME = "3", GENDER=c("F","M")), b = list(trt = "2",
        TIME = "3",GENDER=c("F","M")), type = "average")
```

9.6 Summary

In the ANCOVA model where baseline is accounted for as a covariate, baseline is considered a fixed effect. In the LDA and cLDA models where baseline is considered a response, it is a random effect. The ANCOVA model tends to be the easier and the more common approach. However, when an appreciable number of baseline observations are missing, or when an appreciable number of subjects have a baseline but no post-baseline values, the LDA or cLDA approaches can have advantages.

Fitting just the main effect of the covariate assumes a constant effect at all assessments. This assumption may not be justifiable. Therefore, it is often useful to fit the interaction of covariates with time.

In longitudinal clinical trials, it can also be useful to understand if the effects of the covariate differed by treatment group; that is, to assess subgroup-by-treatment interactions. It is important to consider for categorical covariates, especially when fitting covariate-by-treatment interactions, whether focus should be on the observed versus balanced margins. When fitting a continuous covariate, especially when fitting the covariate-by-treatment interaction, it may be useful to assess treatment contrasts at values of the covariate other than the default of using the mean value.

10

Categorical Data

10.1 Introduction

A comprehensive review of categorical data analyses can be found in Agresti (2002). McCullagh and Nelder (1989) provide specific focus on generalized linear models, which are used extensively in categorical data analyses. This chapter provides an overview of longitudinal categorical analyses.

Many of the principles guiding analyses of continuous outcomes also apply to categorical outcomes. For example, considerations regarding modeling means over time and correlations between repeated measurements are essentially the same as previously outlined for continuous outcomes (see Chapters 7 and 8). Additional similarities include the ability to formulate a longitudinal categorical analysis with treatment contrasts that exactly match the results from an analysis of the endpoint time only. However, analyses of categorical endpoints entail additional complexity compared with continuous endpoints that are typically modeled using linear models with Gaussian error distributions. This additional complexity stems from the (typically) nonlinear relationship between the dependent variable and independent variables and from the nonnormal distribution of errors.

Conceptually, accommodating these aspects is as simple as specifying an appropriate link function to account for nonlinearity and an appropriate distribution for the errors. However, these accommodations necessitate additional computational complexity and intensity, which in turn limits flexibility in implementing analyses.

Moreover, unlike the "linear normal" modeling of continuous outcomes where a single result has both a marginal and a hierarchical (random effects) interpretation, the parameters estimated from marginal and random-effects models with categorical data, and more broadly for any generalized linear mixed model with a nonidentity link function, describe different effects and have different interpretations (Jansen et al. 2006). Therefore, the choice between marginal and random-effect models should ideally be driven by the scientific goals, but the computational complexity and availability of software tools are also a consideration.

Conceptually, the distinction between marginal and random effects models is that marginal models estimate the average response in the population, whereas random effects models estimate responses for the average subject (the subject for which b = 0). In linear mixed-effects models with normally distributed data, the average response and the response of the average subject are the same because the random effects cancel out when taking expectation over the outcome variable. This is due to the additivity of linear models with an identity link and also random effects having a mean and expected value = 0. Hence, fixed effect parameters estimated from a linear mixed-effects model in Gaussian data have both a marginal and hierarchical interpretation. In nonnormal data these two targets of inference are not identical because the function connecting outcome variables and covariates is not linear.

A similar consideration for categorical data analyses is with regard to inclusion of covariates. When a covariate is included, the resultant estimates and inferences are conditional on the covariate. By default, analyses are typically adjusted to the mean value of the covariate. When the association between the response and the covariate is linear, as in Gaussian data, the population average response and the response of the average subject with the mean covariate value are the same. Therefore, in Gaussian data, including versus not including covariates does not influence the target of inference; but in non-Gaussian data, including versus not including the covariate does influence the target of inference because the population average is not equal to the expected value for the subject with the average covariate value. The technical details in the next section help to further clarify these issues.

10.2 Technical Details

10.2.1 Modeling Approaches

Three common modeling approaches to longitudinal categorical data include marginal, random effects, and conditional models.

A marginal model for nonnormally distributed data can be written as

$$h\left(E\left(Y_{ij} \mid X\right)\right) = x_{ij}'ß$$

where $h(.)$ is a link function that creates a linear association between the mean of Y_{ij} (outcome measured on subject *i* on *j*th occurrence) and associated covariate vector x_{ij}.

In marginal models, marginal distributions are used to describe the outcome vector Y, given a set of X predictor variables. The correlation among the components of Y (e.g., repeated measurements on subjects) and fixed effects parameters can be estimated via fully parametric approaches such as likelihood-based analyses, or by working assumptions in the semiparametric GEE framework (Molenberghs and Kenward 2007).

In random-effect models the predictor variables in X are supplemented with a vector of random effects:

$$h\left(E\left(Y_{ij} \mid X, b_i\right)\right) = x_{ij}'ß + z_{ij}'b_i$$

This model has been termed a generalized linear mixed-effect model. It is generalized in the sense that the link function generalized the linear mixed-effects model to a more general class, allowing for nonnormal (e.g., count or binary) data.

In a random-effects model, the fixed effects estimates are conditional upon the random-effects vector. In principle, it is possible to model correlations among components in Y as a function of both random effects and residual correlation. However, in most applications, the computational complexity necessitates assuming that conditional upon the random effects the components of Y are independent. The linear mixed model for continuous data is a special case of this model with an identity link function. The random effects b_i are, as in general linear models for continuous data, assumed to be sampled from a (multivariate) normal distribution with mean 0 and covariance matrix D. With a logit link and normally distributed random effects, the familiar logistic-linear generalized linear mixed-effects model (GLMM) follows (Molenberghs and Kenward 2007).

In conditional models, the distribution of the components of Y are conditional on X and conditional on (a subset of) the other components of Y. In the example below, outcomes are conditional on the previous outcomes:

$$h\left(E\left(Y_{ij} \mid Y_{i,j-1,\ldots,} Y_{i1}, x_{ij}\right)\right) = x_{ij}'ß + \alpha Y_{i,j-1}$$

That is, rather than add random effects, expectations are based on previous outcomes. In clinical trials, interest is often on an overall, or population average treatment effect, not on a treatment effect associated with specific outcome histories. Therefore, conditional models will not be further considered here.

As noted above, linear mixed model analyses exploit the elegant properties of the multivariate normal distribution, resulting in fixed effect parameters having both a marginal and hierarchical (random effects model) interpretation. Given this connection, it is easy to appreciate why the linear mixed model provides a unifying framework for analyses of Gaussian data. However, the connection between the model families does not exist when outcomes are nonnormal (Jansen et al. 2006). Therefore, analysts need different tools for marginal and random-effects analyses of categorical data. However, as described in the next section, computational considerations restrict implementation of analyses, especially likelihood-based analyses.

10.2.2 Estimation

In a generalized linear model (GLM), the log likelihood is well-defined and an objective function for estimation of the parameters is straightforward to construct. In a GLMM, categorical data pose increased complexity over continuous data. These complexities hinder construction of objective functions. Even if the objective function is feasible mathematically, it still can be out of reach computationally (SAS 2013). These complexities and restrictions have led to the development of a number of estimation methods. Many of these methods are based on either approximating the objective function or approximating the model.

Integral approximation methods approximate the log likelihood of the GLMM and submit the approximated function to numerical optimization. The advantage of integral approximation methods is that an actual objective function is optimized. This facilitates likelihood ratio tests among nested models and likelihood-based fit statistics. A significant disadvantage of integral approximation methods for typical clinical trial scenarios is the inability to accommodate residual covariance structures. Hence, the within-subject correlations must be modeled as a function of only random effects. The number of random effects must be small for integral approximation methods to be practically feasible (SAS 2013).

Algorithms to approximate the model can be expressed in terms of Taylor series (linearization) and are hence also known as linearization methods. They employ expansions to approximate the model based on pseudo data with fewer nonlinear components (SAS 2013). For example, one approach is based on a decomposition of the data into the mean and an appropriate error term. All methods in this class differ in the order of the Taylor approximation and/or the point around which the approximation is expanded. More specifically, one approach uses the decomposition

$$Y_{ij} = \mu_{ij} + \varepsilon_{ij} = h^{-1}\left(x_{ij}'\beta + z_{ij}'b_i\right) + \varepsilon_{ij}$$

where h^{-1} is the inverse link function and the error terms have the appropriate distribution (Molenberghs and Kenward 2007).

Several approximations of this model can be considered. The basic idea is to create the so-called pseudo data Y_i^* to which a general linear model can then be fit. Results from this model are then used to update the pseudo data and the linear model is refit to the updated pseudo data. This doubly iterative procedure continues until the desired level of convergence is met (Molenberghs and Verbeke 2005; Molenberghs and Kenward 2007). A specific example is the so-called pseudo-likelihood approach where

$$Y_i^* \equiv W_i^{-1}\left(Y_i - \mu_{ij}\right) + X_i\beta + Z_ib_i \approx X_i\beta + Z_ib_i + \varepsilon_i^*$$

with W_i being a diagonal matrix with entries equal to $v(\mu_{ij})$, and with $\varepsilon * I$ equal to $W_i^{-1}\varepsilon_i$, which still has mean zero. This model is essentially a linear mixed model for the pseudo data (Molenberghs and Kenward 2007).

Advantages of linearization-based methods include a relatively simple form of the linearized model that can be fit based on only the mean and variance in the linearized form. Models for which the joint distribution of outcome variables (repeated measurements) is difficult—or impossible—to ascertain can be fit with linearization-based approaches. Models with correlated errors and a large number of random effects are well-suited to linearization methods. The disadvantages of linearization approaches include the absence of a true objective function for the overall optimization process and potentially biased estimates, especially for binary data when the number of observations per subject is small (SAS 2013).

Generalized estimating equations can circumvent the computational complexity of likelihood-based analyses of categorical data, and is therefore a viable alternative whenever interest is restricted to the mean parameters (treatment difference, time evolutions, effect of baseline covariates, etc.). As introduced in Chapter 5, generalized estimating equations are rooted in the quasi-likelihood ideas expressed by McCullagh and Nelder (1989). Modeling is restricted to the correct specification of the marginal mean function, together with the so-called working assumptions about the correlation structure among the repeated measures.

10.3 Examples

10.3.1 Binary Longitudinal Data

To illustrate analyses of a longitudinal binary outcome, the continuous HAMD17 outcomes from the small example data set were dichotomized as is often done in depression clinical trials based on whether or not improvement from baseline was ≥ 50%, the so-called responder rate analysis. The percentage of responders by treatment and time are summarized below.

Treatment	Time	Percent Responders
1	1	8
2	1	24
1	2	32
2	2	44
1	3	56
2	3	88

The model for binary data can be very similar to that used for the corresponding continuous endpoint. Fixed effects include treatment, time, treatment-by-time interaction, along with the continuous HAMD17 score as baseline covariate and its interaction with time. For hierarchical inference that require explicit fitting of random subject effects, likelihood-based estimation would typically be used. For the present purpose marginal inference is preferred. Therefore, estimation can be either likelihood-based or via generalized estimating equations.

Code fragment 10.1 lists code to fit a pseudo likelihood-based marginal model using SAS. Code fragment 10.2 lists code to fit the same marginal model using generalized estimating equations. Results are summarized in Tables 10.1 and 10.2, respectively. These summaries focus on visit-wise contrasts. As with continuous data, emphasis can also be on the fixed effect parameter estimates, but are not discussed here. Also note that an unstructured correlation matrix was fit in both the pseudo likelihood and GEE analyses. Although fitting of alternative correlation structures is not discussed here, many of the same principles and approaches apply as in continuous data.

TABLE 10.1

Pseudo Likelihood-Based Results for Binary Data from the Small Example Data Set

		Logit Scale		Percent Scale[a]		
Treatment	**Time**	**Estimate**	**SE**	**Estimate**	**SE**	**P Value**
1	1	−2.511	0.738	0.075	0.051	0.166
2	1	−1.282	0.493	0.217	0.083	
1	2	−0.732	0.439	0.325	0.096	0.458
2	2	−0.279	0.414	0.431	0.101	
1	3	0.392	0.425	0.597	0.102	0.023
2	3	2.240	0.683	0.904	0.059	

[a] Results on the percent scale are obtained by using the inverse link function.

TABLE 10.2

Generalized Estimating Equation-Based Results for Binary Data from the Small Example Data Set

		Logit Scale		Percent Scale[a]		
Treatment	**Time**	**Estimate**	**SE**	**Estimate**	**SE**	**P Value**
1	1	− 2.518	0.706	0.075	0.048	0.194
2	1	− 1.293	0.577	0.215	0.097	
1	2	− 0.729	0.423	0.325	0.093	0.456
2	2	− 0.292	0.409	0.428	0.100	
1	3	0.386	0.406	0.595	0.097	0.020
2	3	2.206	0.671	0.901	0.059	

[a] Results on the percent scale are obtained by using the inverse link function.

Results from the pseudo likelihood and GEE approaches were similar, both yielding significant treatment contrasts at Time 3, as was seen for the continuous HAMD scores in previous Chapters. At Time 3, response rates from both analyses were approximately 90% for Treatment 2 and 60% for Treatment 1, reflecting slight differences from the observed percentages due to the adjustment for baseline score.

Dichotomization of continuous outcomes results in a loss of information. However, this will not always translate into "less significant" treatment contrasts. Treatment differences for the dichotomized outcome depend on the distribution of the continuous data relative to the cut point chosen for dichotomization. It is possible that the cut off for dichotomization is chosen at a point that is achieved by many subjects in one group but not another, despite relatively small differences in means. This can happen because of greater variance in one group or as an artifact of chance, especially in a small sample such as this example where results from the dichotomized outcome were actually more significant than from the continuous outcome. The P value for the treatment contrast at Time 3 from continuous data was 0.027 (see Table 7.3), versus 0.023 from pseudo likelihood and 0.020 from GEE analyses of the dichotomized (categorical) data.

10.3.2 Ordinal Model for Multinomial Data

Analyses of the PGI improvement (patient global impression) is used to further illustrate categorical analyses of longitudinal data. The PGI is an ordinal variable with scores that can range from 1 (very much improved) to 7 (very much worse), with 4 meaning no change (see Chapter 4). The frequency of responses in the 5, 6 and 7 categories were rare. Therefore, all scores greater than 4 were recoded as 4 for these analyses.

Code fragment 10.3 lists SAS code to fit a marginal, ordinal model for these multinomial data using GEE. The only differences from Code Fragment 10.2 that was for a binary outcome is use of a cumulative logit link and multinomial error distribution rather than a logit link and a binomial error distribution.

Although software tools generally accommodate a wide variety of correlation structures that can be fit to categorical data, for multinomial data typically independence must be assumed. This strong limitation can be addressed by using empirical standard errors based on the sandwich estimator. Results are summarized in Table 10.3.

First, focus on results at Time 3. The results in Table 10.3 as obtained in default output reflect accumulations over categories. Probabilities for individual categories can be obtained by subtracting adjacent categories. For example, the estimated probabilities for category 3 are 0.501 – 0.209 = 0.292 for Treatment 1 and 0.174 – 0.053 = 0.121 for Treatment 2. Estimated probabilities for category 1 (very much improved) = 1 – prob 2 or worse, which is 0.079 for Treatment 1 and 0.291 for Treatment 2. Both treatments had estimated probabilities for category 2 of approximately 0.4.

TABLE 10.3

Generalized Estimating Equation-Based Results of Ordinal Data from the Small Example Data Set

		Estimated Probabilities		
Time	Category	Treatment 1	Treatment 2	P Value[a]
1	4 or worse	0.522	0.378	
	3 or worse	0.806	0.697	
	2 or worse	0.980	0.964	0.262
2	4 or worse	0.386	0.235	
	3 or worse	0.705	0.539	
	2 or worse	0.965	0.931	0.151
3	4 or worse	0.209	0.053	
	3 or worse	0.501	0.174	
	2 or worse	0.921	0.709	0.014

[a] Results on the original percentage scale are obtained by using the inverse link function.

Therefore, Treatment 1 had greater estimated probabilities in categories 3 and 4 (worse outcomes) and Treatment 2 had a greater estimated probability for category 1. The significant P value (0.014) reflects the differences between treatments across all categories. Similar trends were seen at Time 1 and Time 2; however, as in continuous and binary analyses, improvements and differences between treatments at earlier times were less than at endpoint.

10.4 Code Fragments

CODE FRAGMENT 10.1 SAS Code for a Pseudo Likelihood-Based Analysis of Binary Data from the Small Example Data Set

```
PROC GLIMMIX DATA=ONE PLOTS=ALL METHOD=RMPL;
 NLOPTIONS MAXITER=50 TECHNIQUE=NEWRAP;
 CLASS SUBJECT TRT TIME GENDER ;
 MODEL RESP = BASVAL TRT TIME BASVAL*TIME TRT*TIME /
   DIST=BINOMIAL LINK=LOGIT;
 RANDOM TIME / SUBJECT=SUBJECT RESIDUAL TYPE=UN V VCORR;
 LSMEANS TRT*TIME / diffs ILink;
 ODS OUTPUT LSMEANS=_LSMEANS DIFFS=_DIFFS V=_V VCORR=_VCORR;
RUN;
```

CODE FRAGMENT 10.2 SAS Code for a Generalized Estimating Equation-Based Analysis of Binary Data from the Small Example Data Set

```
PROC GENMOD DATA =ONE DESCENDING;
 CLASS TRT TIME SUBJECT;
 MODEL RESP=BASVAL TRT TIME BASVAL*TIME TRT*TIME
 /LINK=LOGIT DIST=BINOMIAL;
 REPEATED SUBJECT=SUBJECT / TYPE=UN;
 LSMEANS TRT*TIME / DIFFS ILINK;
 ODS OUTPUT LSMEANS=_LSMEANSG;
 ODS OUTPUT DIFFS=_DIFFSG;
RUN;
```

CODE FRAGMENT 10.3 SAS Code for a Generalized Estimating Equation-Based Analysis of Multinomial Data from the Small Example Data Set

```
PROC GENMOD DATA=ONE DESCENDING;
 CLASS TRT TIME SUBJECT;
 MODEL PGI= TRT TIME TRT*TIME / LINK = CLOGIT DIST=MULT;
 REPEATED SUBJECT=SUBJECT / TYPE=IND;
 LSMEANS TRT*TIME / DIFFS ILINK;
RUN;
```

10.5 Summary

Many of the modeling considerations and principles regarding longitudinal analysis of continuous outcomes also apply to categorical outcomes. However, one key difference is with regard to inference. Fixed effect parameters estimated from a linear mixed-effects model in Gaussian data have both a marginal and hierarchical interpretation. In nonnormal data, these are different targets of inference because the link between the mean of the outcome variable and the covariates is not identity. Therefore, separate models are needed for marginal and hierarchical inference in categorical data.

Incorporating an appropriate link function to account for nonlinearity and an appropriate distribution for the errors in categorical data increases computational complexity. This complexity limits the implementation of certain models, especially for likelihood-based estimation. Therefore, generalized estimating equation-based analyses can be particularly useful in categorical data.

11

Model Checking and Verification

11.1 Introduction

Important assumptions required for valid regression-type analyses of continuous outcomes include linearity, normality, and independence (Wonnacott and Winacott 1981). The first assumption is about the true form of the mean function and the last two assumptions are with regard to the error term. Errors (i.e., residuals) are the difference between observed and predicted values. Several options to account for correlation between repeated observations on the same subjects in mixed-effect model analyses were presented in Chapter 7. Options to account for nonlinearity were presented in Chapter 10.

An inherent challenge in model checking—evaluating the mean structure and the errors—is that they are conditional on one another. Therefore, checking assumptions is typically an iterative process that entails refitting the model. For example, the errors may have some type of skewed distribution due to an incorrect mean model. After altering the mean model and refitting the model, the residuals can be rechecked.

11.2 Residual Diagnostics

Outliers are anomalous values in the data that may have a strong influence on the fitted model, resulting in a worse fit for the majority of the data. Outliers typically increase the residual variance, thereby widening confidence intervals and reducing power. Outliers may be due to errors in data collection and recording. These errors can be corrected. Examples include recording weight in pounds rather than kilograms, recording systolic blood pressure as diastolic blood pressure, etc. Therefore, checking for outliers can be a useful part of establishing the integrity of a database.

Outliers not due to correctable errors may result from several causes. For example, if important fixed effects are not included in the model, then sampling is in essence from a mixture distribution. Apparent outliers may also result from sampling from a nonnormal distribution. Or a few outliers may exist because these values are unusual simply due to chance.

Outliers may be detected in simple scatterplots of the data. However, more sophisticated approaches can be useful. Boxplots and the so-called Q–Q or normal probability plots for the residuals may be useful. Signs of nonnormality include skewed (lack of symmetry), light-tailed, or heavy-tailed distributions. Although specific tests for normality exist, these tests may lack power in small data sets, and in large data sets statistically significant departures from normality may have a trivial impact. Therefore, the important issue to address is whether outliers had an important effect on results, not whether outliers or nonnormality existed.

Some general considerations for residual diagnostics include:

- If the residuals are from a normal distribution, normal probability plots should approximate a straight line, and boxplots should be symmetric, with the median and mean close together in the middle of the box.
- If the normal probability plot is generally a straight line with a few points lying off that line, those points are likely outliers.
- If both ends of the normality plot bend above the straight line, the distribution from which the data were sampled may be skewed to the right.
- If both ends of the normality plot bend below the straight line, the distribution from which the data were sampled may be skewed to the left.
- If the right (upper) end of the normality plot bends below the straight line while the left (lower) end bends above that line (an S curve), the distribution from which the data were sampled may be light-tailed.
- If the right (upper) end of the normality plot bends above the straight line while the left (lower) end bends below it, the distribution from which the data were sampled may be heavy-tailed.

Several types of residuals can be calculated. A raw residual is simply the difference between the observed and predicted value. A studentized residual is the raw residual divided by the standard deviation in residuals. A Pearson residual is the raw residual divided by the standard deviation in the observed values.

11.3 Influence Diagnostics

The general idea of quantifying the influence of one or more observations relies on computing parameter estimates based on all data points, removing the case(s) in question from the data, refitting the model, and computing statistics based on the change between the full-data and reduced-data estimations.

Influence statistics can be grouped by their primary target of estimation.

- Restricted likelihood distance is a measure of general change; that is, change in the overall objective function.
- The influence on parameter estimates, such as treatment effects or other fixed effects can be assessed using Cook's D.
- Influence on fitted and predicted values can be assessed using the PRESS residual and PRESS statistic.
- Influence on precision of estimates can be evaluated using the CovRatio and CovTrace tests.

Additional details on these quantities and how they are calculated in mixed-effect models can be obtained in the SAS documentation for PROC MIXED (SAS 2013). An example of how the measures can be used in practice is provided in Section 11.5 using the small example data set.

11.4 Checking Covariate Assumptions

In a simple regression setting, if the assumption of equal variance across values of the dependent variable is correct, the plot of the observed Y values against X should suggest a band across the graph with roughly equal vertical width for all values of X. A pattern to the scatterplot with greater vertical spread at either the right or left end suggests that the variance in the values increases in the direction with greatest vertical spread. In such cases, a transformation of the Y values might be useful.

11.5 Example

A code fragment to implement residual and influence diagnostics in SAS is listed below. Results from the small example data set follow the code fragment.

CODE FRAGMENT 11.1 SAS Code for Implementing Residual and Influence Diagnostics

```
ODS GRAPHICS ON;
PROC MIXED DATA=ONE plot=all;
 CLASS TRT TIME GENDER SUBJECT;
 MODEL CHANGE= TRT TIME BASVAL TRT*TIME BASVAL*TIME /
 INFLUENCE(EFFECT=SUBJECT ITER=5 estimates);
 REPEATED TIME / SUBJECT=SUBJECT TYPE=UN;
 ODS OUTPUT INFLUENCE=INFLUENCE;
RUN;
ODS GRAPHICS OFF;
```

Studentized residuals are plotted in Figure 11.1. The normal probability plot (lower left panel) shows both ends bending above the straight line, suggesting the distribution is skewed to the right. This skewness is also suggested by the plot of the studentized residuals (upper right panel). Pearson residuals (not shown) indicated the same pattern.

Residual plots by treatment, time and treatment-by-time are depicted in Figures 11.2, 11.3, and 11.4, respectively. These plots reinforce the suggestion of some skewness to the distribution of residuals.

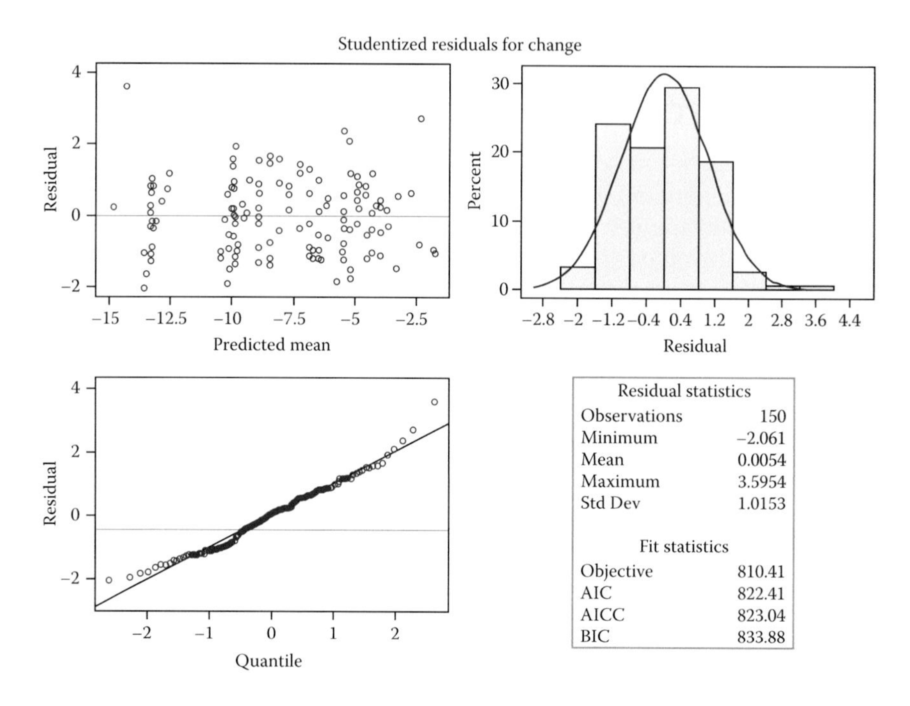

FIGURE 11.1
Residual diagnostics based on studentized residuals from the small example data set.

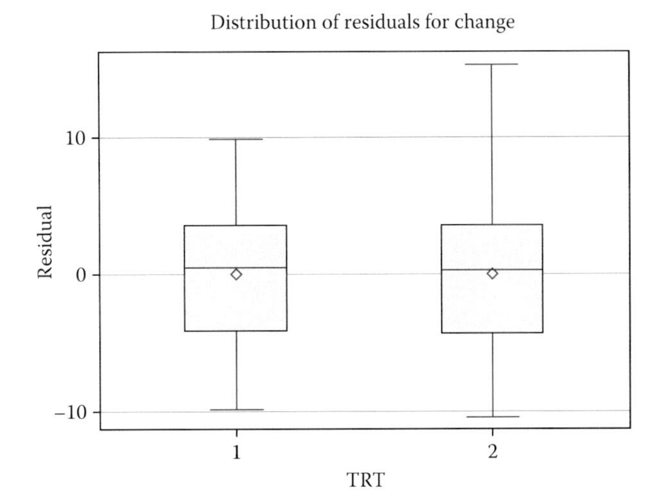

FIGURE 11.2
Distribution of residuals by treatment group from the small example data set.

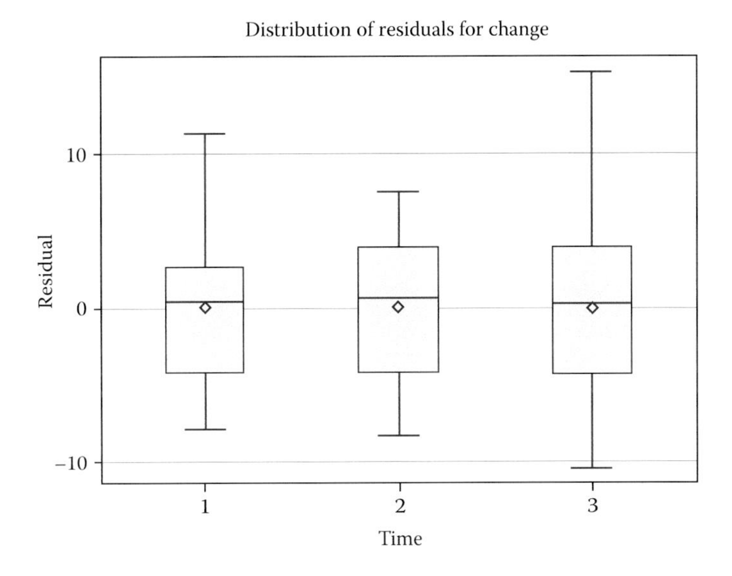

FIGURE 11.3
Distribution of residuals by time from the small example data set.

Restricted likelihood distances are plotted in Figure 11.5. Subject 47 had by far the greatest influence on the overall fit to the model, with Subject 4 standing out to a lesser degree.

To better understand how these influential subjects affected results, influence statistics for fixed effects and covariance parameters are plotted in Figure 11.6. Subjects 4 and especially 47 were appreciably more

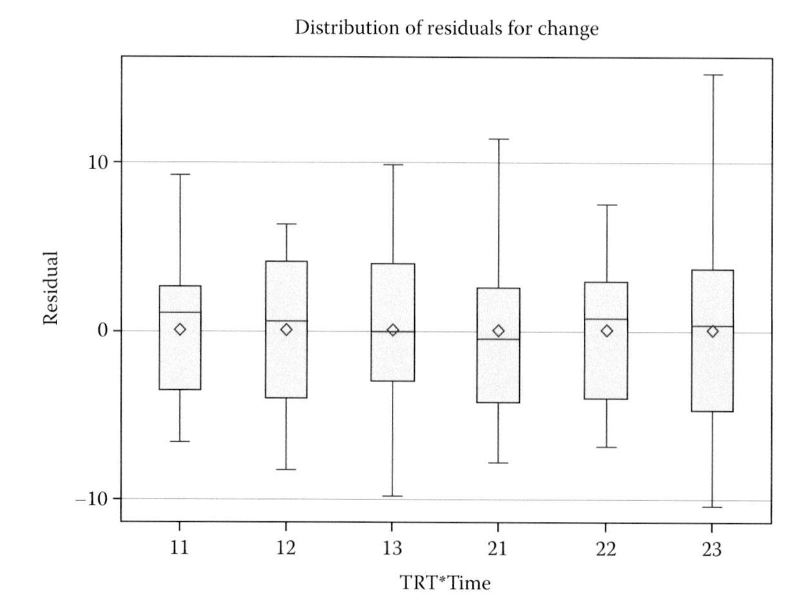

FIGURE 11.4
Distribution of residuals by treatment group and time from the small example data set.

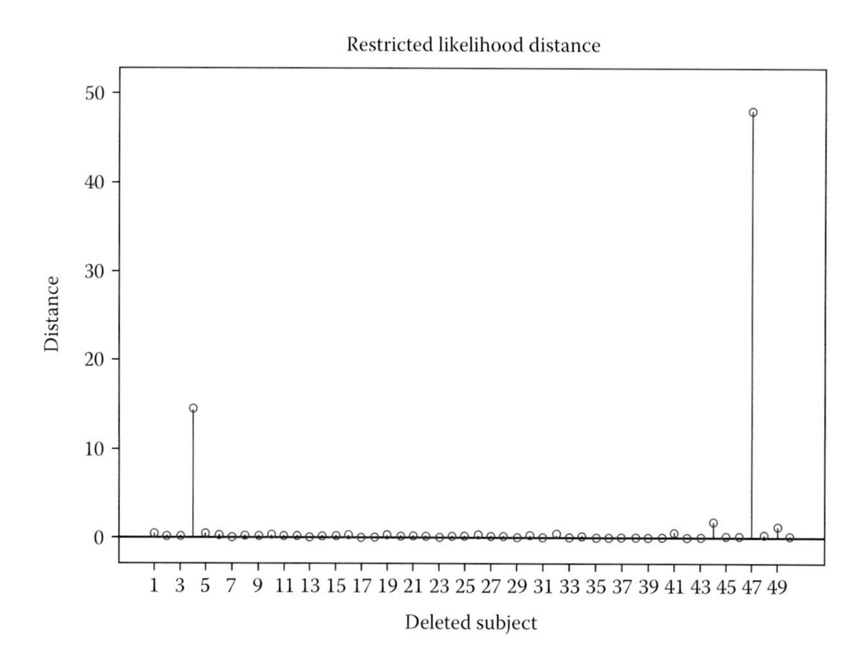

FIGURE 11.5
Plot of restricted likelihood distances by subject from the small example data set.

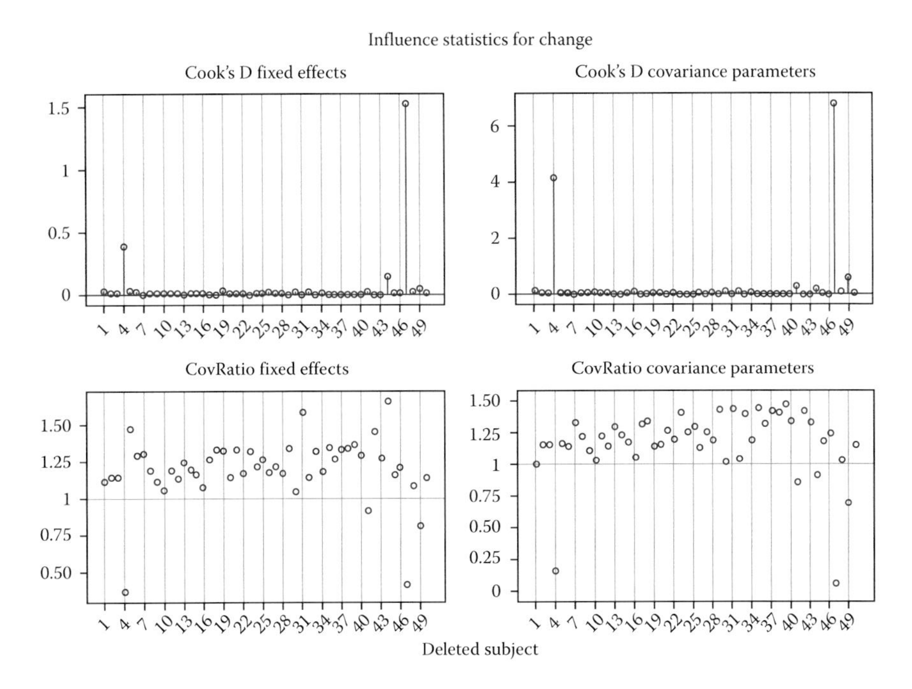

FIGURE 11.6
Influence statistics for fixed effects and covariance parameters from the small example data set.

TABLE 11.1

Comparisons of Endpoint Contrasts from All Data and Data with Influential Subjects Excluded

Data	Endpoint Treatment Contrast	Standard Error	P Value
All data	3.39	1.49	0.0274
Excluding Subject 4	3.54	1.51	0.0234
Excluding Subject 47	4.55	1.31	0.0011

influential than other subjects for fixed effects, covariance parameters, and for precision in those estimates.

Influence statistics for individual fixed effect parameters are also produced by the code in Code Fragment 11.1. However, plots are not shown here. Subject 47 had a large influence on almost every parameter. The influence of Subject 4 was less consistent. Influence statistics for individual covariance parameters are also produced by the code in Code Fragment 11.1. However, plots are not shown here. Deleting Subject 47 reduced variance at Times 2 and 3, and deleting Subject 4 reduced variance at Time 1.

Treatment lsmeans after deleting Subject 47 and Subject 4 are compared to results from including all Subjects in Table 11.1. Excluding Subject 4 slightly increased the treatment contrast, had little effect on the standard error, and resulted in a small decrease to the P value. Deleting Subject 47 resulted in a large increase in the treatment contrast and a decrease in the standard error. Therefore, the T statistic when excluding Subject 47 was much larger and the P value much smaller compared with results from including all subjects.

If these were real data, the consequences of excluding Subject 47 would warrant additional investigation from a clinical perspective. In general, final inferences from confirmatory trials are based on results from including all randomized subjects. However, if this was an early phase or otherwise non-confirmatory study, clinical considerations could warrant basing conclusions on data with Subject 47 excluded. Regardless of the scenario, it is important to know about influential subjects and how they influenced results.

The additional investigations might focus on subject history or other demographic or illness characteristics to verify whether the subject was indeed appropriate for inclusion in the study. If nothing anomalous was discovered, the subject may simply seem unusual because the data set was small and in a larger data set other subjects more similar to Subject 47 may be present.

For this example, results were statistically significant with or without Subject 47 included. Therefore, the anomalous profile of Subject 47 did not alter conclusions about the existence of a treatment effect. However, the difference in magnitude of the treatment effect could still be a consideration.

11.6 Summary

Outliers are anomalous values in the data that may have a strong influence on the fitted model, resulting in a worse fit for the majority of the data. The important issue to address is whether outliers had an important effect on results, not whether outliers or nonnormality existed.

Checking for patterns of residuals, such as associations between residuals and covariates, helps ascertain whether or not the mean function is appropriately specified; that is, are all the important effects fitted and is the modeled form of the association (linear etc.) correct? This emphasizes the iterative nature of model checking in that after identifying such patterns the model would be modified and refit, and the residuals reevaluated.

Another important aspect of model checking is to assess the influence of clusters of observations on model fit. In clinical trials, the clusters of interest usually include subject and investigative site. The general idea of quantifying the influence of clusters relies on computing parameter estimates based on all data points, removing the cases in question from the data, refitting the model, and computing statistics based on the change between the full-data and reduced-data estimations. Again, the main idea is not so much whether or not influential clusters existed, but rather to understand what impact the most influential clusters had on results.

Section III

Methods for Dealing with Missing Data

Missing data is an incessant problem in longitudinal clinical trials. The fundamental problem caused by missing data is that the balance provided by randomization is lost if, as is usually the case, the subjects who discontinue differ with regard to the outcome of interest from those who complete the study. This imbalance can lead to biases in the comparison of the treatment groups.

Fortunately, missing data has been an active area of research, with many advances in statistical theory and in our ability to implement the theory. Section III focuses on statistical methods for dealing with incomplete data. However, missing data is a cross-functional problem that is best dealt with by preventing missing data. Therefore, other aspects of missing data, including trial design and conduct to minimize missing data, were covered in Section I.

The focus in this section is to introduce various methods and their general attributes. How to use these various methods in developing a comprehensive analysis plan is covered in Section IV.

12

Overview of Missing Data

12.1 Introduction

Missing data in longitudinal clinical trials is a complex and wide-ranging topic, in part because missing data may arise in many ways. Intermittent missing data occurs when subjects miss scheduled assessments but attend subsequent visits. Dropout (withdrawal, attrition) is when subjects miss all subsequent assessments after a certain visit. Intermittent missing data are generally less problematic than withdrawal/attrition because, having observed data bracketing the unobserved value makes it easier to verify assumptions about the missing data compared to when no subsequent values are observed.

In addition, values may be missing because a subject is lost to follow-up, with nothing known about treatment or measurements past the point of dropout. Alternatively, a subject may withdraw from the initially randomized study medication and be given an alternative (rescue) treatment, but with no further measurements taken. Or, follow-up measurements may continue after initiation of the rescue treatment. All these and other scenarios may happen within a single trial, with differing implications for analyses (Mallinckrodt and Kenward 2009).

Importantly, missing data may need to be handled differently for different estimands. In addition, the consequences of missing values are situation-dependent. For example, in a clinical trial for rheumatoid arthritis, if a subject is lost to follow-up halfway through the trial, some of the information needed to understand how well the drug worked for that subject is indeed missing. On the other hand, if the subject discontinued for lack of efficacy, it is known the drug was, at least in a global sense, not effective for that subject and no information is missing for that subject relative to global effectiveness. However, other information regarding safety or secondary aspects of efficacy may be hindered by the incompleteness of the data.

The following hypothetical data illustrates the ambiguity missing data can cause. Assume that Treatment 1 is an investigational medicine and Treatment 2 is the standard of care. Results for each subject are categorized as success or failure and the outcomes are summarized in Table 12.1.

TABLE 12.1

Hypothetical Trial Results (Number of Subjects by Outcome Category)

	Treatment 1	Treatment 2
Success	35	40
Failure	35	50
Missing	30	10
Total	100	100

Success rates based on the observed data are 50% (35/70) for Treatment 1 and 44% (40/90) for Treatment 2 (for ease of illustration, significance testing is ignored). Therefore, if it is assumed that presence or absence of the observations was not related to the outcome, then the observed percentages reflect what would have been observed if data were complete, and Treatment 1 would appear to have the greater success rate. In contrast, if it is assumed that all subjects with unknown outcomes were failures, then the success rate would be greater for Treatment 2 (35% vs. 40%).

These results illustrate how missing outcomes can undermine the clarity and robustness of trial conclusions. According to one assumption the success rate for Treatment 1 was greater, but under another assumption Treatment 2 was better. Drawing the proper inference depends on which assumption was most appropriate. However, assumptions about missing data cannot be evaluated from the available data because the data about which the missing data assumptions are made are missing (Verbeke and Molenberghs 2000).

Despite the presence of missing data, a clinical trial may still be valid provided the statistical methods used are sensible (www.ich.org/cache/compo/276–254-1.html). Carpenter and Kenward (2007) define a sensible analysis as one where:

1. The variation between the intervention effect estimated from the trial and that in the population is random. In other words, trial results are not systematically biased.
2. As the sample size increases, the variation between the intervention effect estimated from the trial and that in the population gets smaller and smaller. In other words, as the size of the trial increases, the estimated intervention effect hones in on the true value in the population. Such estimates are called consistent in statistical terminology.
3. The estimate of the variability between the trial intervention effect and the true effect in the population (i.e., the standard error) correctly reflects the uncertainty in the data.

If these conditions hold, then valid inference can be drawn despite the missing data. However, the analyses required to meet these conditions may be different from the analyses that satisfy these conditions when no data are missing. Regardless, whenever data intended to be collected are missing, information is lost and estimates are less precise than if data were complete (Mallinckrodt 2013).

When drawing inference from incomplete data, it is important to recognize that the potential bias from missing data can either mask or exaggerate the true difference between treatments (Mallinckrodt et al. 2008; NRC 2010). Moreover, the direction of bias has different implications in different scenarios. For example, underestimating treatment differences in efficacy is bias *against* an experimental treatment that is superior to control, but is bias *in favor* of an experimental treatment that is inferior to control. This situation has particularly important inferential implications in noninferiority testing.

Underestimating treatment differences in safety is bias in favor of an experimental treatment that is less safe than control, but is bias against the experimental drug that is safer than control.

12.2 Missing Data Mechanisms

In order to understand the potential impact of missing data and to choose an appropriate analytic approach for a particular situation, the stochastic process(es) (i.e., mechanisms) leading to the missingness must be considered. The following taxonomy of missing data mechanisms is now well-established in the statistical literature (Little and Rubin 2002).

Data are missing completely at random (MCAR) if, conditional upon the covariates (e.g., treatment group, baseline severity, investigative site) in the analysis, the probability of missingness does not depend on either the observed or unobserved outcomes of the variable being analyzed.

Data are missing at random (MAR) if, conditional upon the covariates in the analysis and the observed outcomes of the variable being analyzed, the probability of missingness does not depend on the unobserved outcomes of the variable being analyzed.

Data are missing not at random (MNAR) if, conditional upon the covariates in the analysis model and the observed outcomes of the variable being analyzed, the probability of missingness does depend on the unobserved outcomes of the variable being analyzed. Another way to think about MNAR is that if, conditional on observed outcomes, the statistical behavior (means, variances, etc.) of the unobserved data is equal to the behavior had the data been observed, then the missingness is MAR; if not, then MNAR.

With MCAR, the outcome variable is not related to the probability of dropout (after taking into account covariates). In MAR, the observed values of the outcome variable are related to the probability of dropout, but the unobserved outcomes are not (after taking into account covariates and observed outcome). In MNAR the unobserved outcomes are related to the probability of dropout even after the observed outcomes and covariates have been taken into account.

The practical implications of the distinction between MAR and MNAR is best appreciated by example. Consider a clinical trial where subjects are assessed every 4 weeks for 24 weeks, and a subject had clinically meaningful improvement during the first 12 weeks. Subsequent to the Week-12 assessment the subject had a marked worsening and dropped out. If the subject was lost to follow-up and there was no Week-16 observation to reflect the worsened condition, the missingness was MNAR. If the Week-16 observation was obtained before the subject dropped out, it is possible the missingness was MAR (provided the outcomes were incorporated in the analysis model). Note that this example illustrates what happens on average under the two mechanisms. With the stochastic nature of the missingness processes, it is impossible to claim with certainty whether missingness for a particular subject was driven by an MAR or MNAR mechanism.

Mallinckrodt et al. (2008) summarized several key points that arise from the precise definitions of the missingness mechanisms given above. First, given that the definitions are all conditional on the model, characterization of the missingness mechanism does not rest on the data alone; it involves both the data and the model used to analyze them. Consequently, missingness that might be MNAR given one model could be MAR or MCAR given another. In addition, since the relationship between the dependent variable and missingness is a key factor in the missingness mechanism, the mechanism may vary from one outcome to another within the same data set.

Moreover, when dropout rates differ by treatment group, it would be incorrect to conclude on these grounds alone that the missingness mechanism was MNAR and that analyses assuming MCAR or MAR were invalid. If dropout depended only on treatment, and treatment was included in the model, the mechanism giving rise to the dropout was MCAR. This is one example of what some have termed covariate-dependent MCAR (Little 1995; O'Kelly and Ratitch 2014). The distinction between covariate-dependent MCAR and MCAR applies to all covariates, not just treatment.

Given that the missingness mechanism can vary from one outcome to another in the same study, and may depend on the model and method, statements about the missingness mechanism without reference to the model and the variable being analyzed are problematic to interpret. This situational dependence also means that broad statements regarding missingness, and validity of particular analytic methods across specific disease states are unwarranted (Mallinckrodt 2013).

Moreover, terms such as ignorable missingness can also be problematic to interpret. For example, in the case of likelihood-based estimation, if the parameters defining the measurement process (i.e., governing the distribution of both observed and missing outcomes) are independent of the parameters defining the missingness process (this condition sometimes is referred to as the separability or distinctness condition), the missingness is ignorable if it arises from an MCAR or MAR mechanism but is nonignorable if it arises from an MNAR process (Verbeke and Molenberghs 2000).

In this context, ignorable means the missing-data mechanism need not be modeled because unbiased estimates of the parameters governing the measurement process can be obtained from the maximum likelihood analysis of observed data. However, if other forms of estimation are used, missing data may be ignorable only if arising from an MCAR mechanism. Hence, if missing data are described as ignorable or nonignorable, this must be done with reference to both the estimation method and the analytic model (Mallinckrodt 2013).

Informative censoring is yet another term used to describe the attributes of missing data. Censoring is best understood in the context of survival analyses. If the response variable was time to an event, subjects not followed long enough for the event to occur have their event times censored at the time of last assessment. It is often assumed in survival time analyses that what caused a subject to be censored is independent of what would cause her/him to have an event. This assumption is often taken after conditioning on available baseline covariates or strata, such as in a Cox proportional hazards regression model. If the outcome is related to the likelihood of censoring, conditional on available covariates, informative censoring is said to have been present. For example, if subjects discontinue because of poor response to treatment but did not yet have the event of interest, the censoring times indirectly reflect bad outcomes. Thus, the censoring is said to be informative. Analogously, the censoring can be said to be not at random because the statistical behavior or distribution of event times for censored patients is not equal to that of uncensored patients.

However, an important consideration differentiates informative censoring in the survival time setting from the repeated measures setting. In survival time settings, typically there is one observation of the analyzed outcome (event time) per subject; no intermediate observations exist. In longitudinal settings with repeated measures, most subjects will have at least partially observed sequences. With repeated measurements, for censoring (dropout) to be informative, this must be in addition to what is known from the observed outcomes. With no intermediate observations included in the model in the survival time setting, it is more likely censoring would be informative than in an otherwise similar scenario where analyses can condition on the intermediate observations. Simply put, MAR (noninformative censoring) is more likely valid with intermediate observations in a repeated measures setting. In survival time settings, these intermediate observations are often not included in analysis.

Throughout the remainder of this book, missing data are described via the mechanism giving rise to the missingness (Mallinckrodt 2013).

12.3 Dealing with Missing Data

12.3.1 Introduction

Dealing with missing data is of course in part an analytic problem. However, the best way to deal with missing data is to prevent it (NRC 2010; Fleming 2011; Mallinckrodt 2013; O'Kelly and Ratitch 2014). A comprehensive approach to the prevention and treatment of missing data involves three pillars: (1) setting clear objectives and defining the causal estimands; (2) minimizing the amount of missing data; and, (3) defining an appropriate primary analysis supported by plausible sensitivity analyses (Mallinckrodt et al. 2014).

Minimizing missing data was covered in Chapter 3. Objectives and estimands were discussed in Chapter 2. Recall that some estimands can be formulated such that early discontinuation from treatment or initiation of recuse treatment are considered an outcome and do not result in missing data, whereas for other estimands discontinuation or rescue result in missing data. This chapter and Part III of the book focuses on the second situation. The remainder of this chapter introduces key concepts in analysis of incomplete data. Details on specific analyses are covered in subsequent chapters.

12.3.2 Analytic Approaches

Missing data can be dealt with by:

1. Ad hoc (single) imputation approaches (e.g., imputation with last observed values)
2. Ignoring the missing data
3. Accounting for the missing data via principled approaches to imputation, likelihood-based analyses, or weighting the observed values to adjust for the probability of dropout
4. Jointly modeling the outcome variable and the missingness process

Until recently, guidelines for the analysis of clinical trial data provided only limited advice on how to handle missing data, and analytic approaches tended to be simple and ad hoc (Molenberghs and Kenward 2007). Simple and ad hoc methods became popular during a time of limited computing power because they restored the intended balance to the data, allowing implementation of the simple analyses for complete data. However, with the seminal work on analysis of incomplete data by Rubin (1976), including the now common taxonomy of missingness mechanisms, attention began to shift to accounting for the potential bias from missing data.

Nevertheless, widespread use of simple methods for dealing with missing data set historical precedent that fostered their continued acceptance even after alternative methods were well known. In regulatory settings, methods like baseline observation carried forward (BOCF) and last observation carried forward (LOCF) remained popular choices for the primary analysis long after more principled alternatives could be easily implemented with commercial software (Mallinckrodt 2013).

In addition to historical precedent, continued acceptance of LOCF and BOCF despite strong evidence of their shortcomings was also fostered by the belief that these methods led to conservative estimates of treatment effects. Conservative in this context means not favoring the treatment; that is, underestimating the advantage of treatment over control. Hence, even though it became well known that imputing missing data via LOCF or BOCF yielded biased estimates of treatment effects, that bias was considered appropriate for confirmatory clinical trials of medical interventions because the bias was thought to provide protection against erroneous approval of ineffective interventions (Kenward and Molenberghs 2009).

However, as detailed in Chapter 13, the conditions under which LOCF and BOCF yield conservative estimates and maintain control of Type I error rates are not straightforward and cannot be assured at the start of the trial. Not surprisingly, LOCF and BOCF are now generally not seen as suitable for use as a primary analysis (Molenberghs and Kenward 2007; Mallinckrodt et al. 2008; NRC 2010; O'Kelly and Ratitch 2014).

For an analysis to yield unbiased results when ignoring missing data, the missingness must typically arise from an MCAR mechanism. One notable exception to the requirement of MCAR for ignorability is direct likelihood analyses, which can be valid under the far less restrictive assumption of MAR. Part II of this book described many aspects of direct likelihood analyses. Chapter 14 provides further detail on how likelihood-based analyses can ignore missing data that arise from an MCAR or MAR mechanism.

Multiple imputation has several variations, but the key idea is to impute the missing values using a likelihood-based model, combine the actually observed and imputed values to create a complete data set, analyze the now complete data, and repeat the process multiple times. Results are combined across data sets for final inference in a manner that takes into account the uncertainty due to missing data. More details on multiple imputation are provided in Chapter 15.

Inverse probability weighting is another MAR approach wherein a specific model is used to estimate the probability of dropout given the observed data. The inverse of these probabilities are applied to the observed data to create a pseudo-sample reflecting what would have been observed if no data were missing. Chapter 16 includes additional theoretical details and specifics on implementing inverse probability weighting.

Jointly modeling the outcome of interest and the dropout process typically involves MNAR analyses. Chapter 18 includes additional theoretical details and some implementation specifics on MNAR methods.

The analytic conundrum missing data pose is that MCAR is usually not a reasonable assumption, MAR may be reasonable but there is no way to know for certain, and there is no way to be certain that an MNAR method and model is appropriate (Mallinckrodt 2013). A sensible compromise between blindly shifting to MNAR models and ignoring them altogether is to use MNAR methods in sensitivity analyses (Molenberghs and Kenward 2007; Mallinckrodt et al. 2008). Indeed, broad consensus has emerged indicating that the primary analyses of longitudinal clinical trials should often be based on methods that assume MAR, and that robustness of the MAR result should be assessed using sensitivity analyses (Verbeke and Molenberghs 2000; Molenberghs and Kenward 2007; Mallinckrodt et al. 2008; Siddiqui et al. 2009; NRC 2010; Mallinckrodt et al. 2014).

12.3.3 Sensitivity Analyses

Sensitivity analyses can be a single analysis or a series of analyses with differing assumptions. The aim is that by comparing results across sensitivity analyses it becomes apparent how much inferences rely on the assumptions (NRC 2010; Phillips et al. 2016). In longitudinal clinical trials, sensitivity analyses typically focus on inferences regarding the treatment effects. Therefore, a primary aim of sensitivity analyses is to assess how treatment effects vary depending on assumptions about the missing data.

Sensitivity analyses in principle can be used for any analytic assumption. However, it is useful to distinguish between testable and nontestable assumptions. Assumptions regarding covariance between repeated measurements, mean trends over time, distribution of residuals, etc. can be tested from the observed data. In contrast, the fundamental sensitivity task for missing data will often center on the distinction between MAR and MNAR mechanisms; however, a formal data-based distinction between MAR and MNAR is not possible because each MNAR model fit to a set of observed data can be reproduced exactly by an MAR counterpart (Molenberghs and Kenward 2007). Of course, such a pair of models will produce different predictions of the unobserved outcomes, given the observed outcomes.

That is, it is not possible to distinguish MAR versus MNAR in practice (NRC 2010; Mallinckrodt et al. 2014). Therefore, the aim of sensitivity analyses for missing data is typically to evaluate the degree to which inferences are influenced by departures from MAR. Departure from MAR is typically quantified via one or several sensitivity parameters. Unlike parameters that can be estimated from observed data, there is no information in the observed data about the missing data sensitivity parameters. Therefore, the sensitivity parameters are typically chosen by the analyst in order to create a relevant departure from MAR from which results can be compared to the MAR result (Carpenter et al. 2013).

It is important to keep missing data sensitivity analyses within the overall context of assessing uncertainty in clinical trial results. This uncertainty arises from different sources: (1) inherent imprecision in parameters of the model estimated from a finite sample; (2) model selection (e.g., for the mean and covariance functions); and, (3) the level of uncertainty due to incompleteness. Sources 1 and 2 can be assessed from the observed data. What sets missing data apart is that uncertainty from incompleteness cannot be objectively evaluated from observed data. Hence, the need for missing data sensitivity analyses (Molenberghs and Kenward 2007).

12.3.4 Inclusive and Restrictive Modeling Approaches

Collins et al. (2001) describe restrictive and inclusive modeling philosophies. Restrictive models typically include only the design factors of the experiment, and perhaps one or a few covariates. Inclusive models include, in addition to the design factors, auxiliary variables whose purpose is to improve the performance of the missing data procedure.

Recalling the specific definition of MAR provides rationale for inclusive modeling. Data are MAR if, conditional upon the variables in the model, missingness does not depend on the unobserved outcomes of the variable being analyzed. Therefore, if additional variables are added to the model that explains missingness, MAR can be valid; whereas if the additional variables are not included, the missing data would be MNAR.

Ancillary variables can be included in likelihood-based analyses by either adding the ancillary variable as a covariate or as an additional response to create a multivariate analysis. However, the complexity of multivariate analyses and the features of most commercial software make it easier to use ancillary variables via MI. With separate steps for imputation and analysis, post-baseline, time-varying covariates—possibly influenced by treatment—can be included in the imputation step of MI to account for missingness but then not included in the analysis step to avoid confounding with the treatment effects, as might be the case in a likelihood-based analysis.

12.4 Summary

Missing data is an incessant and complex problem in longitudinal clinical trials. Dealing with missing data is in part an analytic problem. However, the best way to deal with missing data is to prevent it. A comprehensive approach to the prevention and treatment of missing data involves setting clear objectives and defining the causal estimands, minimizing missing data, and having an appropriate primary analysis supported by plausible sensitivity analyses.

The potential impact of missing data is dependent on the underlying mechanism. In MCAR, neither the observed nor the unobserved data are related to the probability of dropout. This situation is unlikely in most clinical trial scenarios. There are two ways to think about the less restrictive MAR mechanism: (1) the missingness does not depend on missing data given observed data and (2) the distribution of unobserved future outcomes is the same as the distribution of observed future outcomes, conditional on earlier outcomes. If these conditions do not hold, then data are MNAR.

13

Simple and Ad Hoc Approaches for Dealing with Missing Data

13.1 Introduction

This chapter provides an overview of simple and ad hoc methods of dealing with missing data in longitudinal clinical trials. These methods are generally not recommended for use but are of historic interest and provide a useful starting point from which to differentiate the more principled methods described in subsequent chapters. It is assumed throughout this chapter that the estimand of interest is the treatment effect that would have been estimated in an infinitely large trial with no missing values; that is, estimand 3 as introduced in Table 2.1, the de jure (efficacy) estimand. Focus is on the difference between treatments in mean change from baseline to endpoint.

In this context, the complete data set is a random sample of subjects from the hypothetical infinitely large trial of all subjects. Therefore, evaluation of treatment effects from complete data (even using simple estimators such as the two sample *t*-test comparing unadjusted sample means) provides unbiased estimates of that estimand. In fact, this consideration motivates use of estimates from complete data as valid benchmarks for performance of methods applied to incomplete data. Bias in methods is with respect to the above estimand, understanding that a method with bias for this estimand may provide unbiased results for a different estimand. Methods are illustrated using the small example data set with dropout (see Section 4.3). Results from the various methods applied to the incomplete data are benchmarked against results from the corresponding complete data set.

As detailed in Section 4.3, missing data were created by applying to the complete data an MAR missingness process with the probability of dropout depending on the observed outcomes. Only monotone missingness patterns were generated; that is, if a subject had a missing value at a time = t all assessments at time > t were also missing.

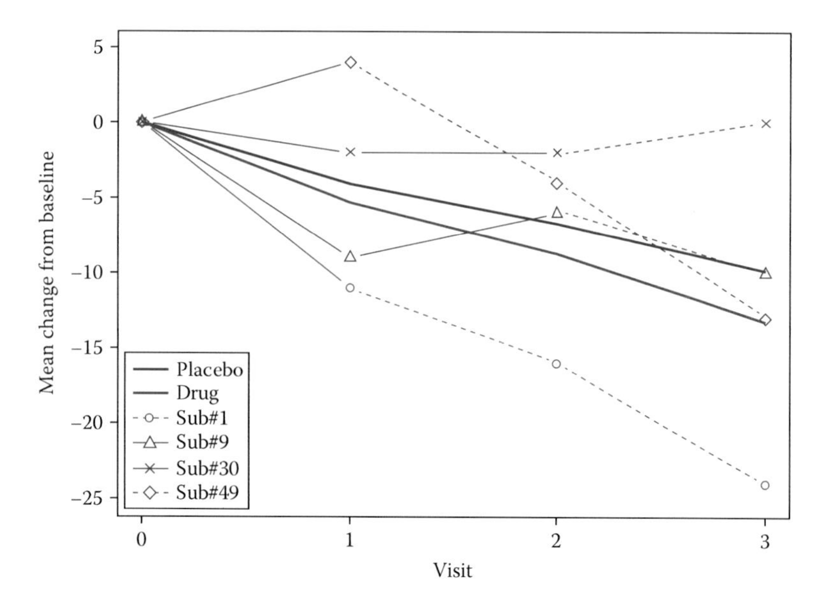

FIGURE 13.1
Response and missing data profiles for four selected patients. Solid lines are the observed outcomes and dotted lines show "unobserved" outcomes from complete data that were deleted to create the incomplete data.

Figure 13.1 illustrates incomplete and complete outcome profiles of four subjects (#1, #9, #30, and #49) that were selected to represent different response and missingness patterns. These subjects are used as case studies to illustrate features of each analytic approach.

13.2 Complete Case Analysis

In complete case analysis (also known as observed case or completers analysis) subjects with one or more missing values for the outcome being analyzed are discarded from the data set. Only subjects with complete data for the outcome being analyzed are included.

Completers analyses have serious drawbacks. The subset of subjects that complete the trial is seldom a random subset. For example, subjects with poor outcomes are often more likely to discontinue. In other words, the missing data seldom arise from an MCAR mechanism. In essence, including only completers creates selection bias. This bias typically causes overestimation of within group effects, particularly at the last scheduled visit.

When the selection process is the same for each treatment arm such that the bias to within-group point estimates is the same, this results in an unbiased estimate of the difference between treatments. However, such an assumption is difficult to justify a priori, especially when comparing active medications to placebo. If for example efficacy differs by treatment and efficacy influences adherence, the amount of selection bias will differ by treatment group, leading to a bias in the treatment contrast when analyzing completers. Moreover, even if the bias in change to last visit cancelled out between treatment groups, other aspects of the analysis are likely biased. For example, the completers are likely a more homogenous group than the initially randomized cohort of subjects, leading to underestimation of variance, which, in turn, leads to standard errors that are too small, confidence intervals that are too narrow, and test statistics that are biased toward inferences that the groups differ.

Setting aside the issue of bias, analyzing only completers results in a problematic loss of information because subjects who discontinued the trial are ignored. The partial information from incomplete sequences can still be valuable in estimating treatment effects. For example, if a subject discontinued just before the last scheduled visit t, his/her observed outcomes up to visit t–1 provide relevant information that could be utilized ("borrowed") for estimating the treatment effect at visit t.

As an illustration, consider the following simple, hypothetical scenario. Assume that the distribution of the change in efficacy scores from baseline to the last scheduled visit is normally distributed with means $\mu_A = -13$ and $\mu_B = -10$ for Drug A and Drug B (a larger negative change indicates greater improvement). Further assume a common standard deviation $\sigma = 5$. Therefore, the true treatment contrast (B–A) for the complete data = 3.

Now assume that subjects discontinue and therefore miss the final assessment with probability 1 if their change score is above the threshold value $k = -10$. The observed data at the last visit will follow a truncated normal distribution within each treatment arm with the mean given by the expression: $\mu - \sigma\phi\left(\frac{k-\mu}{\sigma}\right) \Big/ \Phi\left(\frac{k-\mu}{\sigma}\right)$, where $\phi(.)$ and $\Phi(.)$ are standard normal PDF and CDF, respectively. These new means are about –15.3 for Drug A and –14.0 for Drug B, resulting in a treatment difference of 1.3 versus the difference of 3.0 for the complete data. The truncation causes a shift in the within-group means toward better outcomes. The impact of truncation is not the same in both groups; it is greater in the group with worse efficacy. In real clinical trial scenarios, discontinuations likely result from complex stochastic process(es). However, this simple example illustrates how dropouts due to lack of efficacy would differentially exaggerate observed efficacy within each treatment arm, thus inducing bias (likely dilution) in the contrast between treatments.

Figure 13.2 plots visit-wise least squares means from the small example data set with dropout based on the subset of subjects who completed Time 3 (solid lines) compared to the benchmark from complete (full) data (dotted line). The "complete case" estimates are those at the last visit (Time 3). Estimates were obtained using ANCOVA for visit-wise changes from baseline with treatment and baseline value as covariates in the model.

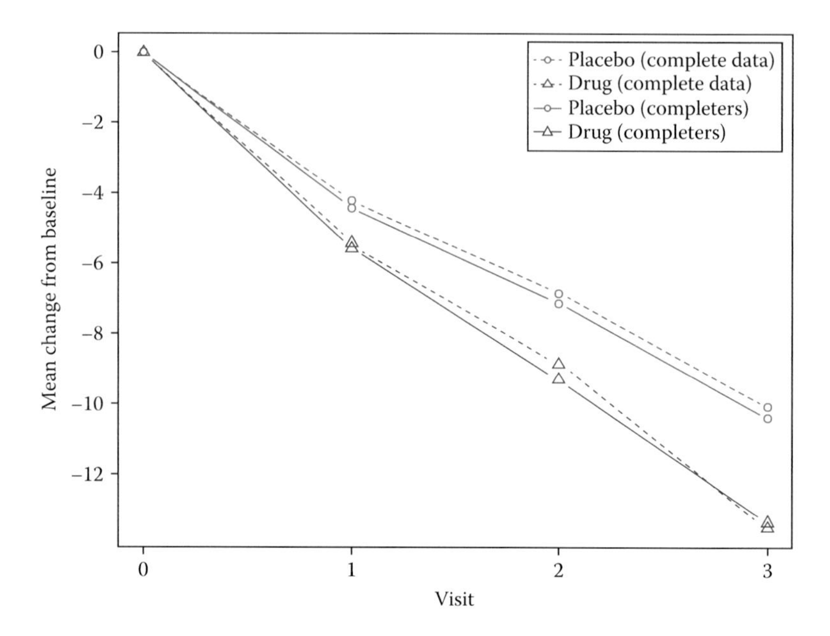

FIGURE 13.2
Comparison of "complete case" analysis with analysis based on complete (full) data.

In this example, visit-wise means for the active treatment arm (Treatment 2) are not affected much by dropouts, whereas in the placebo arm the means for completers consistently deviate from those based on complete data, indicating selection bias and dilution of the treatment contrast at the last visit.

13.3 Last Observation Carried Forward and Baseline Carried Forward

Last observation carried forward (LOCF) and baseline observation carried forward (BOCF) are methods for nonstochastic imputation. For subjects with monotone patterns of missing values, the outcomes are imputed using their earlier observed values. As the names imply, LOCF imputes all missing values for each subject using the last observed value for that subject and BOCF imputes all missing values for each subject using the baseline value for that subject.

Typically, when LOCF and BOCF are used the repeated measures nature of the data is ignored and a single outcome for each subject is analyzed. As initially noted in Chapter 12, use of LOCF and BOCF was in part justified because these methods were thought to provide conservative estimates of treatment effects and/or to be a composite measure of effectiveness that combined aspects of efficacy, safety, and tolerability. However, particularly LOCF can be considered as pursuing different estimands rather than as imputation methods for estimating treatment effects in the sense of a de jure (efficacy) estimand. Focus here is on estimates of efficacy.

If subjects on Drug A discontinue from a trial because of the side effects prior to achieving full benefit from the drug, their last observed values for efficacy outcomes would tend to be worse compared to those that would have been observed had the subjects remained in the trial until the last assessment. Carrying baseline values forward would often be a more conservative imputation because subjects who discontinued at any time, even one visit prior to end of the study, would be considered to have had no change.

Figure 13.3 plots the "visit-wise" LOCF and BOCF estimates by treatment arm as well as the benchmark estimate from the complete data set (shown as dotted line). All estimates are based on an ANCOVA model with treatment and baseline score as covariates. The estimates at visit (Time) 3 are what would be computed as the final LOCF or BOCF estimate of treatment effect. In the example, LOCF and BOCF yield smaller mean changes over time compared with the complete data reference.

Although it seems reasonable to consider LOCF and BOCF as providing conservative estimates of within-group mean changes, the impact on treatment contrasts is less clear. This lack of clarity on the direction of bias from LOCF and BOCF is compounded by the fact that these methods consistently

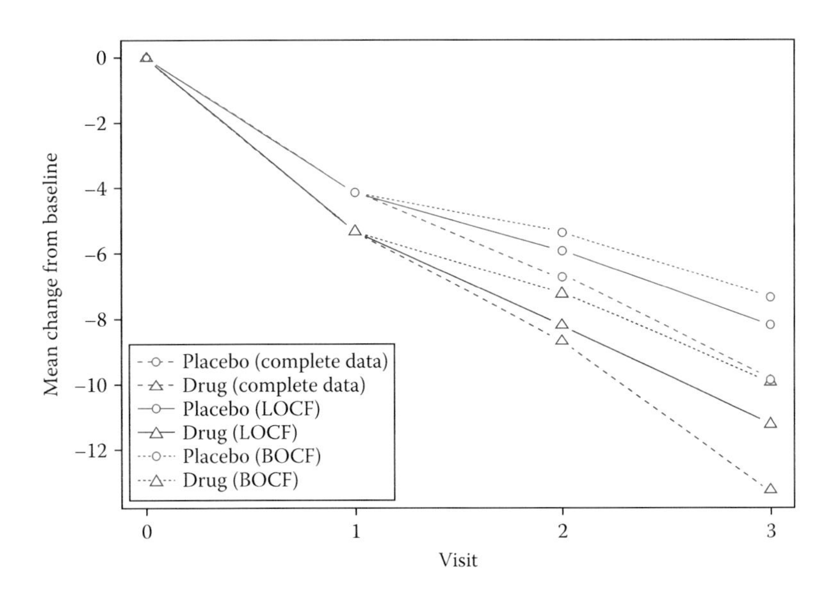

FIGURE 13.3
Mean changes from LOCF and BOCF in data with dropout compared with the analysis of the corresponding complete (full) data.

underestimate the variance. In fact, the power and Type I error rate control provided by LOCF and BOCF when assessing treatment contrasts is difficult to predict (Molenberghs et al. 2004). Many studies have shown that LOCF and BOCF can inflate treatment contrasts and markedly increase the rate of false-positive conclusions (Molenberghs et al. 2004; Lane et al. 2007; Barnes et al. 2008; Mallinckrodt et al. 2008; Sidiqui et al. 2009). Not surprisingly, the expert panel on missing data, convened at the request of FDA, stated that LOCF and BOCF are generally not appropriate means of dealing with missing data (NRC 2010).

Although it is not possible to be certain of the direction of bias, situations in which LOCF and BOCF are likely to overestimate treatment benefit include:

- When dropout in the control group is more frequent.
- When the difference between treatments is greatest at intermediate assessments. This bias would occur even if missingness were completely at random.
- In studies where the treatment goal is to maintain rather than improve outcomes.
- If LOCF and BOCF indeed provided a smaller estimate of the difference between treatments, this would not be conservative for safety outcomes. For example, if a drug causes weight gain, LOCF and BOCF will underestimate the magnitude of this unwanted side-effect.
- In noninferiority (NI) studies the null hypothesis is that the new treatment is worse than the standard treatment by a certain prespecified amount (the noninferiority or Δ margin). Underestimating the difference between treatments in an NI study would be a bias in favor of the experimental arm.
- More generally, underestimating the inferiority of the inferior treatment would not be conservative.

13.4 Hot-Deck Imputation

Another single imputation approach is the so-called *hot-deck* method. Hot deck is of less historical interest, because it was not used as frequently in clinical trials as LOCF and BOCF. However, *hot-deck* imputation is useful to introduce, because it starts the movement toward more principled imputations. In *hot-deck* imputation, values are imputed by borrowing from an appropriate complete case (or *donor* case) that is in some sense similar to the missing case (Molenberghs and Kenward 2007).

Finding the appropriate donor for each subject with missing data involves finding the donor who is most similar. In longitudinal clinical trial data similarity can be based on observed outcomes and baseline covariates. Donors can also be matched based on estimates for the probability of dropout. The donor can be the subject with nonmissing outcomes whose estimated probability of being observed is closest to that of the subject with missing value(s). The model used to assess the probabilities can be fit using a logistic regression of the form $\Pr(R = 1|X,Y_{obs})$.

In general, missingness must arise from an MCAR mechanism for *hot-deck* imputation to yield unbiased estimates of treatment effects. Besides, simple hot-deck methods typically underestimate standard errors of estimated treatment effects. Therefore, *hot-deck* imputation will not usually be valid, but the idea that imputation can be based on borrowed information is central to more principled approaches discussed in subsequent chapters.

13.5 Single Imputation from a Predictive Distribution

The approach illustrated in this section is not of historical interest, because it was not commonly used in clinical trials. However, this approach illustrates some key aspects of the more principled methods of analyzing incomplete data that are discussed in subsequent chapters. The approach takes a data set with missing values and makes it complete by imputing missing observations using a predictive model that is based on data from the longitudinal profiles of all subjects. The imputed-complete data set is then analyzed using a model that would have been appropriate had there been no missing data.

Recall that single imputation approaches do not account for the uncertainty in the imputation, resulting in underestimation of standard errors. Fundamental concepts in accounting for the uncertainty of imputation will be illustrated by introducing randomness in the predicted values; that is, imputed values are drawn from a distribution. Such an approach would be valid under MCAR and MAR if the imputation model properly accounted for the correlations between the repeated measurements within subjects.

A relatively straightforward way to implement this procedure is to first estimate the visit-wise marginal means for each treatment arm and the unstructured covariance matrix by fitting to the data an appropriate direct likelihood model, such as those described in Section II. Then, imputed values can be generated from the conditional normal distribution. A better approach would be to use subject-specific marginal means adjusted for baseline severity and other covariates, but for illustration the simpler imputation model is used here.

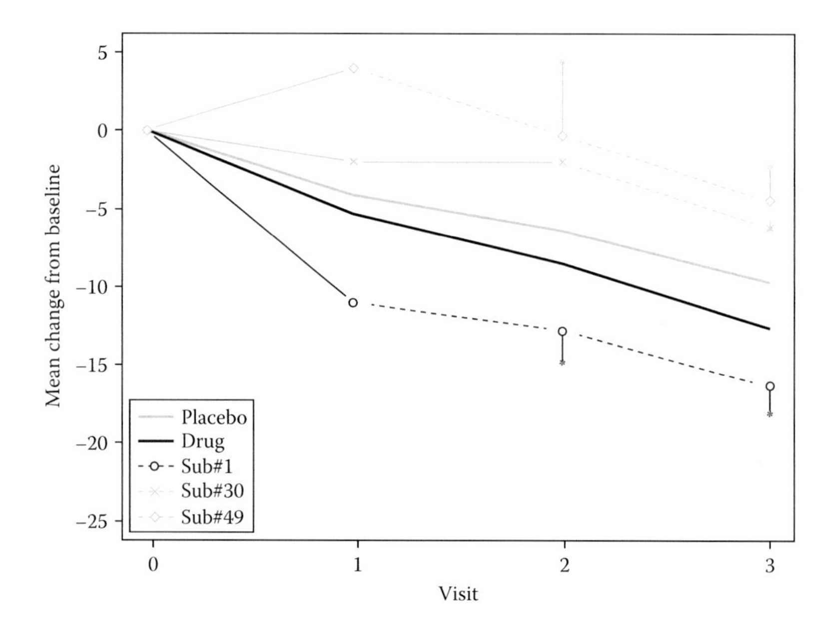

FIGURE 13.4
Illustration of single imputation from a predictive distribution for selected subjects. Subjects #1, #30, and #49 with observed data (solid lines), conditional means (dotted lines), and imputed values (asterisks). Treatment mean profiles (thick lines) are estimated via direct likelihood.

To obtain imputed values for a subject with missing data at Visits (Times) 2 and 3, such as placebo Subject #49 (see Figure 13.4), generate outcomes from the conditional distribution, $f(y_2, y_3 | y_1)$, which is a bivariate normal distribution $N(\mu^*, \Sigma^*)$, with the mean vector μ^* and covariance matrix Σ^* given by

$$\mu^* = (\mu_2, \mu_3) + \frac{1}{\sigma_1^2}\Sigma_{23,1}(y_1 - \mu_1) = (-0.321, -4.454)$$

$$\Sigma^* = \Sigma_{23} - \frac{1}{\sigma_1^2}\Sigma_{23,1}(\Sigma_{23,1})^T = \begin{pmatrix} 9.964 & 7.635 \\ 7.635 & 18.578 \end{pmatrix}$$

where μ_1, μ_2, μ_3 are marginal means at Times 1, 2, and 3 for the placebo arm, Σ_{23} is the 2×2 error covariance matrix for Times 2 and 3, and $\Sigma_{23,1} = (\sigma_{21}, \sigma_{31})$ is a 2×1 vector with covariances between Times 2 and 1, and 3 and 1, respectively.

To obtain imputed values for a subject with missing data at Visit (Time) 3, such as Subject #30 (see Figure 13.4), generate imputed values from the conditional distribution $f(y_3 | y_1, y_2)$ which is univariate normal with the mean μ^* and variance σ^{*2} given by

$$\mu^* = \mu_3 + \Sigma_{3,12}\Sigma_{12}^{-1}(y_1 - \mu_1, y_2 - \mu_2)^T = -6.182$$

$$\sigma^{*2} = \sigma_3^2 - \Sigma_{3,12}\Sigma_{12}^{-1}\left(\Sigma_{3,12}\right)^T = 12.728$$

Predictive distributions for each missing value are obtained by replacing all these elements in the expressions for μ^* and Σ^* by the corresponding estimates from an appropriate likelihood-based analysis, resulting in the numerical values shown in the above equations.

Figure 13.4 plots the observed values and conditional means for the visits when the outcomes were unobserved for Subjects 1, 30, and 49.

The following observations and comments can be made

- The imputation model based on the conditional normal distributions estimated from the observed data likelihood effectively assumes that the distribution of future outcomes given earlier outcomes for subjects with observed future outcomes is the same as for those with missing future outcomes. This is equivalent to an MAR mechanism. Therefore, the point estimates from analysis of completed data with imputed missing values is consistent under MAR.
- The equality of the conditional distributions of missing and observed values given earlier values arises from use of marginal means and covariances estimated from the maximum likelihood analysis of observed data. Had estimates of the marginal means and covariances been obtained from a complete case analysis rather than a maximum likelihood analysis of all observed data, the imputation model would essentially reproduce the complete case analysis inducing similar biases in the final point estimates as the complete case analysis.
- Assuming positive within-subject correlations, which is typically the case, subjects whose observed outcomes were better than their treatment mean would also have conditional means better than the group mean for the future time points. That is, better (worse) than average outcomes at past visits predict better (worse) outcomes at future visits. For example, Subject 1 from the drug-treated group had greater change than the group mean at the time of discontinuation. The conditional means for Subject 1 were greater than the corresponding treatment group means. Similarly, placebo Subjects 30 and 49 were worse than (smaller changes) the corresponding group mean at the time of discontinuation and the projections for outcomes at future visits were worse (smaller changes) than the group means.
- Consistent with the weaker correlations between observations more distant in time, predicted individual conditional means get closer to the group mean (greater shrinkage) as the observation and the prediction time get farther apart. Refer to Section 5.4 for detailed explanation of how variance components influence shrinkage.

- Also consistent with the weaker correlations between observations more distant in time, the conditional distribution has greater variance as the time between the observation and the prediction time get more distant from each other. This makes intuitive sense in that when the source of information (the observed data) is more weakly correlated with what is to be predicted there is greater uncertainty in the prediction. In the example above, the conditional error variances for imputing outcomes at Time 3 using the data from Time 1 and Time 2 was 12.7 and the variance for imputing the Time 3 using only Time 1 was 18.6.

To further explain, consider a simple regression model with a single post-baseline outcome, y_1 regressed on baseline score y_0. Further assume equal variances $\sigma^2 = (\sigma_1)^2 = (\sigma_0)^2$. The conditional mean $E(Y_1|Y_0 = y_0)$ is $\mu_{1|0} = \mu_1 + \rho(y_0 - \mu_0)$. Therefore, the marginal mean μ_1 is adjusted by an additive term $\rho(y_0 - \mu_0)$. Assuming that within-subject error correlation (ρ) between the first and the second time points is positive, the adjustment would be positive or negative depending on whether the observed value y_0 was above or below the mean μ_0. The amount of adjustment is shrunk closer to zero by the factor of $|\rho| \leq 1$. For example, no adjustment would be made if $\rho = 0$ (no within-subject correlation). The conditional variance $\sigma^2(1 - \rho^2)$ is smaller than the unconditional variance σ^2 by a factor $(1 - \rho^2) \leq 1$. However, this factor will get closer to 1 with weaker within-subject correlation, such as when the future and observed time points are farther apart.

Once the missing values have been imputed, a completed data set is obtained and could be analyzed via standard complete data techniques. As previously noted, the point estimates from such an imputation strategy will be correct if the imputation model is based on consistent estimates of means and error covariance from the repeated measures likelihood.

Adding random noise to the predicted values when carrying out imputation (rather than taking the conditional mean for the predicted value "as is") adjusts the variance to account for the uncertainty due to imputation. However, standard errors would still be calculated with imputed values treated as observed values. This effectively assumes a larger sample size than that which was actually observed, resulting in artificially reduced standard errors that reflect greater precision than was actually the case. Although resampling methods (e.g., jackknife or bootstrap) could be used to obtain valid estimates of standard errors, the key concept for the present purpose is that single imputation, combined *with standard estimators of standard errors,* results in invalid inference.

An obvious question is why estimate treatment effects by imputing missing outcomes from a likelihood-based model when treatment effects can be estimated using the same assumptions directly from the likelihood model without imputation? In fact, the method illustrated in this subsection is of little practical value, but it is important for illustrating two key points.

First, imputing from the conditional normal distribution serves as a building block for more principled methods such as multiple imputation. And, as illustrated in Chapter 15, there are situations when breaking the estimation process into two steps: (1) generating a complete data set by imputing missing values and (2) estimating treatment effects from completed data may have advantages over directly estimating treatment effect from a single model applied to incomplete data.

13.6 Summary

The simple and ad hoc methods of dealing with missing data discussed in this chapter are generally not recommended for use. Nevertheless, the methods are of historic interest and provide a useful starting point from which to differentiate the more principled methods described in subsequent chapters. In particular, single imputation from a predictive distribution provides an important stepping stone for understanding multiple imputation and direct-likelihood analyses.

14

Direct Maximum Likelihood

14.1 Introduction

If missing data arise from an MCAR or MAR mechanism, a likelihood-based analysis can yield unbiased estimates and valid inferences from the available data such that the missing data can be ignored. With GEE and least squares estimation, for the missingness to be ignorable, it must arise from an MCAR mechanism. Therefore, the plausibility of ignorable missing data is greater with likelihood-based analyses than with GEE or least squares (Verbeke and Molenberghs 2000).

The technical explanation for why MCAR and MAR missingness can be ignored in likelihood-based analyses (such as those illustrated in Section II) is based on factorization of the likelihood function. This factorization explanation and other technical details are covered in the next section and examples in subsequent sections further illustrate how likelihood-based methods account for missing data.

14.2 Technical Details

Factorization of the likelihood function in this context means that the hypothetical "full" data are split into two parts: the actually observed part and the missing part, which are often described as the measurement process and the missingness process, respectively (Verbeke and Molenberghs 2000).

As a building block to factoring the full data likelihood, consider the observed data for subject i, denoted as an $1 \times n_i$ vector $Y_{i,obs}$, and the observed $1 \times n$ vector of missingness indicators R_i that indicate whether the subject has the outcome observed on jth occasion ($r_{ij} = 1$) or missing ($r_{ij} = 0$). The observed data likelihood can be written as the joint density of the random variables $Y_{i,obs}$ and R_i, $f(y_{i,obs}, r_i | x_i, \theta, \Psi)$, where X is the design matrix for fixed effects (e.g., baseline covariates, treatment, and time), θ is a vector of parameters for the outcome process, and Ψ is a vector of parameters for the missingness process.

The aim in clinical trials is typically to estimate θ, with ψ being of ancillary interest. As such, it would be desirable to partition the joint (log-) likelihood of $(Y_{i,obs}, R_i)$ so as to isolate the portion of the likelihood that is relevant for estimating θ. If such partitioning can be achieved, then the parts of the likelihood associated with missingness parameters are not relevant for maximizing the likelihood with respect to θ—and these missingness parameters could therefore be ignored.

The joint likelihood can be formally written as the product of marginal and conditional distributions

$$f(y_{i,obs}, r_i | x_i, \theta, \Psi) = f(y_{i,obs} | x_i, \theta, \Psi)\, f(r_i | y_{i,obs}, x_i, \theta, \Psi)$$

or on the log-likelihood scale as the sum

$$\log[f(y_{i,obs}, r_i | x_i, \theta, \Psi)] = \log[f(y_{i,obs} | x_i, \theta, \Psi)] + \log[f(r_i | y_{i,obs}, x_i, \theta, \Psi)].$$

In this decomposition, θ and Ψ are present in both pieces of the likelihood in the right-hand side, and thus Ψ is not ignorable. Fortunately, if missingness results from an MCAR or MAR mechanism and the parameters θ and Ψ are functionally separable (the so-called separability condition), a partitioning to isolate the parameters of interest is attainable.

To see how this is possible, consider the full data likelihood that includes both the observed and the missing data. Let a random variable $Y_{i,mis}$ denote the $1 \times (n - n_i)$ component vector of missing data for the ith subject. Although $Y_{i,mis}$ represents data that are not observed, it is a valid random variable representing the potential outcomes for subjects who discontinued from the trial that would have been observed had they remained.

The observed data likelihood can be written as the integral over the $Y_{i,mis}$. Under the integral sign, the joint density can be written as follows:

$$\begin{aligned} f\left(y_{i,obs}, r_i | x_i, \theta, \Psi\right) &= \int f\left(y_{i,obs}, y_{i,mis}, r_i | x_i, \theta, \Psi\right) dy_{i,mis} \\ &= \int f\left(y_{i,obs}, y_{i,mis} | x_i, \theta\right) f\left(r_i | y_{i,obs}, y_{i,mis}, x_i, \Psi\right) dy_{i,mis} \end{aligned}$$

With the introduction of Y_{mis}, the joint likelihood for the full data can be factored into pieces that separate the parameters θ and Ψ because of the assumption that the complete outcome $(Y_{i,obs}, Y_{i,mis})$ does not depend on the missingness parameter Ψ, and the missingness process (R) does not depend on θ *after conditioning on the complete* data. By assuming MAR, the joint distribution of the *observed* data can be factored similarly.

Under MAR, $f(r_i|y_{i,obs}, y_{i,mis}, x_i, \Psi) = f(r_i|y_{i,obs}, x_i, \Psi)$. Therefore, this likelihood factor can be taken outside the integral and the desired factorization of the observed data likelihood is obtained as follows:

$$f(y_{i,obs}, r|x_i, \theta, \Psi) = f(y_{i,obs}|x_i, \theta)\, f(r_i|y_{i,obs}, x_i, \Psi)$$

Now parameter θ is associated only with the likelihood term containing $y_{i,obs}$. Therefore, we could estimate θ (and any functions of treatment effect of our interest) by using only contributions to the observed data likelihood of $y_{i,obs}$, $i = 1, \ldots, N$, because the parts associated with parameters of missingness (Ψ) would not be relevant for maximizing the likelihood with respect to θ.

This elegant proof (Little and Rubin 1987) is general and applies to *any* type of outcome as long as its likelihood can be written. The proof may be appealing to mathematically inclined readers. However, it is not intuitively obvious exactly how the missing data in the context of a longitudinal clinical trial (dropouts) are accounted for in this analytic framework. A more operational and instructive explanation of how direct likelihood methods, and in particular, methods based on an unstructured modeling of time and covariance, yield unbiased estimates under MAR can be given by a factorization of the likelihood for the observed part of the full repeated measures outcome $Y_i = (Y_{i1}, Y_{i2}, \ldots, Y_{in})$.

Consider the small example data set with three post-baseline outcomes, represented for the *i*th subject by the trivariate normal variate $Y_i = (Y_{i1}, Y_{i2}, Y_{i3})$ and further assume that all the missingness is due to dropouts (i.e., the missing data have a monotone pattern). Focus first, for simplicity, on the analysis of a single treatment arm because adding covariates does not change matters in principle. Thus, all time-fixed covariates are denoted collectively as X.

The trivariate normal distribution associated with random variate Y_i can be factored as a product of the conditional distributions that represent a sequence of regressions, where each component of the distribution is regressed on the previous outcomes and baseline scores. Subject indices (*i*) are suppressed for simplicity.

$$f(y|x, \theta) = f(y_1|x, \theta_1)\, f(y_2|x, y_1, \theta_2)\, f(y_3|x, y_1, y_2, \theta_3)$$

Here, parameter θ combines the vector of means and covariance matrix of multivariate normal distribution of Y conditional on X, and parameters θ_1, θ_2, and θ_3 contain regression coefficients and error variances associated with the three univariate conditional normal distributions (regressions): $[Y_1|X]$, $[Y_2|X, Y_1]$, and $[Y_3|X, Y_1, Y_2]$. With multivariate normal distributions, there is a one-to-one relation between parameters in θ and in $(\theta_1, \theta_2, \theta_3)$, therefore, θ can be obtained by simple matrix manipulations with θ_1, θ_2, and θ_3, and vice versa.

It is instructive to think of obtaining maximum likelihood (ML) estimates of θ via sequentially fitting the above regression models, even though that is not how the likelihood maximization procedure is actually implemented in software packages. If the parameters θ_1, θ_2, and θ_3 estimated by the three regression models are unbiased under MAR, then θ would also be unbiased. The key question here is the following: why are the regression models based on observed data unbiased and not adversely affected by the presence of missing data?

Recall that the MAR assumption for monotone missingness patterns can be stated in two equivalent forms: (1) the missingness mechanism does not depend on missing data given observed data and (2) the distribution of unobserved future outcomes is the same as the distribution of observed future outcomes, conditional on earlier outcomes. The second condition means that the future outcomes for subjects who discontinued should be similar to the future outcomes of subjects who continued *if they had the same values of past outcomes, covariates, etc.* As a result of point 2 above, complete data are not needed to estimate any of the three regression models. For example, the model based on fitting $f(y_{3,obs} | x, y_{1,obs}, y_{2,obs}, \theta_3)$ to observed data should estimate the same parameter vector θ_3 as if somehow the model was fit to the actual missing data: $f(y_{3,mis} | x, y_{1,obs}, y_{2,obs}, \theta_3)$. Therefore, failing to observe $y_{3,mis}$ does not bias estimation results for θ_3.

14.3 Example

The small example data set that was introduced in Chapter 4 is used to illustrate how direct likelihood analyses account for missing data. Results are compared to those based on the corresponding complete data set. Selected individual subjects are used for further illustration. Data were analyzed as specified in Code Fragment 8.1, which featured an unstructured modeling of means and covariance. Recall that in this formulation of the mixed-effects model fitting versus not fitting a random intercept has no effect on fixed-effect estimates. The model with the random intercept and unstructured modeling is actually overspecified in that the residual covariance matrix fully captures all the information in the random effects. However, fitting the random intercept is useful here in order to obtain predictions for individual subjects. Therefore, the random intercept was included mindfully that fixed effects would be identical if the random intercept was not included. Results from the data with dropout and the corresponding complete data are summarized in Table 14.1.

Results at Time 1 were similar in complete and incomplete data. Differences in results between complete and incomplete data were greater at Time 3 than at Time 2. This pattern was not surprising, given that no data were missing at Time 1 and more data were missing at Time 3 than at Time 2.

As the amount of missing data increased, standard errors increased. Visit-wise lsmeans for change from baseline were smaller for both treatment groups in the incomplete data than in the complete data. This disparity was

TABLE 14.1

Results from Likelihood-Based Analyses of Complete and Incomplete Data, with a Model Including Baseline as a Covariate

		Complete Data		Incomplete Data	
Treatment	**Time**	**LSMEANS**	**SE**	**LSMEANS**	**SE**
1	1	−4.13	0.91	−4.10	0.91
1	2	−6.70	0.93	−6.42	0.97
1	3	−9.86	1.05	−9.73	1.17
2	1	−5.32	0.91	−5.29	0.91
2	2	−8.70	0.93	−8.52	0.96
2	3	−13.26	1.05	−12.62	1.14
Endpoint Treatment Difference		3.39	1.49 ($p = 0.0274$)	2.90	1.64 ($p = 0.084$)

greater in Treatment 2, thereby yielding a smaller treatment contrast from incomplete data than from complete data.

It is important to interpret the results above as just one realization from a stochastic process. If the comparisons were replicated many times under the same conditions—with missing data arising from an MAR mechanism—the average of the lsmeans and treatment contrasts across the repeated samples would be the same for complete and incomplete data. Standard errors would be consistently greater in incomplete data, however.

To further clarify how missing data are handled in likelihood-based analyses, consider the observed and predicted values for selected subjects summarized in Table 14.2. First, consider the incomplete data for drug-treated (Treatment 2) Subject 1 who was dropped from the study after the first post-baseline visit. Although Times 2 and 3 were not observed, the parameters for the estimated treatment means factor-in the general dependency of Y_2 and Y_3 on Y_1, which can be used to generate predicted outcomes. This is because under MAR the future values of Y_2 and Y_3 for Subject 1 and other subjects who discontinued after Time 1 follow the relationships associated with the conditional distributions of $[Y_2|Y_1]$ and $[Y_3|Y_1,Y_2]$.

For Subject 1, it is predicted that the unobserved outcomes at Times 2 and 3 would have shown continued improvement, and the improvement for Subject 1 would have been greater than the group average. Factors influencing this prediction include the following: (1) the group to which Subject 1 belonged showed continued improvement over time and (2) the positive correlation between the repeated measurements suggested that subjects (such as Subject 1) with outcomes better (worse) than their group mean were likely to remain better (worse) than the group mean in the future.

Recall that the example data were created by first having complete data and then deleting observations according to an MAR mechanism. Therefore, the predicted outcomes from the incomplete data can be compared to

TABLE 14.2

Observed and Predicted Values for Selected Subjects from Analyses of Complete and Incomplete Data

Time	Observed Change	Group Mean	Pred Change	SE Pred	Residual
Subject 1 Complete Data					
1	–11	–5.32	–12.36	2.16	1.36
2	–16	–8.70	–16.12	2.18	0.12
3	–24	–13.26	–19.20	2.27	–4.79
Subject 1 Incomplete Data					
1	–11	–5.29	–10.03	2.70	–0.96
2	.	–8.52	–13.49	3.34	.
3	.	–12.62	–15.39	4.58	.
Subject 30 Complete Data					
1	–2	–4.13	0.20	2.17	–2.20
2	–2	–6.70	–2.32	2.17	0.32
3	0	–9.86	–5.67	2.23	5.67
Subject 30 Incomplete Data					
1	–2	–4.10	–1.34	2.51	–0.65
2	–2	–6.42	–3.62	2.52	1.62
3	.	–9.73	–6.34	3.85	.

the actually observed complete data and to predicted values obtained from the complete data. Predicted values for Subject 1 in the complete data deviate more from the group mean than in the incomplete data. For example, at Time 3, the predicted value for Subject 1 is approximately 6 points above the mean in complete data and only 3 points above the mean with incomplete data. With incomplete data, there is less evidence for the superior improvement of Subject 1; therefore, the above average improvement seen at Time 1 yields a predicted value at Time 3 that is regressed (shrunk) more strongly back to the group mean. The standard errors of the predicted values increase substantially when the corresponding observation was missing. Refer to Section 5.4 for a detailed examination of how variance components in the mixed-effects model influence shrinkage of estimators.

Similar relationships exist for Subject 30, which came from the placebo (Treatment 1) group. However, this subject had smaller improvements than the group mean. In the incomplete data, the predicted values for Subject 30 were less than the group average, reflecting the anticipation of continued below average performance. As with Subject 1, incomplete data resulted in greater shrinkage of predicted values back to the group mean than in complete data. This increased shrinkage with incomplete data is because the evidence for the deviation in performance was weaker with fewer observations.

However, Subject 30 had two observations and the shrinkage in the incomplete data was less than if only one value had been observed. Correspondingly, the standard errors of the predicted values are smaller for Subject 30 than for Subject 1.

14.4 Code Fragments

Given the ignorability properties of direct likelihood, no special adjustments to accommodate missing data are required. All the likelihood-based analyses described in Section II of this book can be implemented exactly to incomplete data.

14.5 Summary

If missing data arise from an MCAR or MAR mechanism, a likelihood-based analysis yields unbiased estimates and valid inferences from the available data such that the missing data process can be ignored. Factorization of the full data likelihood into parts that isolate the missingness parameters from the parameters underlying the outcome process provides the technical explanation for why MCAR and MAR missingness can be ignored in likelihood-based analyses.

A more intuitive explanation for ignorability arises from the definition of MAR. Recall the following two ways to consider MAR: (1) the missingness mechanism does not depend on missing data given observed data and (2) the distribution of unobserved future outcomes is the same as the distribution of observed future outcomes, conditional on earlier outcomes. The second condition means that the future outcomes for subjects who discontinued should be similar to the future outcomes of subjects who continued *if they had the same values of past (observed) outcomes, covariates, etc.* As a result of point 2 above, models can be formulated from only the observed data that yield unbiased estimates of parameters describing the full data.

15

Multiple Imputation

15.1 Introduction

Multiple imputation (MI) is a popular and accessible method of model-based imputation. Standard references for MI include Rubin (1987) and Little and Rubin (2002). Multiple imputation is flexible and therefore has a number of specific implementations. However, the three basic steps to MI are:

1. Impute the missing data (typically) using Bayesian predictive distributions of missing data, conditional on observed data, resulting in multiple (m) completed data sets.
2. Analyze the m completed data sets using an analysis that would have been appropriate for complete data. This results in a set of m estimates (e.g., treatment contrasts).
3. Combine (pool) the m estimates into a single inferential statement by using combination rules (or "Rubin's rules") that account for uncertainty due to imputation of the missing values, therefore providing valid inference.

These steps can be applied to continuous outcomes that follow a normal distribution, categorical outcomes, or time to event (e.g., exponentially distributed) outcomes where missingness is created by censoring.

If MI is implemented using the same imputation and analysis model, and the model is the same as the analysis model used in a maximum likelihood-based (ML) analysis, MI and ML will yield asymptotically similar point estimates. That is, as the size of the data set and the number of imputations in MI increase, results from MI and ML converge to a common estimand for the 2-point estimates. Although ML is somewhat more efficient (smaller standard errors) Wang and Robins (1998), MI is more flexible, the distinct steps for imputation and analysis in MI yields flexibility that, as explained in subsequent sections, can be exploited in a number of situations. A down side to MI is that if interest exists in a number of parameters, the three-step process must be applied for each parameter. Alternatively, multiple parameters can be handled simultaneously using a multiparameter version of the combination rules in step 3, with the additional burden of estimating the variance covariance matrix associated with estimated parameters.

15.2 Technical Details

Point estimates in MI are computed as a simple average of the estimates from the m completed data sets. The precision of these estimates is evaluated using simple formulas that incorporate both between-imputation and within-imputation variability in the calculation of standard errors. In the following, we provide technical details assuming, for simplicity, the test statistics (and associated estimates) are univariate; however, the formulas readily generalize for multivariate statistics.

Let $\hat{\theta}_i$, $i = 1,\ldots,m$ be univariate estimates (e.g., treatment contrasts at the last scheduled visit) obtained by applying an appropriate analysis model to the m completed data set and U_i, $i = 1,\ldots,m$ are their estimated (squared) standard errors. The MI point estimate is

$$\hat{\theta}_{MI} = \frac{\Sigma_{i=1}^{m}\hat{\theta}_i}{m}$$

The total variance is computed by combining the between-imputation variability, $B = (m-1)^{-1}\,\Sigma_{i=1}^{m}(\hat{\theta}_i - \hat{\theta}_{MI})^2$, and the within-imputation variability, $W = m^{-1}\Sigma_{i=1}^{m}U_i$

$$V = W + \left(1 + \frac{1}{m}\right)B$$

Inference on θ is based on the test statistic $T = \frac{\hat{\theta}_{MI}}{\sqrt{V}}$. As with ML, the $\hat{\theta}_{MI}$ estimator is unbiased if missing data arise from an MCAR or MAR mechanism.

The null distribution of T is not normal. Therefore, standard Wald-based inference assuming T has the standard normal null distribution is not valid. This is because for finite $m < \infty$ the total variance V is an inconsistent estimate of the true variance of the point estimator, $var(\hat{\theta}_{MI})$. That is, when the sample size N increases to infinity, NV does not converge to a constant but remains a random variable following a nondegenerate (chi-squared) distribution. This is in contrast to, for example, the variance of a sample mean: $N\left[\widehat{\text{var}}(\bar{x})\right] = \frac{N}{N}\hat{\sigma}^2 \xrightarrow{p} \sigma^2 = const.$

To account for this extra variability, Rubin (1987) proposed using a student's t distribution instead of a normal distribution, with the number of degrees of freedom computed as

$$v = (m-1)\left(1 + \frac{1}{1+m^{-1}}\frac{W}{B}\right)^2$$

The price paid for the generality of the MI estimator is a degree of conservatism (sometimes negligible). This overestimation of variability has three sources (Wang and Robins 1998 and Robins and Wang 2000):

- The asymptotic variance of the MI point estimator (for finite m) exceeds that of the ML estimator
- The standard error of the MI point estimator obtained by Rubin's rules may exceed its true value, the square root of the asymptotic variance (i.e., overestimation of the standard error)
- Inconsistency of Rubin's variance estimator requiring use of the wider confidence intervals based on the t distribution rather than the normal distribution.

The MI procedure outlined above is essentially an extension of the single imputation model using a conditional normal distribution that was introduced in Section 13.5. There are two important differences, however. First, each missing value is imputed *multiple* times, which allows for explicit accounting for uncertainty due to the imputation/missing data. This is accomplished by incorporating the between-imputation variability.

The second difference is more subtle. In MI, imputations are simulated from the Bayesian predictive distribution of missing data given observed data $f(y_{mis}|y_{obs})$ rather than from the density $f(y_{mis} \mid y_{obs}, \hat{\theta})$ with parameters θ estimated at specific values (e.g., by maximum likelihood), as shown in Section 13.5. The predictive distribution is obtained by integrating (averaging) out parameters from the likelihood using the posterior distribution of parameters.

$$f(y_{mis} \mid y_{obs}) = \int f(y_{mis} \mid y_{obs}, \theta) f(\theta \mid y_{obs}) d\theta$$

Therefore, imputed values are sampled from distributions that incorporate uncertainty in estimating model parameters and uncertainty due to sampling data from the estimated model.

As a simple example, when estimating the mean and variance of a univariate normal distribution $N(\theta, \sigma^2)$, MI accounts for uncertainty in the estimated θ and σ^2 as well as uncertainty of sampling missing values from $Y_{mis} \sim N(\hat{\theta}, \hat{\sigma}^2)$.

It is instructive to think of imputing (sampling) from a predictive distribution as a two-stage procedure that is repeated m times. Repeat the following two steps m times for $i = 1,\ldots,m$:

1. Draw a single random sample from the posterior distribution of parameters given observed data $\tilde{\theta}_i \sim f(\theta \mid y_{obs})$.
2. Draw random samples from the observed-data likelihood model $Y_{mis} \sim f(y \mid \tilde{\theta}_i)$ to produce a single completed data set.

The single imputation scheme considered in Section 13.5 essentially implements only the second step for $m = 1$ with $\tilde{\theta}_1$ set to the ML estimate $\tilde{\theta}_1 = \hat{\theta}_{ML}$.

It is useful to consider the consequences of creating m completed data sets using only the second step (i.e., without re-sampling from the posterior of θ). In this approach, point estimates would still be valid, essentially reproducing the ML estimates. However, the total variance V computed using Rubin's rules would be too small because the between-imputation variability would not include the uncertainty due to parameter estimation. As a result, the confidence intervals based on V would be too narrow, failing to maintain the nominal Type I error rates. Such imputation models have been termed *improper* (Rubin 1987).

With complex models, analytic formula for the posterior distribution $f(\theta \mid y_{obs})$ often do not exist and Markov Chain Monte Carlo (MCMC) methods can be used (Tanner and Wong 1987; Schafer 1997).

The MCMC algorithms are widely used in Bayesian inference to sample from joint posterior distributions of parameters when analytical expressions are not available. Sampling from the predictive distribution of missing data can be incorporated within this general approach through data augmentation algorithms. In the Bayesian framework there is no fundamental difference between missing data and parameters; both are unobserved quantities and are dealt with similarly. Although application of MCMC appears different from the two-stage sampling outlined above, they implement sampling from the same target distribution: $f(y_{mis} \mid y_{obs})$.

For example, the Gibbs method alternates between sampling from full conditionals $\tilde{y}_{mis}^{(k+1)} \sim f\left(y_{mis} \mid \tilde{\theta}^{(k)}, y_{obs}\right)$ and $\tilde{\theta}^{(k+1)} \sim f\left(\theta \mid \tilde{y}_{mis}^{(k+1)}, y_{obs}\right)$ through a large number of iterations $k = 0,\ldots,K$, starting with some initial values for parameters $\tilde{\theta}^{(0)}$. As a result, after some initial (burn-in) draws, the samples of $\tilde{y}_{mis}^{(k+1)}$ and $\tilde{\theta}^{(k+1)}$ will be drawn approximately from the unconditional target distributions of $f(y_{mis} \mid y_{obs})$ and $f(\theta \mid y_{obs})$, respectively.

In the context of repeated measures analysis with a multivariate normal model, when the pattern of missingness is arbitrary, generic MCMC sampling must be used for imputation. When the pattern is monotone, sampling can be based on factorization of the joint normal distribution into a sequence of conditionals and using analytical formulas for the posterior distribution of parameters associated with each factor.

For the small example data set with dropout, the factorization of the likelihood is

$$f(y|x,\theta) = f(y_1|x,\theta_1)\, f(y_2|x,y_1,\theta_2)\, f(y_3|x,y_1,y_2,\theta_3)$$

Then, imputation can be organized sequentially

- Draw $\tilde{\theta}_1 \sim f(\theta_1 \mid x, y_1)$ and impute missing values for $Y_1, Y_{mis} \sim f(y_1 \mid x, \tilde{\theta}_1)$ (in the example data set no y_1 are missing and this step is not needed)
- Draw $\tilde{\theta}_2 \sim f(\theta_2 \mid x, y_1, y_2)$ and impute missing Y_2 based on observed and imputed Y_1 with $Y_{mis} \sim f(y_2 \mid x, \tilde{y}_1, \tilde{\theta}_2)$, where $\tilde{y}_1$ indicates that the value can be observed or imputed
- Draw $\tilde{\theta}_3 \sim f(\theta_3 \mid x, y_1, y_2, y_3)$ and impute missing Y_3 based on observed and imputed Y_1 and $Y_2, Y_{mis} \sim f(y_3 \mid x, \tilde{y}_1, \tilde{y}_2, \tilde{\theta}_3)$

Therefore, imputation of missing values is done via estimated Bayesian regression models where parameters are drawn from posterior distributions. In this case of normal linear regression, missing values for y_2 (Time 2) are imputed by sampling values from the regression model $Y_{mis} = \tilde{\beta}_0 + \tilde{\beta}_1 X + \tilde{\beta}_2 \tilde{Y}_1 + e\tilde{\sigma}$, where X is the baseline score, $\tilde{Y}_1$ is observed or imputed value of the change from baseline at Time 1 and $\tilde{\beta}_0, \tilde{\beta}_1, \tilde{\beta}_2, \tilde{\sigma}^2$ are drawn from their respective posterior distributions. Random error e is sampled from the standard normal distribution, $e \sim N(0,1)$. Here we omit details on specification of prior distributions for the parameters of the imputation model and corresponding posterior distributions, which for this case of normally distributed data are fairly straightforward and can be found, for example, in Schafer (1997) or SAS technical documentation for PROC MI.

As an illustration, Figure 15.1 depicts the observed data and the means from 100 imputations using the above sequential Bayesian regression for Subjects 1, 30, and 49 from the small example data set with dropout. The SAS and R code for this analysis is listed in Section 15.8 (Code Fragment 15.1). Results for treatment groups are discussed later. The focus here is on the individual subjects. Thin solid lines depict the observed data and dotted lines depict means of the imputed values for the focus subjects. Thick solid lines depict the treatment group means. The error bars indicate standard deviation of imputed values.

The trajectory for means of the imputed values resembles the conditional means based on a direct likelihood analysis as depicted Figure 13.4 and Table 14.2. Subjects with observed changes that were less than the average of their group have mean imputed values that are less than the corresponding group mean; subjects with observed changes that were greater than the group average have mean imputed values that are greater than the corresponding group mean. Also, similar to the direct-likelihood analysis, the

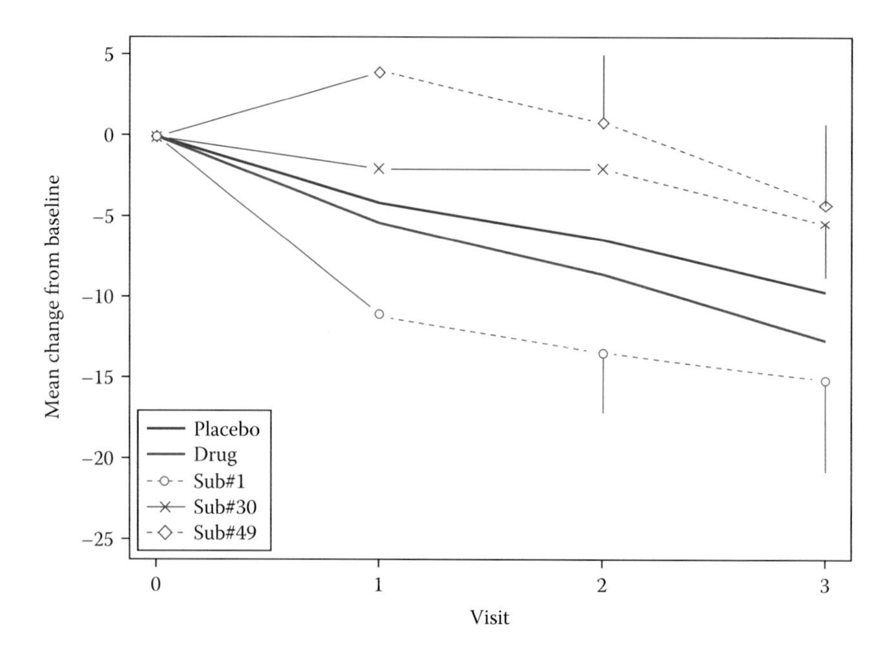

FIGURE 15.1
Illustration of multiply imputed values for Subjects #1, #30, and #49 from the small example data set with dropout. The error bars represent the between imputation variability (standard deviation based on the 100 imputed values at each time point).

standard deviation bars indicate greater variability in imputed values at Time 3 for Subjects 1 and 49, who had only one observed value (at Time 1) compared with Subject 30 who had two observed values.

The concordance between direct-likelihood and MI results is not coincidental; these similarities are expected in all circumstances when the methods are implemented using similar models. Multiple imputation can also be compared with direct Bayesian inference. Rubin (1987) showed that MI is compatible with Bayesian analysis in the sense that the MI point estimate and variance are approximating the posterior expectation and posterior variance of a Bayesian analysis.

In that regard, MI is somewhat circular. First, the Bayesian posterior distribution of parameters is sampled. Next, the distribution of missing values is simulated, and in the end the posterior sample of parameters is discarded. Hence, the posterior distribution of parameters serves merely as an intermediate step in imputation. Alternatively, sampling from posterior distribution could continue and be used for purely Bayesian inference about parameters based on the output from posterior distribution of θ's (and any of their functions).

As noted earlier in this section, when implemented with similar models, MI and ML yield asymptotically similar point estimates, but MI has greater variance and is therefore less efficient, meaning that ML would be somewhat more powerful. However, MI has other advantages, such as when some covariate values are missing. In likelihood-based analyses, if a covariate is missing for a subject, all post-baseline data for that subject are discarded. In MI the missing covariates can be imputed, thereby preserving inclusion of the post-baseline data. An example of imputing missing covariates is provided in Section 15.5.

Other advantages of MI stem from having separate steps for imputation and analysis. This flexibility does not exist in ML because ML has only the analysis step, thereby implying that only the analysis variables can be used to account for the missing data.

In MI, the imputation model can include additional covariates not present in the analysis model. These covariates may be predictive of outcomes and/or the probability of dropout. Meng (1994) and Collins et al. (2001) provide examples of and rationale for these so-called inclusive modeling strategies. An example of inclusive modeling is provided in Section 15.6 and additional details of inclusive modeling were discussed in Section 12.3.4.

The consequences of an analysis model that is richer (has more variables) than the imputation model is very different. Consider an imputation model that does not include treatment. The imputation model in essence assumes no *direct* treatment effect and is capable of capturing *indirect* treatment effect that may be mediated via intermediate outcomes (if included in the model). As a result, imputed outcomes across treatment arms are likely to be more similar than should be the case. Analyses based on such imputed data sets therefore would be biased whenever a direct treatment effect existed (additionally to the effect mediated via intermediate outcomes).

Although the model in the example above is misspecified—in the context of MAR—it can also be thought of as a specific form of MNAR. In the above example, the imputed values systematically deviate from unbiased MAR estimates in a manner that decreases the magnitude of the estimated treatment contrast. This points to what is becoming an important usage of MI—as a convenient tool for conducting sensitivity analyses. The imputation models can be set up to generate specific departures from MAR, thereby fostering a sensitivity analysis for an MAR-based primary analysis. These implementations of MI are considered in Chapter 18 and further illustrated in Chapter 21.

15.3 Example—Implementing MI

15.3.1 Introduction

This section provides details on implementing several multiple imputation strategies using readily available statistical software applied to data from the small example data set with dropout. Focus is on relevant SAS procedures because they are commonly used in practice; however, some examples using R are also provided.

In SAS, multiple imputation can be implemented via the following steps:

1. Use PROC MI to generate m completed data sets.
2. Analyze each data set, resulting in m point estimates and standard errors.
3. Pass the point estimates and standard errors from Step 2 to PROC MIANALYZE that implements Rubin's rules for combining results.

The output from PROC MIANALYZE includes the upper and lower limits of the confidence interval and associated p-value for the two-sided null hypothesis that the parameter is at the specified value (e.g., $\theta = 0$). The parameter of interest for MI inference can be multivariate, although scalar parameters of treatment effects at specific time points will be considered in the examples here.

The procedure outlined above is easy to implement and is a common approach in conducting multiple imputation analysis in SAS. However, variations on the approach are possible and sometimes needed. For example, the first step can be divided into two steps: (1) sampling from posterior distributions of parameters estimated by an appropriate likelihood-based model using a SAS procedure (different from PROC MI); (2) given each posterior draw, impute missing values from the posed imputation model with custom programming code. An example could be imputing missing counts (such as in the analysis of recurrent events) from a Bayesian Poisson regression, which can be fitted separately using SAS PROC GENMOD with the BAYES statement. In some situations (in particular, when modeling growth curves in repeated measures data) multiple draws from posterior predictive distributions can be conveniently obtained via SAS PROC MCMC (available from SAS Version 9.3). Performing MI using the above procedures is not covered as we focus here on imputation from general multivariate distributions via PROC MI.

In some cases (particularly, for nonparametric and semiparametric models) sampling from posterior distributions can be replaced with nonparametric bootstrap. For example, data can be sampled with replacement, resulting in m bootstrap samples from the original data. Posterior draws $\tilde{\theta}_1, \tilde{\theta}_2, \ldots, \tilde{\theta}_m$ are mimicked with parameter estimates from bootstrap samples $\hat{\theta}_1^*, \ldots, \hat{\theta}_m^*$. The imputed values are then generated from conditional distributions, $Y_{mis} \sim f\left(y \mid \hat{\theta}_i^*\right), i = 1, \ldots, m$.

As an example, consider imputing time to event for a subject censored at time t_{cens}. Imputations can be based on Kaplan-Meier estimates of a survival distribution computed for m bootstrap samples: $\tilde{T} \sim \hat{S}_i^*\left(t \mid t > t_{cens}\right), i = 1, \ldots, m$.

Bootstrap is also often used in conjunction with hot-deck procedures. As stated in Chapter 13, single hot-deck imputation is generally not valid because it fails to fully account for uncertainty due to missing data. However, using approximate Bayesian bootstrap (such as in "Monotone Propensity Score Method" implemented in SAS PROC MI) allows constructing more valid hot-deck procedures. First observed values are sampled with replacement (stratified by the propensity of missingness) to generate sets of "donors". Then missing values are replaced by resampling from "donors" within propensity score groups that have similar probability of missingness. In this case, the bootstrap is used to mimic sampling from predictive posterior distribution of missing data.

Using bootstrap to mimic posterior sampling of parameters—or the predictive distribution of missing data—was termed "approximate Bayesian bootstrap" in Little and Rubin (1987, section 14.5). This should not be confused with standard uses of bootstrap as a method for obtaining standard errors and confidence intervals (e.g., via percentile or ABC methods). For example, 95% confidence interval for the treatment contrast θ can be constructed in the familiar manner of using the 2.5% and 97.5% percentiles of the bootstrap distribution of the MI point estimator $\hat{\theta}_{MI}$ as the confidence interval bounds.

Bootstrap confidence intervals are more computationally intensive than the usual confidence intervals based on Rubin's rules, but can be useful when the latter have questionable validity. When using the bootstrap for confidence intervals, multiple imputation should be carried out on each bootstrap sample and the MI point estimate computed from the m completed data sets. Efron (1994) presented different methods of using bootstrap with missing data and in conjunction with multiple imputation. However, the following details focus only on the traditional three-step process for MI that does not include bootstrapping.

Example SAS code to implement MI for the small example data set with dropout is provided in Code Fragment 15.1 (Section 15.8). The most commonly used R package for MI is *mice*. Example R code to implement MI is provided in Code Fragment 15.2.

15.3.2 Imputation

To use PROC MI, the data should be prepared in the so-called "multivariate" (or "wide" or "horizontal") format with data from each time point in a separate column. Longitudinal data are typically stored as a "stacked" (or "long") data set, which is the format anticipated by SAS PROC MIXED. Converting data from the stacked format to the wide format can be accomplished by using SAS PROC TRANSPOSE. The transposed data set is passed to PROC MI and missing data are imputed using a multivariate normal model with treatment fitted as a covariate or imputations done separately by treatment.

The example data have a monotone missingness pattern. Therefore, a Bayesian regression for multivariate normally distributed data can be used, thus avoiding the MCMC methods that are needed for imputing data with arbitrary missingness patterns. Checking whether the pattern is monotone can be conveniently done by running PROC MI with parameter NIMPUTE = 0. Table 15.1 shows the missing data patterns by treatment group that are produced as default output from PROC MI. The output makes it easy to see that the response patterns in the example data are indeed monotone. If a subject has a missing value at a given visit, all subsequent observations are also missing.

TABLE 15.1

Missing Data Patterns for the Small Example Data Set with Dropout

		Variables[a]					
Treatment	Group	Basval	Yobs1	Yobs2	Yobs3	Freq	Percent
	1	X	X	X	X	18	72.0
1	2	X	X	X	.	2	8.0
1	3	X	X	.	.	5	20.0
2	1	X	X	X	X	19	76.0
2	2	X	X	X	.	3	12.0
2	3	X	X	.	.	3	12.0

[a] "X" indicates presence of the outcome score at baseline (Basval) and three post-baseline visits (Yobs1, Yobs2, Yobs3). "." indicates the value is missing. "Groups" identifies the distinct patterns present in the data set.

The order of variables listed in the VAR statement of PROC MI should correspond to the order of imputations. For the example data, the order of variables corresponds to the assessment times. Alternatively, the sequential orientation can be made explicit using multiple statements. The code for this explicit specification is also provided in Code Fragment 15.1. The explicit specification is not needed for this example, but provides flexibility that can be utilized in other situations that will be illustrated in subsequent examples.

In this example, data are imputed by treatment arm. This is equivalent to having a single imputation model that includes treatment, treatment-by-visit and all treatment-by-covariate interactions. However, having separate imputation models by treatment arm is simple and yields the same result as the more parameter-rich single, saturated imputation model (with the minor difference that separate covariance structures would be fitted when using by-treatment processing, whereas a single pooled error covariance matrix will be used in case of a single imputation model).

The number of imputations (specified by the parameter NIMPUTE) chosen for this example is 1000. In the early MI literature it was recommended that as few as $m = 5$ imputations was sufficient to achieve good precision of MI estimates. This recommendation was based on the argument of relative efficiency of MI estimates compared to that based on maximum likelihood estimates. However, this recommendation was later challenged. The decrease in power due to small m may substantially exceed that expected from the theoretical argument based on relative efficiency (Graham et al. 2007). With modern computing power, generating hundreds and even thousands of imputations can be done in reasonable time. The case for using a small number of imputations is obsolete. For a summary of recent literature on choosing the number of imputations see van Buuren (2012, pp. 49–50).

As a practical tool for selecting a reasonable number of imputations, the MI point estimates can be plotted against the number of imputations, as done in Figure 15.2 for the small example data set with dropout. This plot allows visual

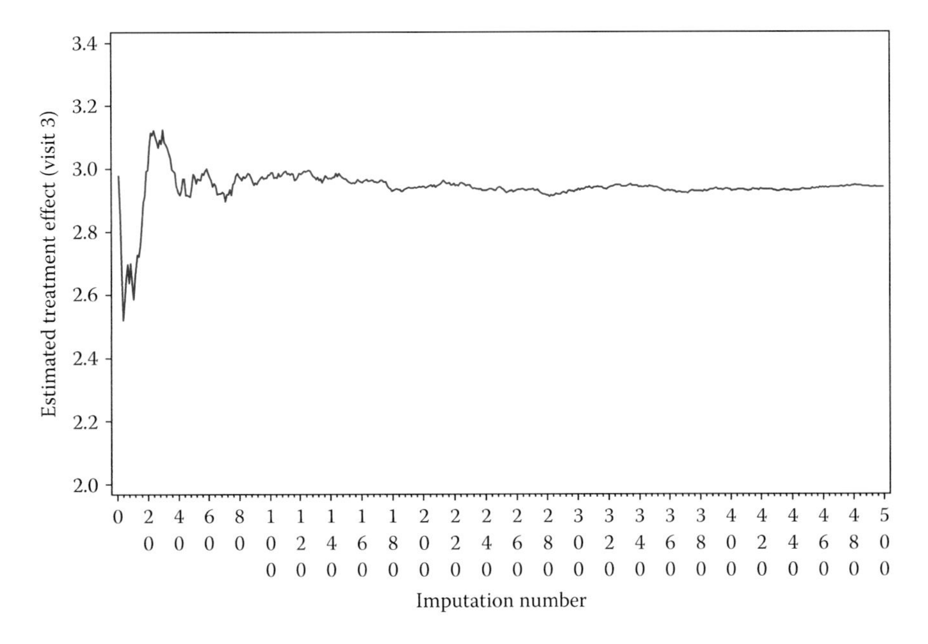

FIGURE 15.2
MI estimator $\hat{\theta}_m$ for the treatment contrast at visit 3 computed over the first m completed data sets versus the number of imputations (m).

assessment of the stability of MI estimator $\hat{\theta}_m$ for smaller m and its "convergence" to $\hat{\theta}_\infty$. In Figure 15.2 after $m_0 = 200$, the point estimator is stable, which ensures the *reproducibility* of MI analyses for this data set with $m \geq m_0$. The sufficient number of imputations will of course vary from one data set to another. In all examples for this Chapter, $m = 1000$, although this may be larger than needed.

In PROC MI, the output data set has the same "multivariate" structure as the input data set. However, the now completed multiple data sets are *stacked* and the variable named _Imputation_ (assuming values 1,..., <*nimpute*>) is automatically generated to indicate to which data set each observation belongs. Figure 15.3 shows a fragment of the imputed (completed) data set. Imputed values can be clearly discerned in this example as they have a larger number of decimal points. Sometimes auxiliary variables (with values 0 and 1) that indicate whether values were actually observed or imputed may be needed. This should be done by writing custom SAS code prior to calling PROC MI.

15.3.3 Analysis

After completing the imputation step, an appropriate analysis model can be applied to each completed set. For longitudinal data, as in the example data set, it is natural to consider applying the same direct likelihood analysis of repeated measures via PROC MIXED to each completed data set as

	Imputation	trt	subject	basval	Yobs1	Yobs2	Yobs3
1	1	1	2	20	−6	−5.371893093	−10.27327664
2	1	1	5	12	−6	−3	−9
3	1	1	6	14	−6	−10	−10
4	1	1	8	21	−2	−9	−9
5	1	1	9	19	−9	−6	−12.78127318
6	1	1	13	20	−9	−12	−13
7	1	1	14	19	−6	−12	−16
8	1	1	16	19	−3	−11	−17
9	1	1	18	23	−7	−10	−15
10	1	1	19	26	−5	−5	−11
11	1	1	24	20	1	−1	−6
12	1	1	25	22	0	−4	−9
13	1	1	27	21	−1	−2	−3
14	1	1	28	21	−2	−2	−2
15	1	1	30	19	−2	−2	−6.425250822
16	1	1	32	24	−10	−14	−20
17	1	1	34	21	−2	−1	−6
18	1	1	36	20	−4	−7.120718604	−14.13814589
19	1	1	38	22	−3	−5	−6
20	1	1	40	18	−5	−6.057750783	−2.045101917
21	1	1	42	15	0	−2	−8
22	1	1	43	19	−3	−6.167970307	−10.26103763
23	1	1	45	20	−9	−11	−9
24	1	1	48	17	−10	−14	−14
25	1	1	49	23	4	4.4830432444	2.5435936604
26	2	1	2	20	−6	−11.29465031	−11.65938348
27	2	1	5	12	−6	−3	−9
28	2	1	6	14	−6	−10	−10
29	2	1	8	21	−2	−9	−9
30	2	1	9	19	−9	−6	−16.37321523
31	2	1	13	20	−9	−12	−13
32	2	1	14	19	−6	−12	−16

FIGURE 15.3
Fragment of complete data set produced by PROC MI.

for the analysis of incomplete data. While this analysis approach is useful for assessing the longitudinal response profiles, it is also now possible to implement a simple visit-wise ANOVA or ANCOVA if interest is only on the cross-sectional contrasts. This is possible because imputation fully accounts for the missing data (if assumptions hold true) and there is no benefit from further accounting for the missing data via a repeated measures analysis.

When applying the analysis model to imputed data it is useful to take advantage of SAS "BY-processing" capability using the "by _Imputation_"

	Imputation	Label	Estimate	StdErr	DF	tValue	Probt	time
267	67	trt effect at vis 3	−1.7813	1.4729	47	−1.21	0.2325	3
268	68	trt effect at vis 3	−3.4297	1.4091	47	−2.43	0.0188	3
269	69	trt effect at vis 3	−3.1104	1.5551	47	−2.00	0.0513	3
270	70	trt effect at vis 3	−2.3183	1.5762	47	−1.47	0.1480	3
271	71	trt effect at vis 3	−2.5356	1.4717	47	−1.72	0.0915	3
272	72	trt effect at vis 3	−4.4898	1.6927	47	−2.65	0.0109	3
273	73	trt effect at vis 3	−2.9977	1.4591	47	−2.05	0.0455	3
274	74	trt effect at vis 3	−3.4374	1.5221	47	−2.26	0.0286	3
275	75	trt effect at vis 3	−1.8695	1.7225	47	−1.09	0.2833	3
276	76	trt effect at vis 3	−3.6741	1.5684	47	−2.34	0.0234	3
277	77	trt effect at vis 3	−3.5779	1.4950	47	−2.39	0.0207	3
278	78	trt effect at vis 3	−3.8548	1.5870	47	−2.43	0.0190	3
279	79	trt effect at vis 3	−3.5465	1.4240	47	−2.49	0.0163	3
280	80	trt effect at vis 3	−4.0039	1.7441	47	−2.30	0.0262	3
281	81	trt effect at vis 3	−4.0162	1.4955	47	−2.69	0.0100	3
282	82	trt effect at vis 3	−4.0411	1.3845	47	−2.92	0.0054	3
283	83	trt effect at vis 3	−3.5701	1.4470	47	−2.47	0.0173	3
284	84	trt effect at vis 3	−2.3854	1.3850	47	−1.72	0.0916	3

FIGURE 15.4
Fragment of results from the analyses of multiply imputed data sets to be used as input for PROC MIANALYZE.

statement in the analysis procedure. If a repeated measures analysis of the imputed data is desired, an additional data manipulation step is needed to transpose the PROC MI output data set back to the "stacked" format required with repeated measures data in PROC MIXED. In this example, the simple ANCOVA model is implemented to analyze the Time 3 variable (Yobs3 in the imputed data set). The point estimates and standard errors from the analyses of some of the imputed data sets are shown in Figure 15.4.

15.3.4 Inference

The last step in MI is to combine estimates and standard errors to obtain a single inferential statement. Code Fragment 15.3 shows the SAS code for PROC MIANALYZE to accomplish this step. The "by time" statement is used here because the input data set contains treatment contrasts for Time 2 and Time 3. Note that Time 1 did not have missing values; therefore, all estimates for the treatment contrast at Time 1 obtained from the multiply imputed data set are identical and, of course, it does not make sense to run PROC MIANALYZE for Time 1. The results are shown in Table 15.2.

The lsmeans, treatment contrasts, and standard errors from the MI analysis of the incomplete data are, as expected, similar to the corresponding results from direct likelihood (see Table 14.1). Compared with the complete data, the

TABLE 15.2

Treatment Contrasts and Least-Squares Means Estimated by Multiple Imputation from the Small Example Data Set with Dropout

		Complete Data		Incomplete Data (MI), $m = 1000$	
Treatment	**Time**	**LSMEANS**	**SE**	**LSMEANS**	**SE**
1	2	−6.70	0.93	− 6.36	1.01
1	3	−9.86	1.05	− 9.61	1.19
2	2	−8.70	0.93	− 8.50	0.99
2	3	−13.26	1.05	− 12.56	1.23
Endpoint Treatment Difference		3.39	1.49 (p = 0.0274)	2.95	1.73 (p = 0.0971)

MI results show a smaller treatment contrast, larger standard errors, and a larger *P*-value for the endpoint treatment contrast. It is important to interpret these results as just one realization from a stochastic process. If the comparisons were replicated many times under the same conditions—with missing data arising from an MAR mechanism—the average of the lsmeans and treatment contrasts across the repeated trials would be (approximately) the same for complete and incomplete data. Standard errors would be consistently greater in incomplete data, however.

15.3.5 Accounting for Nonmonotone Missingness

Thus far, only monotone missingness has been addressed. When the pattern of missing data is nonmonotone, PROC MI with the addition of the MCMC statement can be used. To illustrate these procedures, intermittent missingness was introduced into the example data by deleting some outcomes at Time 2 for subjects that had no other missing data. The Time 2 data were deleted for three subjects in the treated group (2) and for two subjects in the placebo group (1).

The top panel (a) of Code Fragment 15.4 (Section 15.8) provides an example of PROC MI code for imputation from a multivariate normal distribution using MCMC. Missing values are imputed from a single chain of the MCMC algorithm. Recall that MCMC samples converge to the target posterior distribution as the number of samples becomes large. Therefore, to ensure that the draws occur sufficiently close to the target distribution, a number of initial samples are skipped. This skipping is specified in the number of burn-in iterations (NBITER = 200). Also because of serial correlation in sampled values within the same chain, a thinning period should be specified as the number of iterations between imputations in a chain. In the example, (NITER = 100) and PROC MI skips 100 samples after each imputation. The values NBITER = 200 and NITER = 100 are defaults that would be used if these options are omitted but are explicitly specified here for illustration.

The various MCMC diagnostics (e.g., autocorrelation plots) should be inspected. Imputations should be rerun with increased values of NBITER and

NITER if issues exist with MCMC convergence (see PROC MI help for more details). The example code explicitly specified that the initial values for the MCMC chain are posterior modes of parameters obtained by the EM (expectation-maximization) algorithm, with the maximum number of iterations set at MAXITER = 200. This number should be increased if the EM algorithm fails to converge within the specified limit. Nonconvergence is more likely in data sets with larger fractions of missing data or if there are sparse patterns of missing values. The SAS log file includes a warning if convergence was not achieved.

The MCMC approach may be rather cumbersome. It (typically) requires more computing time compared with regression methods. The additional layer of approximation inherent in MCMC requires monitoring for convergence to the desired target distributions. In contrast, the regression methods for monotone data sample *directly* from the target distributions and so there is no worry about convergence.

Often, only a few intermittently missing values cause the patterns to deviate from monotone as a result of a few patients with missed outcomes while remaining in the study. In these situations it is efficient to first impute the intermittent missing values using PROC MI to complete the pattern to monotone; then, methods for monotone missingness can be applied, such as the Bayesian regression from the previous example.

The SAS code for implementing this two-stage imputation strategy is presented in the bottom panel (b) of Code Fragment 15.4 (Section 15.8). Two runs of PROC MI are required. The first run produces partially completed data sets, each having a monotone pattern of missing values. The second run takes the output data set from the first run as input, processed by _Imputation_, and completes each data set with a single imputation from Bayesian regression for monotone data.

15.4 Situations Where MI Is Particularly Useful

15.4.1 Introduction

This section outlines situations when MI-based analyses provide certain advantages compared to direct likelihood (ML) or present a reasonable analytic strategy in absence of appropriate direct likelihood methods. Detailed examples are provided in subsequent sections.

15.4.2 Scenarios Where Direct Likelihood Methods Are Difficult to Implement or Not Available

One general area where MI can be particularly useful is situations where direct likelihood methods are hard to implement or not available. Several scenarios when this may be the case for analysis of clinical data are outlined below.

Missing baseline covariates make direct likelihood methods (e.g., via SAS PROC MIXED) sub-optimal because all subjects with a missing covariate are discarded from the analysis. In contrast, MI can be used to impute baseline covariates jointly with outcome variables (see Section 15.5 for examples).

Repeated categorical outcomes are hard to analyze using direct likelihood methods because—in contrast to multivariate normal distributions for repeated continuous outcomes—multivariate distributions for binary or count data do not have simple and natural formulations. Details on analyses of incomplete categorical data are provided in Chapter 19. Imputing missing categorical data is relatively easy, especially for data with monotone missingness when sequential imputation strategies can be applied.

For outcomes of mixed types (continuous and categorical), MI can be implemented either by sequential imputation (for monotone patterns of missing data) or in the case of arbitrary missingness by repeatedly sampling from full conditional distributions (van Buuren 2007). The method of "fully conditional specification" (FCS) is implemented in the R package *mice* (Multivariate Imputation by Chained Equations; van Buuren and Groothuis-Oudshoorn 2011) and recently in SAS PROC MI (via FCS statement available from SAS Version 9.3 and later).

Unlike joint modeling, FCS specifies the multivariate distributions through a sequence of conditional densities of each variable given the other variables. With FCS it is even possible to specify models for which no joint distribution exits — a situation referred to as incompatibility. Although incompatibility is not desirable, in practice it is a relatively minor problem, especially if the missing data rate is modest (van Buuren 2012, p. 112).

15.4.3 Exploiting Separate Steps for Imputation and Analysis

Other situations where MI is particularly useful are those in which the separation of the imputation and analysis stages can improve efficiency (compared to direct likelihood methods).

Recall that the original motivation for MI in Rubin (1978) was for analysis of complex surveys where the *imputer* had access to more information than the *analyst*. The idea was that once the missing data has been imputed using the richer set of data, completed data sets with a limited number of variables would be made publicly available for analysts. Several clinical trial situations are considered where the imputation model can be based on more information than is included in the analysis model.

Sometimes clinical endpoints specified in the primary analysis are *derived* outcomes based on underlying outcomes. In such situations, an efficient MI strategy could include four steps:

1. Impute missing data for the underlying outcome measures.
2. Compute derived outcomes from the completed data sets.
3. Analyze completed data.
4. Combine (pool) results for inference.

An example of a derived variable is the analysis of "clinical response," defined as x% improvement in some continuous scale (or a combination of several scales). Imputing the underlying continuous measures may improve efficiency compared to analysis (or imputation and analysis) of the binary outcome.

As noted in Section 15.3.4, MI can utilize auxiliary variables in the imputation model that help predict the outcome and/or the dropout process. These auxiliary variables may not be available or are undesirable for use in analysis model (Meng 1994; Collins et al. 2001). For example, the analysis model should not include intermediate outcomes or *mediators* of treatment effect, which would result in diluting the estimated treatment effect in a likelihood-based analysis. Classic examples of such variables would be time-varying post-baseline variables that are influenced by treatment, such as secondary efficacy outcomes.

The following situations are examples of inclusive imputation strategies that can be useful.

- Pretreatment covariates (demographic and illness characteristics), and perhaps their interactions with treatment, are included in the imputation model. The selection of covariates can be based on their ability in predicting the outcome or in predicting dropout. This can be evaluated in separate modeling steps and a subset of covariates can be selected from a broader set of candidate covariates using appropriate model selection techniques such as stepwise selection, LASSO, or other machine learning methods.
- Post-baseline time-varying covariates. Inclusive imputation models can be used to *jointly* impute two related outcomes, such as two efficacy scales, Y1 and Y2. This may be two clinical rating scales that reflect different aspects of the disease and "borrowing" from Y2 may improve imputation of Y1. An example is given in Section 15.6, where joint imputations of the clinician-rated HAMD severity scale and a patient-reported outcome scale (Patient Global Impression of Improvement) are conducted. The basic idea is that incorporating both the clinician's and patient's perspective on response may help explain subsequent HAMD outcomes and/or better inform the missingness process.
- When the outcome of interest is collected at sparse visit intervals or only at the last scheduled evaluation whereas other outcomes are observed more frequently. Examples include efficacy and safety scales collected at scheduled time points and spontaneously recorded outcomes (occurrences of hospitalizations, adverse events).

An approach that at first may seem counterintuitive but can be useful is to use safety assessments to help impute efficacy outcomes. Suppose that dropouts are predicted by both previous outcomes and future (unobserved outcomes) so the missingness is MNAR. Then MI using only earlier outcomes is inadequate and may result in biased estimates. However, suppose that conditional on both recent safety assessments (occurrence of specific adverse events) and earlier efficacy outcomes the dropouts *do not* depend on future outcomes. This may be the case when AEs are early signs/predictors of emerging changes (sudden worsening, say) in the outcome that cannot be predicted from the efficacy outcome alone. In this scenario, adding safety assessments in the imputation model may help satisfy the MAR assumption.

15.4.4 Sensitivity Analysis

The flexibility of separate analysis and imputation steps can be used to create relevant departures from MAR, thereby facilitating a sensitivity analysis for an MAR primary analysis. Alternatively, the same imputation approaches can be conceptualized as modeling plausible outcomes after treatment discontinuation or switching treatment when assessing an effectiveness estimand. Such MNAR analyses can be implemented via MI by controlling the imputation procedures or done by manipulating imputed outcomes prior to data analysis. Extensive examples are provided in Chapters 18 and 19.

It is important to appreciate the point raised earlier in this chapter that when implemented in similar manners, MI and ML have similar assumptions and yield similar results. Therefore, MI implemented similarly to ML is not a sensitivity analysis. The point here is that something "different" is done during the imputation step that facilitates the sensitivity assessment.

15.5 Example—Using MI to Impute Covariates

15.5.1 Introduction

In the small example data set with missing values, there were no missing baseline values. In well-conducted clinical trials, missing data in baseline covariates are usually minimal. However, occasionally some subjects may have missing baseline values. In addition, analysis models may include stratification covariates or other covariates that could be missing. In such scenarios the chance that at least one covariate is missing for a given subject can be appreciable (say 5–10%). In these situations, typical likelihood-based analyses are not optimal because subjects with missing covariates are excluded from the analysis, resulting in loss of efficiency and potentially biased estimates.

15.5.2 Implementation

Multiple imputation provides several strategies for imputing missing covariates. An obvious route is to use a two-stage strategy similar to that demonstrated in Section 15.3 for data with nonmonotone missingness. First, MCMC-based imputation is used to impute missing covariates. Then the missing post-baseline values can be imputed to create the complete data sets. The SAS code for imputing covariates and missing post-baseline covariates in a scenario with baseline severity and three covariates (X1, X2, and X3) is presented in Code Fragment 15.5 (Section 15.8). The approach is similar to that in Code Fragment 15.4, thereby illustrating that only minor modification is required to impute missing covariates.

Another potential strategy may be to impute only missing baseline covariates using MCMC (PROC MI) and then applying a direct likelihood repeated measures analysis to multiple data sets with imputed baseline covariates and using Rubin's combination rules as we would normally do when imputing all missing values. Results from this MI approach can be compared with the analysis where all subjects with missing covariates were excluded in order to isolate the impact of missing baseline covariates on the estimated treatment effect and associated standard errors. Imputing missing covariates should improve efficiency and lead to smaller standard errors when compared to deleting records with missing covariates. Also, if baseline covariates are not missing completely at random, estimates of the treatment effect may be biased if subjects with missing covariates are excluded.

To illustrate the efficiency of multiply imputing covariates alone, artificial missingness in baseline severity was created in the small example data set with dropout by deleting the baseline scores of five subjects who had unfavorable outcomes in HAMD changes at the last scheduled visit. Lsmeans and treatment contrasts from a direct likelihood analysis (SAS PROC MIXED) of the 45 subjects with nonmissing baseline scores in the small example data set with dropout are compared to results from MI of the missing covariates in Table 15.3. The left-side columns are results from the direct likelihood analysis that excluded subjects with missing covariates. The right-side columns are results based on the same repeated measures model fitted to data sets with baseline scores imputed using all available outcome variables (via PROC MI, MCMC statement with IMPUTE=MONOTONE option). As mentioned, normally both baseline and post-baseline values would be imputed. However, the approach used here is valid under MAR and allows explicit assessment of the impact of having to exclude subjects with missing covariates in the likelihood-based analysis.

The results with MI of the missing covariates, as expected, had smaller standard errors. Excluding the five patients with missing baseline scores also resulted in approximately a one-half point increase in the endpoint treatment contrast. Of course, this is just one contrived example from a small example data set. It is not possible to know how including versus not including subjects with missing covariates will impact point estimates in actual clinical trial scenarios. However, regardless of scenario, including subjects with missing covariates increases the plausibility of MAR and reduces the standard

TABLE 15.3

Treatment Contrasts and Least-Squares Means with and without Imputation of Missing Covariates in the Small Example Data Set with Dropout

		Covariates Missing[a]		Covariates Imputed[b]	
Treatment	**Time**	**LSMEANS**	**SE**	**LSMEANS**	**SE**
1	1	−4.08	0.90	−4.21	0.94
1	2	−6.55	1.05	−6.56	1.00
1	3	−9.79	1.21	−9.78	1.12
2	1	−6.05	0.92	−5.25	0.94
2	2	−9.05	1.05	−8.45	0.98
2	3	−13.36	1.21	−12.79	1.09
Endpoint Treatment Difference		3.56	1.71 (p = 0.0443)	3.01	1.56 (p = 0.0606)

[a] Direct likelihood analysis with five subjects having missing covariates who are therefore excluded from the analysis.
[b] Direct likelihood analysis after multiple imputation of missing baseline covariates.

errors compared with excluding those subjects and allows following the ITT principle in terms of including all randomized subjects in the analysis.

This hypothetical example also helps to illustrate why imputation models for covariates should include post-baseline outcomes. Including post-baseline outcomes for imputing covariates may at first seem counterintuitive in that the model is predicting the past from the future. However, the approach can be justified theoretically and was also shown to be appropriate in simulation studies (Crowe et al. 2009).

The imputation model does not have to be a causal model. In fact, if the missingness mechanism is such that subjects with poorer outcomes are more likely to have missing baseline scores, failing to include future outcomes when imputing baseline covariates may result in biased estimates of the fixed effects associated with these covariates.

Whether this bias would translate into biased estimates of treatment contrasts is not a clear-cut issue. Treatment may seem independent of baseline covariates due to randomization, in which case bias in estimates of covariates would not bias treatment contrasts. However, an incorrect imputation model (provided it includes post-baseline measures) may induce correlation between the treatment variable and covariates. Treatment contrasts could be biased indirectly through the biased estimates of the fixed effects associated with covariates. See Section 5.3.1 for examples and illustration of how changes that directly affect one parameter also indirectly affect another parameter—that is, correlation between estimates of fixed effect parameters.

In general, the imputation model should be compatible with the analysis model. That is, if an effect is included in the analysis model it should also be used in the imputation model.

15.6 Examples—Using Inclusive Models in MI

15.6.1 Introduction

Section 12.3.4 introduced and contrasted inclusive and restrictive modeling frameworks. This section provides an example of an inclusive imputation strategy for the small example data set with dropouts. In this example, as elsewhere in this book, the primary outcome of interest is change in the HAMD scale. The difference here is that the Patient Global Impression of Improvement (PGIIMP) scale is used in addition to HAMD scores to "improve" the imputation of the missing HAMD scores.

Recall from the descriptions in Chapter 4 that the HAMD is a clinician-rated symptom severity score that focuses explicitly on specific symptoms and combines responses on the 17 individual items into a total score. The PGIIMP scale is a patient-rated measure of global improvement taken at each post-baseline visit. The PGIIMP assesses patient's overall feeling since they started taking medication and ranges from 1 ("very much better") to 7 ("very much worse"). The process used to delete data to create the small example data set with dropout was such that if a HAMD value was deleted, the corresponding PGIIMP value was also deleted.

The clinical and statistical justification for this inclusive strategy stems from the PGIIMP reflecting *patients'* overall perspective, which may capture aspects not fully captured by the *clinician*-rated HAMD scale.

15.6.2 Implementation

The first step in jointly imputing HAMD and PGIIMP using SAS PROC MI is to transpose data for both outcomes from the "stacked" to the "horizontal" format. That is, the output data set has three columns for changes in HAMD (CHG1, CHG2, CHG3) and three columns for PGIIMP1, PGIIMP2, PGIIMP3 that correspond to post-baseline Times 1, 2 and 3. Columns are also included for baseline severity on the HAMD and treatment group. There are no baseline assessments for PGIIMP because it is inherently a measure of change.

The next step is to check for monotonicity of missingness patterns on *both* outcomes. For this purpose, the following order of the outcome variables is assumed: CHG1 PGIIMP1 CHG2 PGIIMP2 CHG3 PGIIMP3. Table 15.4 displays the missing data patterns produced by SAS PROC MI that indicate the joint patterns are indeed monotone. One patient with a HAMD score at Time 3 had a missing Time 3 PGI–Improvement (Group 2, Treatment 2 in Table 15.4). The pattern is still monotone because PGIIMP3 goes after CHG3 in the ordering of variables. Imputation of values for PGIIMP3 is not needed because focus is on HAMD and PGIIMP3 does not inform imputation for CHG3. Hence, the PGIIMP3 column could be omitted with no impact on HAMD results.

TABLE 15.4

Missingness Patterns for Joint Imputation of Changes in HAMD and PGI–Improvement

				Missing Data Patterns					
Group	**Basval**	**CHG1**	**PGIIMP1**	**CHG2**	**PGIIMP2**	**CHG3**	**PGIIMP3**	**Frequency**	**Percent**
Treatment = 1 *(Placebo)*									
1	X	X	X	X	X	X	X	18	72.00
2	X	X	X	X	X			2	8.00
3	X	X	X	.	.	.	.	5	20.00
Treatment = 2 *(Treatment)*									
1	X	X	X	X	X	X	X	18	72.00
2	X	X	X	X	X	X	.	1	4.00
3	X	X	X	X	X	.	.	3	12.00
4	X	X	X	.	.	.	.	3	12.00

Note: "X" indicates presence of the outcome score at baseline (Basval). "." indicates the value is missing. "Groups" identifies the distinct patterns present in the data set.

Two imputation approaches can be considered. All outcomes can be treated as continuous and sequential Bayesian regression for multivariate normal data used to impute both HAMD changes and PGI–Improvement. In this approach, it is possible to impute missing values for PGIIMP that are outside the scales range of 1 to 7. Therefore, the validity of applying a normal distribution to categorical PGIIMP data may be questioned. Schafer (1997) showed that imputation is fairly robust to some deviations from multivariate normality. Also, Lipkovich et al. (2014) provide simulation evidence in favor of using a multivariate normal distribution for imputing categorical data.

The second approach avoids assuming multivariate normality for PGI–Improvement. The process is to sequentially implement: (1) linear regression to impute changes in HAMD conditional on earlier HAMD changes and on PGI–Improvement and (2) ordinal logistic regression to impute missing PGIIMP values conditional on earlier (observed or imputed) HAMD changes and PGIIMP scores.

Implementing this second approach in SAS PROC MI requires specifying PGIIMP1 and PGIIMP2 as class variables in both linear and logistic regression models. Recall that a PGIIMP score of 4 corresponds to "no change," and scores > 4 indicate worsening. In these data, PGIIMP scores > 4 are uncommon. Therefore, all scores > 4 were combined with scores of 4 (i.e., recoded as "level 4") and the rescaled PGI scores for Time 1 and Time 2 were named PGIIMPGR1 and PGIIMPGR2, respectively.

The SAS code to implement the imputation strategy using multivariate normal is provided in the top panel (a) of Code Fragment 15.6 (Section 15.8) and the code to implement the normal-ordinal model is in the bottom panel (b). In PROC MI, it is possible to sample from truncated marginal distributions when imputing PGIIMP2 scores, thereby ensuring the scores are within the scale range 1 to 7. However, this approach was shown to be inferior to nontruncated imputation (Lipkovich et al. 2014). Therefore, truncation is not used here.

Imputation of categorical outcomes by an ordinal logistic model is similar in spirit to imputation by linear regression (explained in Section 15.2). Code Fragment 15.6 implements Bayesian ordinal logistic regression fitted separately for each treatment arm to predict PGIIMP scores at Time 2 given PGIIMPGR1 (class variable), CHG1 (continuous variable) and baseline HAMD score (continuous variable). Then, for a single draw from the posterior distribution of model parameters, the probability for each of the four categories, P1, P2, P3, P4 (adding up to 1), is estimated and imputed values are generated as a multinomial random variable.

For example, the probability of category "2" is computed as the difference Prob(PGIIMP2="2")=Prob(PGIIMP2≤"2")–Prob(PGIIMP2≤"1") whereas Prob(PGIIMP2≤"2") and Prob(PGIIMP2≤"1") are directly estimated from the assumed logistic model

$$logit\left[\text{Prob}(Y_i \le l_k)\right] = a_k + \sum x_{ij}\beta_j$$

TABLE 15.5

Treatment Contrasts and Least-Squares Means Estimated by Multiple Imputation: Changes in HAMD Using Joint Model for HAMD and PGIIMP

		Incomplete Data (MI) (Joint Multivariate Normal Model)		Incomplete Data (MI) (Joint Modeling using Normal Model for HAMD and Ordinal Logistic for PGIIMP)	
Treatment	**Time**	**LSMEANS**	**SE**	**LSMEANS**	**SE**
1	2	−6.37	1.02	−6.35	1.01
1	3	−9.72	1.22	−9.76	1.38
2	2	−8.45	0.99	−8.59	1.00
2	3	−12.41	1.20	−12.63	1.30
Endpoint Treatment Difference		2.69	1.71 (p = 0.1248)	2.87	1.90 (p = 0.1393)

where Y_i denotes the PGI Improvement score for the ith patient, l_k, $k = 1,\ldots,3$ correspond to the categories "1", "2", "3" of the outcome variable, and x_{ij} represents the observed or imputed score for the jth covariate. The time dimension and specific covariate structure (including for this case BASVAL and CHG1) is suppressed to simplify notation.

Results from the two models are summarized in Table 15.5. The treatment contrasts from the normal and logistic-normal imputation models were 2.69 and 2.87, respectively. Recall the treatment contrast from "standard" MI in Table 15.2 was 2.95. It is important to interpret these results as an illustration. The intent is to show the potential usefulness of, and the process for, inclusive multiple imputation models. Results from this small example data set do not inform expectation of results for actual clinical trial scenarios.

The Code Fragment 15.7 illustrates using the R package MICE for multiply imputing continuous outcomes jointly with categorical PGIIMP scores.

15.7 MI for Categorical Outcomes

As explained in Chapter 10, likelihood-based analyses can be difficult to implement for categorical outcomes. Therefore, multiple imputation provides an important framework for MAR-based analyses of categorical data.

See Chapter 19 for a general discussion of accounting for categorical missing data. This discussion includes multiple imputation examples for analysis of a binary outcome derived from an underlying continuous scale and for an ordinal categorical variable.

15.8 Code Fragments

CODE FRAGMENT 15.1 SAS Code for Multiple Imputation Analysis. Creating Completed Data Sets with PROC MI Using Monotone Imputation

```
/* transpose original data resulting in WIDE data with
   outcome columns Yobs1 Yobs2 Yobs3 corresponding to
   post-baseline visits 1,2,3 */
 PROC SORT DATA=ALL2; BY TRT SUBJECT BASVAL; RUN;
 PROC TRANSPOSE DATA=ALL2 OUT= ALL2_TRANSP2 (DROP=_NAME_)
   PREFIX=YOBS;
   BY TRT SUBJECT BASVAL;
   VAR CHGDROP;
   ID TIME;
 RUN;

/* check whether pattern is monotone */
 PROC MI DATA = ALL2_TRANSP2 NIMPUTE =0;
   BY TRT;
   VAR BASVAL YOBS1 YOBS2 YOBS3;
 RUN;

/* perform multiple imputation for monotone data */
 PROC MI DATA = ALL2_TRANSP2 OUT = ALL2_MIOUT NIMPUTE=1000
   SEED=123;
   BY TRT;
   MONOTONE METHOD=REG;
   VAR BASVAL YOBS1 YOBS2 YOBS3;
 RUN;

/* multiple imputation of monotone data with explicit model
   statement*/
 PROC MI DATA = ALL2_TRANSP2 OUT = ALL2_MIOUT_2
   NIMPUTE=1000 SEED=123;
   BY TRT;
   VAR BASVAL YOBS1 YOBS2 YOBS3;
   MONOTONE REG (YOBS1 =BASVAL);
   MONOTONE REG (YOBS2 =YOBS1 BASVAL);
   MONOTONE REG (YOBS3 =YOBS2 YOBS1 BASVAL);
 RUN;
```

CODE FRAGMENT 15.2 Example R Code for Multiple Imputation Analysis of Continuous Outcome with Arbitrary Missingness: Change from Baseline on HAMD

```
library(mice)
# assumes transposed data set in multivariate format
head(hamdchng)

    trt   basval  CHG1   CHG2   CHG3
1    1      20     -6     NA     NA
2    1      12     -6     -3     -9
3    1      14     -6    -10    -10
4    1      21     -2     -9     -9
5    1      19     -9     -6     NA
6    1      20     -9    -12    -13

# performs MI, using imputation sequence: CHG2, CHG3
imp<-mice(hamdchng, seed=123,visitSequence=c(4,5))

# creates data with imputed sets stacked (if need to look
  at data)
# columns are trt, basval CHG1, CHG2,CHG3
stacked<-complete(imp,"long",)

# fits a linear model for changes in HAMD at vis3 to each
completed set
fit<-with(imp, lm(CHG3~trt+basval))

# pooles inference using Rubin's rules
est<-pool(fit)
summary(est)
```

CODE FRAGMENT 15.3 SAS Code for Multiple Imputation Analysis.* Combined Inference Using PROC MIANALYZE

```
/* combined inference for estimated treatment contrasts */
 ODS OUTPUT PARAMETERESTIMATES=ES_MI;
 PROC MIANALYZE DATA=ES_MI_M ;
   BY TIME;
   MODELEFFECTS ESTIMATE;
   STDERR STDERR;
 RUN;
/* combined inference for lsmeans */
 ODS OUTPUT PARAMETERESTIMATES=LS_MI;
 PROC MIANALYZE DATA=LS_MI_M ;
   BY TIME TRT;
```

* Code Fragment 15.3 assumes that data analysis was ran on imputed data and the estimates and associated standard errors of time- specific treatment contrast are saved in SAS data set ES_MI_M.

```
  MODELEFFECTS ESTIMATE;
  STDERR STDERR;
 RUN;
```

CODE FRAGMENT 15.4 SAS Code for Multiple Imputation Analysis. Imputing Data from Nonmonotone Pattern Using MCMC

```
a) /* using MCMC to impute data from non-monotone patterns */

PROC MI DATA = ALL2_TRANSP3 OUT = ALL2_MIOUT NIMPUTE=1000
  SEED=123;
 BY TRT;
 MCMC CHAIN=SINGLE NBITER=200 NITER=100 INITIAL=EM (ITPRINT
   MAXITER=200);
 VAR BASVAL YOBS1 YOBS2 YOBS3;
RUN;

b) /* using MCMC to first complete data to monotone and
   then perform a single imputation to each monotone set by
   Bayesian regression to produce complete data sets */

PROC MI DATA = ALL2_TRANSP3 OUT = ALL4_MIOUT NIMPUTE=1000
SEED=123;
 BY TRT;
 MCMC IMPUTE = MONOTONE;
 VAR BASVAL YOBS1 YOBS2 YOBS3;
RUN;

PROC SORT DATA=ALL4_MIOUT; BY _IMPUTATION_ TRT; RUN;
PROC MI DATA = ALL4_MIOUT OUT = ALL5_MIOUT NIMPUTE =1 SEED
  =123;
 BY _IMPUTATION_ TRT;
 MONOTONE METHOD=REG;
 VAR BASVAL YOBS1 YOBS2 YOBS3;
RUN;
```

CODE FRAGMENT 15.5 SAS Code for Multiple Imputation Analysis. Imputing Data for Baseline Covariates Using MCMC

```
/* using MCMC to first impute baseline covariates X1, X2,
X3, basval and other missing values deviating from monotone
pattern and then perform a single imputation to each
monotone sets by Bayesian regression to produce complete
data sets */

PROC MI DATA = ALL2_TRANSP3 OUT = ALL4_MIOUT NIMPUTE=1000
  SEED=123;
 BY TRT;
 MCMC IMPUTE = MONOTONE;
 VAR X1 X2 X3 BASVAL YOBS1 YOBS2 YOBS3;
```

```
RUN;
PROC SORT DATA=ALL4_MIOUT; BY _IMPUTATION_ TRT; RUN;
PROC MI DATA = ALL4_MIOUT OUT = ALL5_MIOUT NIMPUTE=1
  SEED=123;
 BY _IMPUTATION_ TRT;
 MONOTONE METHOD=REG;
 VAR X1 X2 X3 BASVAL YOBS1 YOBS2 YOBS3;
RUN;
```

CODE FRAGMENT 15.6 SAS Code for an Inclusive Multiple Imputation Strategy: Joint Imputation of Changes in HAMD and PGIIMP

```
 a) Imputing from joint multivariate normal distribution

PROC MI DATA = ALL3_TRANSP OUT = ALL3_MIOUT NIMPUTE=1000
  SEED=123;
 BY TRT;
 MONOTONE METHOD=REG;
 VAR BASVAL CHG1 PGIIMP1 CHG2 PGIIMP2 CHG3 ;
RUN;

 b) multiple imputation using normal regression for changes
   in HAMD and ordinal logistic regression for PGIIMP*/
PROC MI DATA = ALL3_TRANSP OUT = ALL3_MIOUT NIMPUTE=1000
  SEED=123;
 BY TRT;
 CLASS PGIIMPGR1 PGIIMPGR2;
 VAR BASVAL CHG1 PGIIMPGR1 CHG2 PGIIMPGR2 CHG3;
 MONOTONE REG (CHG1=BASVAL);
 MONOTONE LOGISTIC (PGIIMPGR1 =CHG1 BASVAL);
 MONOTONE REG (CHG2= PGIIMPGR1 CHG1 BASVAL);
 MONOTONE LOGISTIC (PGIIMPGR2= CHG2 PGIIMPGR1 CHG1 BASVAL/
   DETAILS);
 MONOTONE REG (CHG3= PGIIMPGR2 CHG2 PGIIMPGR1 CHG1 BASVAL);
RUN;
```

CODE FRAGMENT 15.7 Example of R Code for an Inclusive Multiple Imputation Strategy: Joint Imputation of Changes in HAMD and PGIIMP

```
#### joint imputation of continuous and
  categorical(ordered) outcomes

hamdpgi<-widedata[,c("trt","basval","CHG1","PGIIMPGR1","CHG
  2","PGIIMPGR2","CHG3")]

# make PGIIMP ordered factors
hamdpgi$PGIIMPGR1<-ordered(hamdpgi$PGIIMPGR1)
```

```
hamdpgi$PGIIMPGR2<-ordered(hamdpgi$PGIIMPGR2)

imp<-mice(hamdpgi, seed=123,visitSequence=c(5,6,7))
# fits linear model for change in HAMD at Time 3 to each
  imputed data set
fit<-with(imp, lm(CHG3~trt+basval))

# pooled inference using Rubin's rules

est<-pool(fit)
summary(est)
```

15.9 Summary

Multiple imputation (MI) is a popular and accessible method of model-based imputation. The three basic steps to MI include imputation, analysis, and inference. These steps can be applied to outcomes with a variety of distributions, including normally distributed, categorical, and time to event (e.g., with piece-wise exponential hazard) outcomes.

If MI is implemented using the same imputation and analysis model, and the model is the same as the analysis model used in a maximum likelihood-based (ML) analysis, MI and ML will yield asymptotically similar point estimates, but ML will be somewhat more efficient. However, with distinct steps for imputation and analysis, MI has more flexibility than other methods. This flexibility can be exploited in a number of situations.

Scenarios where MI is particularly useful include those when covariates are missing, when data are not normally distributed such that likelihood-based analyses are difficult to implement, and when inclusive modeling strategies are used to help account for missing data. Multiple imputation is also very useful for sensitivity analyses. See Chapter 18 for further details on using MI for sensitivity analyses.

16

Inverse Probability Weighted Generalized Estimated Equations

16.1 Introduction

Although inverse probability weighting (IPW) can be applied in a variety of settings, focus here is on using IPW in conjunction with generalized estimating equations (GEEs) to construct weighted GEE (wGEE). Technical details on estimating parameters via GEE were presented in Section 5.5.3. A standard reference for wGEE is Robins et al. (1995).

GEEs are nonlikelihood-based equations and parameter estimates (e.g., of treatment effect) are biased under MAR (Robins et al. 1995). The stronger assumption of MCAR is required because the root of the estimating equation expectation is not equal (in general) to the true parameters underlying the outcome process, unless the missingness is MCAR. The requirement of MCAR stems from the parameters of the working correlation matrix in GEE being estimated based on what is essentially a complete case analysis. Only subjects that were observed at both visits t_1 and t_2 contribute to the estimate of within-subject correlation between visits $t_1$and t_2. When within subject correlations are not used in computing point estimates (the case of "independent working correlation structures"), bias under MAR is even more apparent since GEE point estimates of treatment effect at each time point are merely treatment contrasts evaluated for complete cases at a given evaluation visit.

The bias in GEE from MAR missingness can be removed by incorporating weights into the GEE (wGEE). The weights are based on the inverse probability of observing the dropout patterns that were present in the data. The idea of weighting can be traced back to the well-known Horvitz and Thompson (1952) inverse probability (IP) estimator.

16.2 Technical Details—Inverse Probability Weighting

16.2.1 General Considerations

The motivation behind IPW is to correct for bias caused by nonrandom selection (dropout). Assume interest is in computing the expected value of discrete random variable, Y, in a finite population of N elements, and Y can assume only two possible values: y_1 and y_2. The population mean is computed as a weighted average

$$\mu = E(Y) = \frac{N_1 y_1 + N_2 y_2}{N}$$

Now assume that a selection mechanism is applied to the population that removes some elements y_1 with probability of selection $\pi_1 = 1/2$, while not affecting the selection of y_2 ($\pi_2 = 1$). Therefore, only $\frac{N_1}{2}$ occurrences of y_1 are expected to be observed, while N_2 occurrences of y_2 are observed. Assume that the relative frequencies of y_1 and y_2 in the population equal these expected values (i.e., ignoring the randomness in the dropout process). Then, when estimating the population mean based on the mean from incomplete data ("observed case" or "complete case" estimator, $\hat{\mu}_{cc}$) the expectation of this estimator is

$$E(\hat{\mu}_{cc}) = \frac{\frac{1}{2} N_1 y_1 + N_2 y_2}{\frac{1}{2} N_1 + N_2}.$$

Of course, this estimator is biased because in general $E(\hat{\mu}_{cc}) \neq E(Y)$. In this example, the selection probabilities are known and adjustments for the selection bias can be made by associating y_1 and y_2 with weights computed as the inverse of their respective selection probabilities, $w_1 = \frac{1}{\pi_1} = 2, w_2 = \frac{1}{\pi_2} = 1$. Thus

$$E(\hat{\mu}_{\text{IPW}}) = \frac{\frac{1}{2} N_1 y_1 w_1 + N_2 y_2 w_2}{\frac{1}{2} N_1 w_1 + N_2 w_2} = \frac{\frac{1}{2} N_1 y_1 2 + N_2 y_2 1}{\frac{1}{2} N_1 2 + N_2 1} = \frac{N_1 y_1 + N_2 y_2}{N} = E(Y)$$

With $\pi_1 = 1/2$ the inverse is 2/1, which amounts to essentially counting each observed value of y_1 twice because the probability of observing each instance of y_1 from the population is 1/2. If $\pi_1 = 2/3$, then each occurrence of y_1 would be given a weight of 3/2 = 1.5. In actual clinical trial data the probabilities are unknown and must be estimated from sample data.

If the selection probability for elements y_1 were $\pi_1 = 0$ then all y_1 are missing and IPW cannot be used. Hence, an important requirement of IPW is that all possible values of the outcome variable have nonzero probability of being in the observed population. If some values have very low probabilities it is unlikely that these values would be observed in a sample. In such cases IPW may lead to bias (if some values are not observed in the sample) and/or high variance (if some values are observed but have low estimated probabilities resulting in very large weights).

To illustrate a general use of IPW, let y_i, $i = 1,..., N$ denote realizations of an outcome variable Y in a complete data set, $y_{i,obs}$, $i = 1,..., N_1$ and r_i is the observed values of missingness indicator variable R so that for subject i.

$$y_i = \begin{cases} y_{i,obs}, if \quad r_i = 1 \\ y_{i,mis}, if \quad r_i = 0 \end{cases}$$

Assume that the true selection probabilities (or probabilities of nonmissingness) are known, $\pi_i = \Pr(R_i = 1)$. Note that in general π_i may be a function of y_i; therefore, π_i's are conditional probabilities $\pi_i = \Pr(R_i = 1 | Y = y_i)$. The IPW estimator can be defined as

$$\hat{\mu}_{\text{IPW}} = \frac{1}{N} \sum_{i=1}^{N_1} y_{i,obs} \frac{1}{\pi_i}$$

Equivalently, the expression can be written in terms of the complete data outcome as

$$\hat{\mu}_{\text{IPW}} = \frac{1}{N} \sum_{i=1}^{N} y_i r_i \frac{1}{\pi_i}$$

Although some values of y_i are not observed, the product $y_i r_i$ is fully observed. To show that $\hat{\mu}_{\text{IPW}}$ is an unbiased estimator of $\mu = E(Y)$ its expectation with respect to the joint distribution of Y and R is needed. The law of conditional iterated expectations can be exploited to allow decomposition of the joint expectation as $E_{Y,R}() = E_Y\{E_{R|Y}()\}$. Then

$$\begin{aligned} E(\hat{\mu}_{\text{IPW}}) &= \frac{1}{N} \sum_{i=1}^{N} E(Y_i R_i) \frac{1}{\pi_i} = \frac{1}{N} \sum_{i=1}^{N} \frac{1}{\pi_i} E\left(Y_i E_{R|Y} R_i\right) \\ &= \frac{1}{N} \sum_{i=1}^{N} \frac{1}{\pi_i} \Pr\left(R = 1 | Y = y_i\right) E(Y_i) \\ &= \frac{1}{N} \sum_{i=1}^{N} \frac{\pi_i}{\pi_i} E(Y_i) = \frac{1}{N} \sum_{i=1}^{N} E(Y_i) = E(Y) = \mu \end{aligned}$$

Therefore, as seen from the third line, assigning weights that are the inverse of the probability of selecting the observations recovers the mean expected in the complete data. In practice, the weighted sum of observed values is divided by the sum of weights rather than by N.

$$\hat{\mu}_{\text{IPW}} = \frac{1}{\sum_{i=1}^{N_1} \frac{1}{\pi_i}} \sum_{i=1}^{N_1} y_{i,obs} \frac{1}{\pi_i}$$

In expectation, these are equivalent:

$$E\left(\sum_{i=1}^{N_1} \frac{1}{\pi_i}\right) = E\left(\sum_{i=1}^{N} \frac{R_i}{\pi_i}\right) = E\left(\sum_{i=1}^{N} \frac{\pi_i}{\pi_i}\right) = N.$$

Therefore, the relative subject-specific weights (summing up to 1) can be defined as

$$\hat{\mu}_{\text{IPW}} = \sum_{i=1}^{N_1} y_{i,obs} w_i$$

$$w_i = \frac{\frac{1}{\pi_i}}{\sum_{i=1}^{N_1} \frac{1}{\pi_i}}$$

Once IPW estimates of the expected outcome for each treatment group $\left(\hat{\mu}_{\text{IPW}}^{(t)}, t = 0,1\right)$ are obtained, treatment effects can be estimated as, $\hat{\theta}_{\text{IPW}} = \hat{\mu}_{\text{IPW}}^{(1)} - \hat{\mu}_{\text{IPW}}^{(0)}$.

As an initial illustration, consider estimating treatment effect via inverse probably weighting of the completers (subjects with no missing data) in the small example data set with dropout. For this illustration, subjects are considered to have only one observation, the Time 3 assessment. The IPW weights are not known, but can be estimated using logistic regression. For this example probability of dropout was estimated using a model applied to data pooled across visits with the dropout indicator as the response variable. Predictor variables included change from baseline at the previous visit, baseline score, and treatment. The inverse weights estimated from this model were applied to the subset of subjects that completed the trial (sometimes called inverse probability weighted complete case or IPWCC estimator) in order to estimate the mean that would have been observed if all patients had completed.

For this example, the probabilities of completing the trial are computed as a product of conditional probabilities of completing each of the visits. That is,

$$\pi_i = \Pr(R_{1i} = 1)\ \Pr(R_{2i} = 1 | R_{1i} = 1)\ \Pr(R_{3i} = 1 | R_{1i} = 1, R_{2i} = 1)$$

Because all subjects completed the first post-baseline visit it is assumed the $\Pr(R_{1i} = 1) = 1$. Estimates of conditional probabilities are obtained as functions of observed outcomes and other baseline covariates (e.g., using logistic regression) as will be shown in detail in the next sections.

Weighting removes selection bias by giving larger weight to outcomes that are underrepresented in the observed data compared to what would have been observed if there were no dropouts. Conversely, smaller weights are given to observed values that are "overrepresented." Typically, as is the case with the small example dataset with dropout, subjects with poorer efficacy are less likely to be observed. Therefore, subjects with poor outcomes are underrepresented in the observed data and their weight should be larger compared to those who had larger improvements.

As expected, weights estimated from the small example data set are larger for subjects with worse outcomes (changes from baseline closer to zero) and smaller for subjects with better outcome (larger negative changes from baseline). The left panel of Figure 16.1 illustrates this relationship. The right panel is a plot of visit-wise mean changes from baseline for subjects who completed the trial divided into two strata; the first stratum is subjects whose estimated weights were less than the median and the second stratum is subjects with weights larger than the median. The figure clearly shows subjects with larger weights had worse marginal means than those with smaller weights.

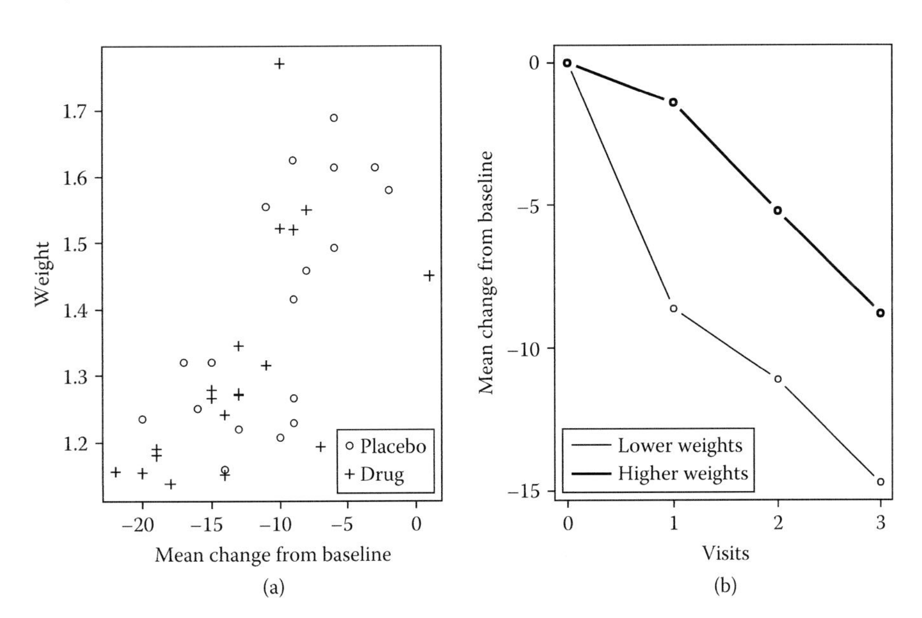

FIGURE 16.1
Relationship between weights and changes from baseline for completers. (a) Scatter plot of subject weights versus changes from baseline to visit 3 and (b) right panel is mean change profiles for completers with weights larger than median (thick line) and lower than the median (thin line).

16.2.2 Specific Implementations

The previous section illustrated IPW for an ANCOVA model with a single outcome per subject. Inverse probability weighting is now considered in the context of repeated measures analysis via weighted GEE. Inverse probability weights are commonly calculated in one of the two ways. Either one weight is given per subject and applied to all visits, thus reflecting the probability of the observed dropout pattern; or, each subject gets a unique weight at each visit, thus reflecting the visit-wise probabilities of dropout.

Robins and Rotnitzky (1995) proposed inverse probability weights that change by visit (observation-level weighting). The weights can be incorporated in the working covariance model as the elements of a diagonal $n_i \times n_i$ weight matrix W_i

$$V_i = \phi A_i^{\frac{1}{2}} W_i^{-\frac{1}{2}} R(\alpha) W_i^{-\frac{1}{2}} A_i^{\frac{1}{2}}$$

The weights are computed for each subject at each time point in a manner similar to how the weights for the last visit were computed in the weighted analysis of completers in the previous section. For example, Subject 9 had two completed visits; hence the matrix W is a 2 × 2 diagonal matrix with weights based on estimated probabilities as follows (subject index omitted whenever it does not cause confusion)

$$w_1 = \frac{1}{\hat{\pi}_1}, w_2 = \frac{1}{\hat{\pi}_2}$$

$$\hat{\pi}_1 = \Pr\left(R_1 = 1 | x\right)$$

$$\hat{\pi}_2 = \widehat{\Pr}(R_1 = 1 | x)\, \widehat{\Pr}\left(R_2 = 1 | R_1 = 1, x, y_1\right)$$

Here again $\hat{\pi}_1 = 1$, and correspondingly, $\hat{\pi}_2 = \widehat{\Pr}(R_2 = 1 | R_1 = 1, x, y_1)$, because no dropouts had occurred prior to the first post-baseline visit. [Note we use $\Pr(R_2 = 1 | R_1 = 1, x, y_1)$ as a shorthand for $\Pr(R_2 = 1 | R_1 = 1, X = x, Y_1 = y_1)$]. The weights can change from visit to visit reflecting the changing probability of a subject remaining in the study given the previous data.

Fitzmaurice et al. (1995) proposed subject-level weighting wherein a single weight is computed for each subject that is used at every visit (repeated for all diagonal elements of the W_i matrix). The weight is an inverse of the estimated probability $\hat{\pi}^{(d)}$ of observing the dropout pattern d that was actually observed for that subject. Here the pattern $d = 1,..., T + 1$ indicates the *next* time point after patient was observed for the last time. That is, for a subject who was last seen at time t, $d = t + 1$. For completers, $d = T + 1$, where T indicates the last scheduled visit.

The working covariance model is then expressed as

$$V_i = \hat{\pi}_i^{(d)} \phi A_i^{\frac{1}{2}} R(\alpha) A_i^{\frac{1}{2}}$$

As a result, the weighted estimating equations are obtained from the original estimating equations simply by multiplying each subject's contributions to the estimating equations by the inverse probability of his/her observed dropout pattern $w_i = 1/\hat{\pi}_i^{(d)}$.

To illustrate, for a subject that completed all the scheduled visits, the weight is computed exactly as weights for completers at the last visit were computed in the previous section. That is,

$$\hat{\pi}^{(d)} = \widehat{\Pr}(R_1 = 1|x)\, \widehat{\Pr}(R_2 = 1|R_1 = 1, x, y_1)\, \widehat{\Pr}(R_3 = 1|R_1 = 1, R_2 = 1, x, y_1, y_2)$$

For subjects who did not complete the trial, the probability of the observed pattern is computed as the probability of that subject remaining in the trial until the last observed visit and discontinuing right after. As an example, for Subject 9, the probability of the observed dropout pattern is computed as

$$\hat{\pi}^{(d)} = \widehat{\Pr}(R_1 = 1|x)\, \widehat{\Pr}(R_2 = 1|R_1 = 1, x, y_1)\left[1 - \widehat{\Pr}(R_3 = 1|R_1 = 1, R_2 = 1, x, y_1, y_2)\right]$$

16.3 Example

With the building blocks of IPW in place, a wGEE analysis of the small example dataset with dropout can be considered. The goal is to estimate treatment effects using a weighted GEE model, with weights reflecting the selection probability; that is the probability of completing all three visits. This example uses the approach of Fitzmaurice et al. (1995) introduced in 16.2.2. Subject weights are computed based on inverse probability of observed dropout pattern $\hat{\pi}_i^{(d)}$.

After estimating the probabilities $\hat{\pi}_i$, the weights are computed as $w_i = \dfrac{1}{\hat{\pi}_i^{(d)}}$.

The weights are then included in the dataset as additional variable and the weighted analysis is conducted, for example, via SAS PROC GENMOD (SAS 2013). The weights are data-dependent, but the analysis assumes the weights are known, similar to the assumption that variance components are known in a standard mixed-effects model analysis. The robust sandwich estimates of standard errors provided by the GEE are still valid, although conservative (Robins et al. 1995). Resampling methods can be used to obtain non conservative estimates.

It is important to recognize that wGEE provides valid estimates under MAR, assuming that the model for dropout is correctly specified. As previously noted, estimating weights can be challenging when some of the true probabilities of observed patterns are close to 0. This can result in large weights and unstable estimates of treatment effects. Truncation and stratification can be used to stabilize weights. Also more stable versions of weights have been proposed (Hernàn et al. 2000).

SAS code for obtaining subject-level and observational-level inverse probability weights are listed in Section 16.4 (Code Fragment 16.1). SAS code to implement wGEE analyses via PROC GENMOD using the calculated IPW weights is listed in Section 16.4 (Code Fragment 16.2), followed by a code fragment for experimental procedure PROC GEE that is available in SAS/STAT 13.2 (SAS 2013) wherein the weights are obtained as part of the PROC.

Results for the wGEE analyses using subject-level weights are compared to results from an unweighted GEE and results from complete data in Table 16.1. It is important to interpret these results as just one realization from a stochastic process. If the comparisons were replicated many times under the same conditions—including missing data arising from an MAR mechanism—the average of the lsmeans and treatment contrasts across the repeated samples would be asymptotically equal for complete data, incomplete data analyzed via direct likelihood, MI, or wGEE with an appropriate dropout model. Standard errors would be consistently greater in incomplete data.

The wGEE analysis yielded a point estimate for the treatment contrast at Time = 3 in-between the result obtained from the analysis of complete cases

TABLE 16.1

Results from GEE and wGEE Analyses of the Small Example Data Set

		Complete Data		GEE Incomplete Data		wGEE Incomplete Data	
Treatment	**Time**	**LSMEANS**	**SE**	**LSMEANS**	**SE**	**LSMEANS**	**SE**
1	1	−4.13	0.91	−4.10	0.76	−4.38	0.83
1	2	−6.70	0.93	−6.70	1.04	−5.64	0.87
1	3	−9.86	1.05	−10.17	1.11	−9.58	1.08
2	1	−5.32	0.91	−5.29	0.97	−4.88	0.88
2	2	−8.70	0.93	−8.29	0.96	−6.09	1.10
2	3	−13.26	1.05	−13.10	1.27	−12.71	1.28
Endpoint Treatment Difference		3.39	1.49 (p = 0.0274)	2.92	1.73 (p = 0.0905)	3.13	1.71 (p = 0.0670)

and from complete data. As expected, the standard error for the Time 3 treatment contrast from wGEE with incomplete data was larger than the standard error from complete data and slightly larger than the standard error from the direct likelihood analysis of incomplete data (see Table 14.1). The relaxed distributional assumptions of GEE results in a slightly less efficient analyses than likelihood-based methods.

16.4 Code Fragments

CODE FRAGMENT 16.1 SAS Code for Obtaining Inverse Probability Weights

```
  /* Create change at previous visit variable and dropout
     indicator variable */
 PROC SORT DATA=ALL2; BY SUBJECT TIME; RUN;
 DATA FOR_WGEE;
  SET ALL2;
  RETAIN DROP CHANGE_LAG1;
  BY SUBJECT TIME;
  IF FIRST.SUBJECT THEN DO;
    DROP=0;
      CHANGE_LAG1=.;
  END;
  IF DROP=1 THEN DELETE;
  IF CHGDROP=. THEN DROP=1;
  OUTPUT;
  CHANGE_LAG1=CHGDROP;
 RUN;

 /* Logistic regression analysis to obtain probabilities of
 dropping, Pr(DROP=1)*/
 PROC LOGISTIC DATA=FOR_WGEE DESC;
  CLASS TRT;
  MODEL DROP=TRT BASVAL CHANGE_LAG1;
  OUTPUT OUT =PRED P=PRED;
 RUN;

 /* Calculate and merge weights into data set */
 DATA WEIGHTS_SUB (DROP=WEIGHT_OBS PB_OBS)
    WEIGHTS_OBS (DROP=WEIGHT_SUB PB_SUB);
 SET PRED;
 BY SUBJECT TIME;
 RETAIN PB_SUB PB_OBS;
 IF FIRST.SUBJECT THEN DO;
```

```
  PB_OBS =1; /* PROB. OF OBSERVING SUBJECT AT GIVEN TIME
    - FOR OBSERVATIONAL WEIGHTS */
  PB_SUB =1; /* PROB. OF OBSERVED DROPOUT PATTERN - FOR
    SUBJECT WEIGHTS */
END; ELSE DO;
  IF DROP THEN PB_SUB =PB_SUB * PRED; ELSE PB_SUB =PB_SUB
    *(1-PRED);
  PB_OBS =PB_OBS * (1-PRED);
END;

WEIGHT_OBS=1/PB_OBS ;
  OUTPUT WEIGHTS_OBS;
  IF LAST.SUBJECT THEN DO;
    WEIGHT_SUB =1/PB_SUB;
    OUTPUT WEIGHTS_SUB;
  END;
RUN;

PROC SORT DATA=FOR_WGEE; BY SUBJECT; RUN;
PROC SORT DATA=WEIGHTS_SUB; BY SUBJECT; RUN;

DATA FOR_WGEE;*
  MERGE FOR_WGEE
    WEIGHTS_SUB (KEEP=SUBJECT WEIGHT_SUB);
  BY SUBJECT;
RUN;
```

CODE FRAGMENT 16.2 SAS Code for Weighted GEE Analysis Using the PROC GENMOD

```
  ODS OUTPUT ESTIMATES=ES_CHDR_WGEE_IND
      LSMEANS=LS_CHDR_WGEE_IND;
PROC GENMOD DATA=FOR_WGEE (WHERE=(CHGDROP NE .));
  CLASS TRT TIME SUBJECT;
  MODEL CHGDROP= BASVAL TRT TIME TRT*TIME /LINK=ID
    DIST=NORMAL;
  WEIGHT WEIGHT_XXX1;
  REPEATED SUBJECT=SUBJECT /TYPE=IND;
  ESTIMATE "TRT EFFECT AT VIS 3" TRT -1 1 TRT*TIME 0 0 -1 0 0 1;
  LSMEANS TRT*TIME;
RUN;
```

1. Use WEIGHT_SUB for subject-level weights and WEIGHT_OBS for observation-level weights

* Here we show creating analysis data set for wGEE using subject weights. Analysis data with observation-level weights is created similarly by merging with WEIGHTS_OBS data set.

CODE FRAGMENT 16.3 SAS Code for Weighted GEE Analysis Using the Experimental PROC GEE

```
PROC GEE DATA=ALL2 DESC PLOTS=HISTOGRAM;
 CLASS SUBJECT TRT TIME;
 MISSMODEL PREVY TRT BASVAL / TYPE=SUBLEVEL;
 MODEL CHGDROP = BASVAL TRT TIME TRT*TIME BASVAL*TIME /
   DIST=NORMAL LINK=ID;
 REPEATED SUBJECT=SUBJECT / WITHIN=TIME CORR=IND;
RUN;
```

16.5 Summary

Although GEE is valid only under MCAR, inverse probability weighting (IPW) can correct for MAR, provided an appropriate model for the missingness process (dropout) is used whereby missingness depends on observed outcomes but not further on unobserved outcomes. The weights are based on the inverse probability of dropout and in effect create a pseudo-population of data that would have been observed with no missing data in an infinitely large trial.

Weighting can be at the subject level, with one weight per subject reflecting the inverse probability of observing the dropout pattern; or, weighting can be at the observation level, with one weight per subject per visit that reflects the changing probability of dropout as outcomes evolve over time.

As with standard GEE, in wGEE no assumptions about the correlation structure are required and therefore wGEE yields semi-parametric estimators. The wGEE estimates are generally not as efficient as maximum likelihood (parametric) estimators obtained using the correct model, but they remain consistent whereas maximum likelihood estimators from a misspecified parametric model are inconsistent.

17

Doubly Robust Methods

17.1 Introduction

Common references for the emerging area of doubly robust (DR) methods include Carpenter et al. (2006) and Tsiatis (2006). The genesis of DR methods can be seen by building from the properties of weighted generalized estimating equations (wGEEs), which are briefly reviewed below.

Although GEE is valid only under missing completely at random (MCAR), inverse probability weighting (IPW) can correct for missing at random (MAR), provided an appropriate model for the missingness process (dropout) is used whereby missingness depends on observed outcomes but not further on unobserved outcomes (Molenberghs and Kenward 2007). The wGEEs yield semi-parametric estimators because they do not model the entire distribution of the outcome values. These semi-parametric estimates are generally not as efficient as maximum likelihood estimators obtained using the correct model, but they remain consistent when maximum likelihood estimators from a misspecified parametric model are inconsistent (Molenberghs and Kenward 2007).

Therefore, a motivation for DR methods is to improve the efficiency of wGEEs by augmenting the estimating equations with the predicted distribution of the unobserved data, given the observed data (Molenberghs and Kenward 2007). Although augmentation is motivated by efficiency, it also introduces the property of double robustness.

To understand double robustness, consider that efficient IPW estimators require three models: (1) a substantive (analysis) model that relates the outcome to explanatory variables and/or covariates; (2) a model for the probability of observing the data (usually a logistic model of some form); and (3) a model for the joint distribution of the partially and fully observed data, which is compatible with the substantive model (1) (Molenberghs and Kenward 2007).

If model (1) is wrong, for example, because a key confounder is omitted, then estimates of all parameters will typically be inconsistent. The intriguing property of augmented wGEE is that if either model (2) or model (3) is wrong, but not both, the estimators in model (1) are still consistent (Molenberghs and Kenward 2007). However, DR methods are fairly new with few rigorous simulation studies or real data applications in the literature. Refer Robins et al. (1995), Carpenter et al. (2006), Tsiatis (2006) and Daniel and Kenward (2012) for additional details.

17.2 Technical Details

In Section 16.2, inverse probability estimation was explained starting with the simple case of estimating the sample mean of an outcome variable Y when some of its values y_i, $i = 1,...,N$, are missing (indicated with $r_i = 0$). Subsequently, IPW was extended to repeated measures. A similar approach is used here, with the ideas of DR estimation building on the results of Chapter 16.

To fix ideas, assume that missingness is MAR and the probability that Y is missing does not depend on unobserved vales of Y, given covariates $\mathbf{X}$ (that includes various pretreatment covariates). Recall that an unbiased estimate of treatment means can be obtained using the inverse probability estimator:

$$\hat{\mu}_{\text{IPW}} = \frac{1}{N}\sum_{i=1}^{N} y_i r_i \frac{1}{\pi_i}$$

where π_i are probabilities of having observed outcome (known or estimated from available data). Note that under MAR (for this example) $\pi_i = \pi(x_i) = \Pr(R = 1|X = x_i)$ is a known or estimated function of covariates; therefore, we can write $\pi = \pi(x)$. The consistency of the IPW estimator follows from the assumption that the model for probability of missingness was correctly specified. If that is not the case, probabilities $\hat{\pi}_i$ estimated from an incorrect model will converge (as N becomes large) to some "misspecified" function $\ddot{\pi}(x)$. As a result, the estimate of population mean would in general be biased. The *augmented inverse probability weighted estimator* of sample mean $\hat{\mu}_{\text{AIPW}}$ aims to protect against bias due to misspecification of the weight by combining IPW with an outcome (or imputation) model $m(x)$

$$\hat{\mu}_{\text{AIPW}} = \frac{1}{N}\sum_{i=1}^{N} \tilde{y}_i = \frac{1}{N}\sum_{i=1}^{N}\left\{\frac{r_i}{\hat{\pi}_i} y_i - \left(\frac{r_i}{\hat{\pi}_i} - 1\right)\widehat{m}_i\right\}.$$

We emphasize that this requires estimation of models for (1) probability of being observed and (2) outcome value (whether missing or observed) by placing hats over $\hat{\pi}_i$ and $\widehat{m}_i$. Therefore, the estimator is an average of N "augmented values", $\tilde{y}_i, i=1,...,N$. Note that, unlike the IPW estimator, the augmented IPW (AIPW) estimator receives nonzero contribution from patients with missing values ($r_i = 0$), specifically such patients contribute with their imputed or predicted value, $\widehat{m}_i$, estimated from the outcome model $m(x)$.

The AIPW estimator is often written in the following alternative forms that can be easily obtained from the original one by re-arranging terms:

$$\hat{\mu}_{\mathrm{AIPW}} = \frac{1}{N}\sum_{i=1}^{N}\left\{\frac{r_i}{\hat{\pi}_i}y_i - \left(\frac{r_i}{\hat{\pi}_i} - 1\right)\widehat{m}_i\right\} = \frac{1}{N}\sum_{i=1}^{N}\left\{\frac{r_i}{\hat{\pi}_i}\left(y_i - \widehat{m}_i\right) + \widehat{m}_i\right\}$$

$$= \frac{1}{N}\sum_{i=1}^{N}\left\{y_i + \left(\frac{r_i}{\hat{\pi}_i} - 1\right)\left(y_i - \widehat{m}_i\right)\right\}.$$

The last representation is particularly useful for demonstrating the *double robustness* property of the AIPW estimator: the estimator is consistent as long as at least one of the two models is correctly specified. To illustrate, assume that the sample size is large so that the estimators $\hat{\pi}_i$ and $\widehat{m}_i$ converge (in probability) to their large sample counterparts, whether they are correctly or incorrectly specified functions of observed data.

Also assume that the model for probability of missingness is correctly specified, $\pi(x)$ and the outcome model is a (possibly) misspecified function $\ddot{m}(x)$. Applying the law of conditional iterated expectations to a joint distribution of random variables R, X, Y as $E_{R,X,Y} = E_{X,Y}\{E_{R|X,Y}()\}$, the expectation of individual augmented values can be written as follows (after factoring out $Y - \ddot{m}(X)$, which is a constant conditional on X and Y):

$$E\left(\tilde{Y}\right) = E(Y) + E\left\{E\left(\frac{R}{\pi(X)} - 1 \mid X, Y\right)\left(Y - \ddot{m}(X)\right)\right\}$$

$$= \mu + E\left\{\left(\frac{E(R \mid X, Y)}{\pi(X)} - 1\right)\left(Y - \ddot{m}(X)\right)\right\}$$

$$= \mu + E\left\{\left(\frac{\pi(X)}{\pi(X)} - 1\right)\left(Y - \ddot{m}(X)\right)\right\}$$

$$= \mu + 0$$

The second term vanishes regardless of what $E_{XY}\left(Y - \ddot{m}(X)\right)$ may be because under MAR $E(R|X = x, Y = y) = \Pr(R = 1|X = x) = \pi(x)$, resulting in consistent estimation of the population mean μ.

Similarly, assuming that the model for probability of missingness is possibly misspecified $\ddot{\pi}(x)$ and for outcome model the true function $m(x)$ is estimated, after applying the law of conditional iterated expectations

$E_{R,X,Y} = E_{R,X}\{E_{Y|R,X}()\}$, the expectation of individual augmented values can be written as follows

$$E(\tilde{Y}) = E(Y) + E\left\{\left(\frac{R}{\ddot{\pi}(X)} - 1\right)E(Y - m(X)) \mid R, X)\right\}$$
$$= \mu + E\left\{\left(\frac{R}{\ddot{\pi}(X)} - 1\right)\left(E(Y \mid X, R) - m(X)\right)\right\}$$
$$= \mu + E\left\{\left(\frac{R}{\ddot{\pi}(X)} - 1\right)\left(m(X) - m(X)\right)\right\}$$
$$= \mu + 0$$

Again, the second term vanishes in expectation because under MAR the distribution of outcomes conditional on observed data is the same for subjects with observed ($R = 1$) and unobserved ($R = 0$) outcome values; hence, $E(Y|X = x, R = r) = E(Y|X = x) = m(x)$.

To summarize, the idea of DR estimation is to combine the strengths of two models: for probability of missingness and for imputing missing values. Both models can be estimated under the assumption of MAR utilizing observed patient-level data which, however, may be undesirable or awkward to include in the direct maximum likelihood-based modeling of the parameter of interest (e.g., treatment contrast at specific time point). The DR estimation via AIPW results in two types of gain: (1) protection against one of the two models being misspecified (doubly robustness) and (2) increased efficiency. While intuitively the increase in efficiency may appear a natural outcome of using additional information (predicted values for subjects with missing outcomes), it relies on sophisticated theory of semi-parametric estimation (Robins and Rotnitzky 1995; Tsiatis 2006), which is outside the scope of this book.

Despite its intuitive appeal the DR estimators also received a great deal of criticism, its opponents arguing that in situations when both models may be "slightly" misspecified (a typical situation with real data) the doubly robustness property may not translate in any gain, especially given inherent instability of IPW. For example, as argued in Kang and Schafer (2009), "two wrong models are not better than one" (see also a different view in Cao et al. 2009 and Tsiatis et al. 2011 who proposed improved DB estimators).

As in the case of IPW, AIPW estimator previously introduced in the context of estimating population means gives rise to AIPW-based (generalized) estimating equations. Their general form is quite simple, it starts with IPW estimated equations (Chapter 16) and adds some function of the data with zero expectation

$$\sum_{i=1}^{N}\left\{\frac{r_i}{\pi_i}U(y_i, x_i, |\theta) - \left(\frac{r_i}{\pi_i} - 1\right)\phi(y_i, x_i)\right\} = 0$$

Like the AIPW estimator of population mean, the AIPW estimating equations have two terms: one is based on contributions from observed data only (inversely weighted by π_i) and the second is based on contributions from both observed and unobserved cases. The zero mean function $\phi(y, x)$ is then constructed to have minimal variance following semi-parametric theory of Robins and Rotnitzky (1995), resulting in conditional expectation of the score function $U(y_i, x_i, | \theta)$ on the observed data Y_{obs}, X, that can be loosely termed "imputation model". However, particular implementations, especially extensions for longitudinal data, are not straightforward and selection of the best augmented function may be not obvious (see Karpenter and Kenward 2006 for applying DR estimators in the context of missing covariate and Tsiatis et al. 2011 for modeling longitudinal outcomes).

17.3 Specific Implementations

Specific implementation of AIPW requires the selection of (1) a substantive model of interest; (2) a missing data model for computing IPW; and (3) an outcome (imputation) model. In the context of data analysis from clinical trials, the substantive model would be the one for evaluating the treatment effect (e.g., treatment contrast at the last scheduled visit). The missingness process can be modeled using logistic regression. The outcome model typically would be estimated using repeated measures analysis. Both (2) and (3) can be modeled using "inclusive" strategies, incorporating a large number of potentially relevant covariates, whereas model (1) is typically focused on the primary estimand (parameter) of interest.

Consider a simple application of AIPW estimating equations in the context of the small example data set that has three post-baseline visits, which is a natural extension of the example of the IPW estimator of treatment effect in completers (IPW complete-case, or IPWCC) from Section 16.2.1 (see Seaman and Copas 2009, for other implementation).

Here, the substantive model (1) will be an ANCOVA for outcome at Time 3 with terms for intercept, baseline covariate (Y_0) and treatment indicator (Z),

$$E(Y_3 | Z, Y_0) = \beta_0 + \beta_1 Z + \beta_2 Y_0.$$

Let x_i be a row vector comprising the constant 1 and two covariates: $x_i = \{1, Y_{i0}, Z_i\}$. A possible augmented estimating equations can be

$$\sum_{i=1}^{N} \left\{ \frac{r_i}{\hat{\pi}_{i3}} x_i^T \left(y_{i3} - x_i^T \beta \right) - \left(\frac{r_i}{\hat{\pi}_{i3}} - 1 \right) \hat{E}\left(X_i^T \left(Y_{i3} - X_i^T \beta \right) | x_i, y_{i1}, y_{i2} \right) \right\} = 0$$

Here (similarly to computing IPW weights for completers for the example shown in Section 16.2), the probability of being observed at the last visit $\hat{\pi}_{i3}$ is estimated as a function of baseline and available post-baseline data

$$\pi_3(x_i, y_{i,obs}) = \Pr(R_{i3} = 1 | R_{i2} = 1, x_i, y_{i1}, y_{i2}) \Pr(R_{i2} = 1 | x_i, y_{i1})$$

The probabilities in the chain product can be estimated from two separate logistic regressions for dropouts at Times 2 and 3 (recall that there are no dropouts in the first post-baseline visit, $\Pr(R_{i1} = 1) = 1$).

Solving the above augmented estimating equations can be challenging. Let $\hat{m}_{i3} = \hat{E}(Y_{i3} | x_i, y_{i1}, y_{i2})$. It is easy to see that the equations can be written by rearranging terms as

$$\sum_{i=1}^{N} \left\{ \frac{r_{i3}}{\hat{\pi}_{i3}} x_i^T \left(y_{i3} - \hat{m}_{i3} \right) + x_i^T \left(\hat{m}_{i3} - x_i^T \beta \right) \right\} = 0$$

If the outcome model $m_3(x, y_1, y_2)$ is correctly specified, the first term vanishes in expectation and the roots of the equations (in expectation) must be the true values of the parameter vector β. With some particular choices of estimated mean function $\hat{m}_3$, the elements of the first term (shown below as a 3×1 vector S) can be made *exactly* equal to zero which, as seen shortly, would greatly simplify the estimation of parameter β

$$S = \sum_{i=1}^{N} \left\{ \frac{r_{i3}}{\hat{\pi}_{i3}} x_i^T \left(y_{i3} - \hat{m}_{i3} \right) \right\} = 0$$

Obviously, $S = 0$ can be enforced by choosing $\hat{m}_{i3}$ to be the solution of the above-mentioned IPW estimating equations. However, note that $\hat{m}_{i3}$ is sought as a function of a broader set of covariates *including all observed post-baseline outcomes*, not just those included in the covariate set X. To this end, m_{i3} is estimated as $\hat{m}_{i3}^{IPW} = \hat{m}_3(x_i, y_{i1}, y_{i2})$ by using the weighted estimating equations as a linear function in X, Y_1, and Y_2

$$\sum_{i=1}^{N} \left\{ \frac{r_{i3}}{\hat{\pi}_{i3}} \left(x_i, y_{i1}, y_{i2} \right)^T \left(y_{i3} - m_3\left(x_i, y_{i1}, y_{i2} \right) \right) \right\} = 0$$

Now that the elements of S are made exactly zero, the original augmented equations for estimating β's simplify to (unweighted) estimating equations

$$\sum_{i=1}^{N} x_i^T \left(\hat{m}_{i3}^{IPW} - x_i^T \beta \right) = 0$$

where $\hat{m}_{i3}^{IPW}$ are predicted outcomes at post-baseline visit 3 for each subject, either with observed or missing outcomes.

However, one caveat is that the predictive model m_3 includes as covariates (possibly missing) intermediate outcomes at Time 2, Y_2. Now, we can apply (recursively) the same idea and use similar weighted estimating equations for estimating $\widehat{m}_{i2}^{IPW}$

$$\sum_{i=1}^{N}\left\{\frac{r_{i2}}{\widehat{\pi}_{i2}}\left(x_i, y_{i1}\right)^T\left(y_{i2}-m_2\left(x_i, y_{i1}\right)\right)\right\}=0$$

Here, $\widehat{\pi}_{i2}$ is the estimated probability of the i-th subject not missing at Time 2. Since no outcomes Y_1 are missing at Time 1, our "recursion" stops here and we will be able to compute $\widehat{m}_{i3}^{IPW}=\widehat{m}_3\left(x_i, y_{i1}, y_{i2}\right)$, $i=1,\ldots,N$, where the missing values for Y_2 will be replaced with predicted $\widehat{m}_{i2}^{IPW}=\widehat{m}_2\left(x_i, y_{i1}\right)$.

This gives rise to the following general algorithm, suggested by Vansteelandt et al. (2010) for analysis of data with missing covariates and very similar to that implemented for repeated measures recently in O'Kelly and Ratitch (2014, section 8.4, pp. 377–378).

1. Compute subject-specific probabilities of being observed at the specific time point $\widehat{\pi}_{it}(x_1, x_2)$ using a full set of covariates partitioned into two subsets: X_1 (intended for modeling treatment effect) and X_2 (including baseline and post-baseline variables observed prior to the time point t when treatment assessment is made).
2. Predict outcome $\widehat{m}_{it}^{IPW}(x_1, x_2)$ at time point t for all subjects, whether observed or missing the outcome, using the full set of covariates and inverse probability weights from Step 1 (e.g., via appropriate generalized linear model). If some post-baseline covariates in the set X_2 are missing, iterate Steps 1 and 2 to impute them taking advantage of monotone patterns of missing data.
3. Use predicted values $\widehat{m}_{it}^{IPW}$ from Step 2 as new responses to fit a generalized linear model (GLM) on covariates from the set X_1 and obtain estimates of the coefficients.
4. Compute standard errors for coefficients of the model in Step 3 via bootstrapping the entire modeling strategy (Steps 1–3).

Details of this analytic strategy are illustrated in the next section using application to the example data set.

17.4 Example

In this section, DR estimation outlined in Section 17.3 is applied to the small example data set to evaluate the treatment effect at the last scheduled visit.

This analysis involves the following steps (the SAS code is included in Section 17.5).

1. Estimating probabilities of discontinuation (and remaining on treatment) at Times 2 and 3 using logistic regression models. Specifically, the model for probability $\hat{\pi}_{i2} = \widehat{\Pr}\left(R_{i2} = 1 \mid x_i, y_{i1}\right)$ of remaining on treatment by Time 2 included terms for baseline severity score, changes in outcome from baseline at Time 1, treatment indicator and all interactions of treatment with other covariates. Only subjects who completed the first post-baseline visit contributed to this estimate (which in our case were all randomized subjects). Probability of remaining on treatment at Time 3 was estimated as a product of conditional probabilities $\hat{\pi}_{i3} = \hat{\pi}_{i2} \times \widehat{\Pr}\left(R_{i3} = 1 \mid R_{i2} = 1, x_i, y_{i1}, y_{i2}\right)$, where the second conditional probability was estimated from a separate logistic regression with terms for the baseline score, changes from baseline at Times 1 and 2, treatment indicator and all treatment-by-covariate interactions. Only subjects completing the first two post-baseline visits contributed to this model.
2. Imputing missing values for the changes in outcome variable at Time 2 with its predicted values from the linear regression model $m_2(x_i, y_{i1})$ estimated using inverse probability weights, $w_i = 1/\hat{\pi}_{i2}$, with the same terms that were used for modeling $\hat{\pi}_{i2}$ (although this is not essential).
3. Fitting a linear regression model for completers (patients with non-missing outcomes at visit 3) $m_3\left(x_i, y_{i1}, y^*_{i2}\right)$ with weights, $w_i = 1/\hat{\pi}_{i3}$, and with the same terms that were used for modeling $\hat{\pi}_{i3}$. Missing outcomes for changes from baseline to Time 2 were replaced with predicted values from the previous step (which is emphasized in the notation with an asterisk, y^*_{i2}).
4. Finally, we use predicted values $\widehat{m}_{i3}, i = 1, \ldots, N$, obtained at previous step as "new data" to fit an ANCOVA model with baseline score and treatment indicator as covariates.
5. The point estimate for the treatment contrast from the model in #4 is the final estimate of treatment effect at Time 3 (shown in Table 17.1), $\hat{\theta}_{AIPW}$. Clearly, the standard errors and p-values reported by ANCOVA (on the basis of full sample of N subjects) are severely biased downward, as they do not account for the estimation done in previous steps, in particular, the uncertainty due to imputation of missing values.
6. We obtain valid standard errors and confidence intervals by bootstrap (shown in Table 17.1). Each bootstrap sample of size N is formed by sampling with replacement subject records (rows) of the observed $N \times p$ data matrix. Any subject irrespective of his/her missingness pattern has the same probability $1/N$ to be selected

TABLE 17.1

Estimating Treatment Contrast and Least-Squares Means Using a Doubly Robust AIPW Method for Completers (Bootstrap-Based Confidence Intervals and Standard Errors)

		Complete Data			Incomplete Data (AIPWCC)		
Treatment	Time	LSMEANS	SE	95% CI	LSMEANS	SE	95% CI
1	3	−9.86	1.05	(−11.98, −7.75)	−9.70	1.11	(−11.62, −7.17)
2	3	−13.26	1.05	(−15.37, −11.14)	−12.58	1.26	(−15.19, −10.23)
Endpoint Treatment Difference		3.39	1.49	(0.39, 6.39)	2.88	1.71	(0.18, 6.82)

in each draw and may appear multiple times in each bootstrap data set. We form 2000 bootstrap data sets, and each gives rise to the same analysis Steps 1–5 as were applied to the observed data (including re-fitting models for computing weights) resulting in point estimates $\hat{\theta}_{\text{AIPW}}^{(b)}, b = 1,\ldots,2000$, which is the bootstrap distribution of our AIPW estimate. A valid estimate of standard error can be obtained as the standard deviation of the bootstrap distribution. We further construct a 95% confidence interval by using the percentile method; that is, by taking as confidence limits the 2.5% and 97.5% percentile points of the bootstrap distribution. Other more sophisticated methods for bootstrap intervals can be used (e.g., BCa, bias-corrected and accelerated bootstrap intervals, available in SAS %BOOTCI macro and R package *boot*). Because the example data set is rather small, in some bootstrap samples modeling probability of discontinuation using logistic regression may be challenging because of quasi-complete or even complete separation making maximum likelihood estimation of parameters not possible. In many situations, this can be fixed by using a variant of penalized regression known as Firth's (1993) penalized likelihood (available in SAS logistic regression procedure). A small number of particularly unfortunate bootstrap samples (e.g., with no missing values) can be skipped.

17.5 Code Fragments

Here, we implemented a simple version of AIPW estimator similar in spirit to Vansteelandt et al. (2010). To obtain bootstrap-based standard errors, we used %BOOT and %BOOTCI macros available at http://support.sas.com/kb/24/982.html. These macros require that the computation of estimates subjected to bootstrapping was implemented by the user in a separate macro called %ANALYZE. To facilitate "by-processing" when computing bootstrap distribution of estimates, %BYSTMT macro is called within each procedure and data step inside %ANALYZE macro. The code may be not most efficient and specific to the data set at hand but easy to follow and (as we hope) generalize to other examples the reader may encounter.

CODE FRAGMENT 17.1 SAS Code for Implementing Augmenting Inverse Probability Weighting

```
 %macro analyze(data= , out= );
/* predicting prob of dropping at vis 2 */
   ODS LISTING CLOSE;
   PROC LOGISTIC DATA=&DATA DESC;
   %BYSTMT;
   MODEL R2 =TREAT BASVAL YOBS1 TREAT*YOBS1 TREAT*BASVAL/
     FIRTH MAXITER=100 ;
   OUTPUT OUT =PREDR2 P=PROB_V2;
 RUN;

/* predicting prob of dropping at vis 3 */
   PROC LOGISTIC DATA=PREDR2 DESC;
   %BYSTMT;
   MODEL R3 =TREAT BASVAL YOBS1 YOBS2 TREAT*YOBS1
     TREAT*YOBS2 TREAT*BASVAL/FIRTH MAXITER=100 ;
   OUTPUT OUT =PREDR3 P=PROB_V3;
 RUN;

/* computing weights at vis 2 and 3 */
   DATA WEIGHTS_OBS ;
    SET PREDR3;
    %BYSTMT;
    IF R2 =0 THEN DO;
      WEIGHT2=1/(1-PROB_V2);
    END;
    IF R3 =0 THEN DO;
      WEIGHT3=1/(1-PROB_V2)*1/(1-PROB_V3);
    END;
 RUN;

/* predict missing outcomes for vis 2 using IPW model*/
   PROC GENMOD DATA=WEIGHTS_OBS ;
    %BYSTMT;
    MODEL YOBS2= TREAT BASVAL YOBS1 TREAT*BASVAL
    TREAT*YOBS1;
    WEIGHT WEIGHT2;
   OUTPUT OUT=PREDY2 PRED=PRED_Y2;
 RUN;
```

```
/* replace missing values for vis 2 with predicted */
   DATA PREDY2;
    SET PREDY2 ;
   %BYSTMT;
    IF YOBS2= . THEN YOBS2=PRED_Y2;
 RUN;

/* predict outcomes for vis 3 using IPW model */
   PROC GENMOD DATA=PREDY2;
   %BYSTMT;
   MODEL YOBS3= TREAT BASVAL YOBS1 YOBS2 TREAT*BASVAL
     TREAT*YOBS1 TREAT*YOBS2;
   WEIGHT WEIGHT3;
   OUTPUT OUT=PREDY3 PRED=PRED_Y3;
 RUN;

ODS OUTPUT LSMEANS=LSDR1
      ESTIMATES=ESDR1;
PROC GENMOD DATA=PREDY3;
   %BYSTMT;
   CLASS TREAT;
   MODEL PRED_Y3= BASVAL TREAT;
   LSMEANS TREAT;
   ESTIMATE "DR ESTIMATE OF TRT" TREAT -1 1;
 RUN;

PROC TRANSPOSE DATA=LSDR1 OUT= LSMEANS_TRANSP (DROP=_NAME_)
   PREFIX=LSMEANS;
   %BYSTMT;
   VAR ESTIMATE;
   ID TREAT;
 RUN;

   DATA &OUT;
    MERGE ESDR1 (KEEP=MEANESTIMATE &BY RENAME=(MEANESTIMATE
      =TRTDIFF3))
      LSMEANS_TRANSP;
   %BYSTMT;
   RUN;
   ODS LISTING;
%MEND;

/* construct analysis data with single record per subject */
 PROC TRANSPOSE DATA=DATALONG OUT= DATAWIDE (DROP=_NAME_)
   PREFIX=YOBS;
   BY TRT SUBJECT BASVAL;
   VAR CHGDROP;
   ID TIME;
 RUN;
```

```
 DATA FOR_ANALYSIS;
   SET DATAWIDE;
   R2=(YOBS2=.);
   R3=(YOBS3=.);
   TREAT=(TRT="2");
RUN;

/* applying analyze macro to observed data */
 %LET BY=;
   %ANALYZE(DATA=FOR_ANAL, OUT=OUT_EST);

   %BOOT(DATA=FOR_ANAL, ALPHA=.05, SAMPLES=2000,
     RANDOM=123, STAT = TRTDIFF3 LSMEANS0 LSMEANS1,
     CHART=0, BIASCORR=1);

   %BOOTCI(METHOD=PERCENTILE);
```

17.6 Summary

One motivation for DR methods is to improve the efficiency of wGEEs by augmenting the estimating equations with the predicted distribution of the unobserved data, given the observed data. This augmentation also introduces the property of double robustness.

Efficient IPW estimators require three models: (1) a substantive (analysis) model that relates the outcome to explanatory variables and/or covariates of interest; (2) a model for the probability of observing the data (usually a logistic model of some form); and (3) a model for the joint distribution of the partially and fully observed data, which is compatible with the substantive model (1).

With augmented wGEEs if either model (2) or model (3) is wrong, but not both, the estimators in model (1) are still consistent. If model (1) is wrong, then estimates of all parameters will typically be inconsistent.

DR methods are fairly new and our understanding of how to best apply these methods in clinical trial scenarios is emerging.

18

MNAR Methods

18.1 Introduction

Analyses in the MNAR framework try in some manner to model or otherwise take into account the missingness process and its impact on outcomes of interest. However, moving beyond MAR to MNAR poses fundamental problems. In MAR, it is assumed that the statistical behavior of the unobserved data is the same as it had been observed, such that the unobserved data can be predicted from the observed data. Of course, the characteristics and statistical behavior of the missing data are unknown (Mallinckrodt 2013). Therefore, it is impossible to know if MAR is valid and it is impossible to know if any specific MNAR model is correct.

Moving beyond MAR to MNAR can only be done by making assumptions. Conclusions from MNAR analyses are therefore conditional on the appropriateness of the assumed model (Verbeke and Molenberghs 2000). While dependence on assumptions is not unique to MNAR analyses, an important feature of MNAR analyses (as with MAR analyses) is that (some of) the assumptions are not testable (Molenberghs et al. 1997) because the data about which the assumptions are made are missing (Laird 1994). Hence, no individual MNAR analysis can be considered definitive and multiple MNAR models can yield the same fit but imply very different dropout processes (Verbeke and Molenberghs 2000; Molenberghs and Kenward 2007). Therefore, MNAR methods are evolving to be used as sensitivity analyses more so than as primary analyses (Mallinckrodt 2013; Molenberghs et al. 2015).

18.2 Technical Details

18.2.1 Notation and Nomenclature

General classes of MNAR methods arose from different factorizations of the likelihood functions for the joint distribution of the outcome variable and the indicator variable for whether or not a data point was observed, which are often described as the measurement process and the missingness process, respectively (Verbeke and Molenberghs 2000). In this context, outcome variable indicates the hypothetical "complete" data, which are split into two parts: the actually observed part and the missing part. The "full data" consist of the complete data and missingness indicators. The following terminology is used to describe and compare the methods.

Subject $i = 1,\ldots, N$ is to be measured at times $j = 1,\ldots, n$

Y_{ij} is the random variable measured on Subject i at time j, where j can take on the values $1,\ldots, n$

R_{ij} is an indicator random variable taking on the value of 1 if Y_{ij} is observed, 0 otherwise.

Group Y_{ij} into a vector $Y_i = (Y_{i,obs}, Y_{i,mis})$

$Y_{i,obs}$ contains Y_{ij} for which $R_{ij} = 1$,

$Y_{i,mis}$ contains Y_{ij} for which $R_{ij} = 0$.

Group R_{ij} into a vector R_i that is commensurate with Y_{ij} such that all 1s are paired with the $Y_{i,obs}$ and the 0s are paired with the $Y_{i,mis}$

D_i is the time of dropout

Ψ = Parameters describing the missingness process

θ = Parameters describing the measurement process

18.2.2 Selection Models

A standard reference for selection models is Diggle and Kenward (1994). For a more recent reference, see Molembergh et al. (2015, chapter 4).

In selection models, the joint distribution of the ith subject's outcomes (Y_i) and the missingness indicators (R_i) is factored as the marginal distribution of Y_i and the conditional distribution of R_i given Y_i.

$$f(y_i, r_i|\theta, \Psi) = f(y_i|\theta)f(r_i|y_{i,obs}, y_{i,mis}, \Psi)$$

A selection model can be thought of as a multivariate model, where one variable is the continuous efficacy outcome from the primary analysis and the second variable is the binary outcome for dropout modeled via logistic regression (Mallinckrodt 2013). In ignorable models, it is assumed that the missingness process is independent of the measurement process (conditional on the measurements). An MNAR selection model explicitly ties together the measurement and missingness processes as the outcome variable (Y) from the measurement model is a predictor variable in the dropout (missingness) model (Mallinckrodt 2013).

Parametric selection models can be fit to observed data, even though there is no empirical information about the association between the values of R

(0 or 1) and Y_i. By definition, Y_i is missing in all instances when $R_i = 0$. The parametric and structural assumptions imposed on the full data distribution allow the model to be fit. However, the appropriateness of the model and its assumptions cannot be verified from the data (Verbeke and Molenberghs 2000). Interestingly, Molenberghs et al. (2015) demonstrated that multiple selection models can be fit to the same data, yielding the same fit to the data, but implying different dropout processes, which in turn alter parameters describing the observed data. In other words, there is no definitive selection model that can be fit to a data set.

An example of a selection model used in a sensitivity analysis context is provided in Chapter 21.

18.2.3 Shared-Parameter Models

Standard references for shared-parameter models include Wu and Carroll (1988) and Wu and Bailey (1989). In a shared-parameter model, a set of latent variables, latent classes, and/or random effects is assumed to drive both the Y_i (measurement) and D_i (missingness, in this case time to dropout) processes. An important version of this model further asserts that, conditional on the latent variables, Y_i and D_i are independent. A shared-parameter model can be thought of as a multivariate model, where one variable is the continuous efficacy outcome from the primary analysis and the second is (typically) a proportional hazards time to event analysis for dropout (Mallinckrodt 2013).

Specifically, the full data likelihood can be factored similarly to a selection model as the product of the marginal outcome distribution $f(y_i \mid b_i)$ and the conditional distribution of D_i given Y_i and b_i (for simplicity, the dependence on fixed parameters associated with these distributions is suppressed).

$$f(y_i, d_i, b_i) = f(y_i \mid b_i) f(d_i \mid y_i, b_i) f(b_i)$$

$$= f(y_i \mid b_i) f(d_i \mid b_i) f(b_i)$$

Note that dependence of dropout on Y_i in the last equation can be dropped because of the assumption that the outcome and dropout processes are conditionally independent given the shared random effects, b.

Therefore, the dropout and measurement models are linked by having the same random effects in both the outcome and dropout models. As in selection models, there are again untestable assumptions, namely that conditional on the latent (i.e., unobserved) random effects, Y_i and D_i are independent. This assumption is untestable because Y_i is missing in each instance when D_i is prior to the end of the trial.

18.2.4 Pattern-Mixture Models

Standard references for pattern mixture models (PMMs) include Little (1993, 1994, 1995). PMMs as originally proposed were based on the reverse factorization of the full data likelihood as compared with the selection model factorization. In PMMs, the full data likelihood is the product of the measurement process conditional on the dropout pattern and the marginal density of the missingness process.

$$f(y_i, r_i | \theta, \Psi) = f(y_i | r_i, \theta) f(r_i | \Psi)$$

As originally proposed, PMMs fit a response model for each pattern such that the observed data are a mixture of patterns weighted by their respective probabilities. Results are pooled over the various patterns for final inference. These models can be viewed from an imputation perspective in which missing values Y_{mis} are imputed from their predictive distribution.

PMMs in this imputation context are by construction under-identified, that is, over-specified. For example, in the small example data set with dropout, say the goal is to estimate the difference between treatments at Time = 3. Although more dropout patterns are possible, only the three monotonic dropout patterns were actually present; that is, there were no intermittent missing data. Hence, the three patterns were last observations at Time 3 (completer), last observation at Time 2, and last observation at Time 1. Missing values for Time 3 can be imputed separately for each of the two noncompleter dropout patterns. However, information must be borrowed because there is no information about Time 3 within the noncompleter groups. This problem can be resolved through the use of identifying restrictions wherein inestimable parameters of the incomplete patterns are set equal to (functions of) the parameters describing the distribution of other patterns (Molenberghs and Kenward 2007).

Three specific and common identifying restrictions all use data from subjects that remained in the study at time *t* to identify the distribution for those subjects that discontinued (NRC 2010). These restrictions are:

- CCMV: Complete Case Missing Values, where information is borrowed from the completers group.
- NCMV: Neighboring Case Missing Values, where information is borrowed from the nearest dropout pattern.
- ACMV: Available Case Missing Values, where information is borrowed from all patterns in which the information is available.

ACMV is important because it corresponds to MAR, thereby providing a benchmark from which deviations can be judged (Mallinckrodt 2013).

Although not commonly seen thus far in the literature, it is also possible to define patterns by reason for dropout rather than time of dropout; or, as described in the next section, patterns can be defined by treatment group using the so-called controlled imputation approaches (Carpenter et al. 2013; O'Kelly and Ratitch 2014).

18.2.5 Controlled Imputation Approaches

Recently, another family of methods referred to as controlled imputation has been discussed in the literature and used in practice (Mallinckrodt 2013). Little and Yao (1996), Carpenter and Kenward (2007), Ratitch and O'Kelly (2011), Carpenter et al. (2013), Ayela et al. (2014) and Lipkovich et al. (2016) proposed imputation approaches that can be thought of as specific versions of PMMs. The common idea in each of these approaches is to construct a principled set of imputations that are controlled in a manner that creates a specific departure from MAR.

Controlled imputation approaches benefit from having assumptions—such as specific departures from MAR—that are transparent and therefore easy to understand and debate. This is an important feature given that accounting for departures from MAR must be purely assumption driven. Therefore, controlled imputation approaches are especially useful for sensitivity analyses and are therefore explained in some detail, with example analyses in the following Section 18.4.

Two general families of controlled imputation can be considered. In the delta-adjustment approach, it is assumed that subjects who discontinued had outcomes that were worse than otherwise similar subjects that remained in the study. The difference (adjustment) in outcomes between dropouts and those who remain can be a shift in mean or slope, an absolute value, or a proportion. The adjustment is referred to as delta (Δ). The delta-adjustment can be implemented in manners resulting in increasing, decreasing, or constant departures from MAR. Recent references for delta-adjustment methods include O'Kelly and Ratitch (2014) and Molenberghs et al. (2015, chapter 19).

The second general approach to controlled imputation is the so-called reference-based imputations. In this family of approaches, after dropout (or discontinuation of randomized study drug, or initiation of rescue medication), values are imputed by making qualitative reference to another arm in the trial (Molenberghs et al. 2015, chapter 19). In other words, deviations from MAR are created by assuming that after deviating from the initially randomized treatment (either via dropout, discontinuation of study drug, and/or initiation of rescue medication), imputed values take on the characteristics of a reference group.

The intent for sensitivity analyses is to generate a conservative estimate of an MAR-based estimand. This approach can be especially useful when the reference arm can be seen as a worst plausible case departure from MAR for the treatment group (Mallinckrodt et al. 2014). In some instances, reference-based imputation has been proposed as the primary approach to estimating effectiveness that reflects change in or discontinuation of treatment (Mallinckrodt et al. 2014).

Reference-based imputations can be implemented in a manner such that the transition to the reference arm is immediate or gradual, or the deviation from reference at the time of discontinuation can be maintained. A common approach is for missing values of drug-treated subjects to be imputed such that the post-deviation imputed values take on the statistical behavior of placebo-treated subjects. That is, the benefit of the drug is assumed to immediately disappear if study drug is discontinued (and/or rescue medication is initiated).

18.3 Considerations

Review papers that describe in detail, compare, and critique selection models, and shared parameter models and PMMs by identifying restrictions include Little (1995), Hogan and Laird (1997), Little and Rubin (2002), Diggle et al. (2002), Fitzmaurice et al. (2004), and Molenberghs and Kenward (2007). The NRC guidance on prevention and treatment of missing data summarizes the advantages and disadvantages of selection models and PMMS as follows (NRC 2010).

The basic idea behind selection models is intuitive: specify a relationship between the probability of discontinuation and the outcome of interest, including the unobserved outcomes. However, operationalizing that idea can be problematic. The predictive distribution of missing responses is typically intractable, making it difficult to understand exactly how the missing observations are being treated for a given selection model. This is especially the case given that the outcomes and probability of discontinuation are linked on the logit scale. Moreover, selection models are sensitive to parametric assumptions about the full data distribution. This concern can be alleviated to some degree via semi-parametric selection models. Many of these same comments can be applied to shared-parameter models.

Like selection models, PMMs start from an intuitive premise: conditional on the observed data, subjects with complete data have different outcome distributions than subjects with incomplete data. PMMs with identifying restrictions are transparent with respect to how missing observations are being imputed because the within-pattern models specify the predictive distributions directly.

However, PMMs can be computationally difficult. Ironically, this issue is especially problematic when, as would be hoped, the rates of missing data are low such that the parameters associated with sparse patterns cannot be estimated reliably. In addition, although the identifying restrictions are transparent, it is not necessarily easy for nonstatisticians to understand exactly what they imply about the missing values.

One of the NRC expert panel's recommendations (NRC 2010) was that methods for handling missing data be explained in protocols in a manner easily understood by clinicians. Others have questioned if, and if so, how this can be done. For example, Permutt (2015b) stated:

> No doubt there are clinicians who understand the assumptions of inverse probability weighting, pattern mixture models, and multiple imputation along with clinicians who do not. However, much of the language in the NRC report is inaccessible to many of the clinicians who serve as study investigators or who evaluate new drug applications. Furthermore, a general understanding of the methods does not suffice: what is required is to understand, so as to evaluate their plausibility, the specific assumptions being made by a specific model with specific covariates in a specific setting.

For example, consider trying to explain to clinicians how the various MNAR methods work. It is known that all methods rely on untestable assumptions. But explaining exactly what those assumptions are in a selection model, shared-parameter model, or even a PMM with traditional identifying restrictions (e.g., ACMV, CCMV, NCMV) is not straight-forward. Simply put, it is hard to understand exactly how these methods treat missing data, especially for nonstatisticians.

Therefore, for sensitivity analyses of confirmatory trials in a regulatory setting, selection models, shared-parameter models, and PMMs with traditional identifying restrictions may have limited utility.

Transparency and ease of understanding are far easier with delta-adjustment and reference-based imputations. For example, in a reference-based imputation, it is easier to understand the implications of assuming that drug-treated patients after early discontinuation of study medication have outcomes similar to placebo-treated patients; or, for delta-adjustment, that drug-treated patients after early discontinuation have outcomes worse than otherwise similar drug-treated patients who did not dropout by an amount equal to delta.

These advantages over earlier MNAR methods are leading to a wider use of controlled imputations, especially in regulatory settings (Permutt 2015b). Therefore, means to implement controlled imputations are covered in the next section.

18.4 Examples—Implementing Controlled Imputation Methods

18.4.1 Delta-Adjustment

Typically, only the experimental arm is delta-adjusted while the control arm is handled using an MAR-based approach. However, it is easy to delta-adjust each arm, using the same or different deltas. Whether or not to apply different dropout models by treatment arm is an important consideration for all MNAR approaches, not just delta-adjustment.

The magnitude of the deviation from MAR in an MNAR model is generally proportional to the amount of missing data. Therefore, unless dropout rates vary widely between treatments, fitting the same MNAR model to all treatment groups will typically have a relatively small effect on treatment contrasts. However, different MNAR models for each treatment arm provides greater opportunity for changes to estimated treatment contrasts compared with the corresponding MAR result. Delta-adjustment has thus far typically been implemented by applying delta to only the drug-treated arm(s) of the trial, leaving the control arm unadjusted.

Two general families of delta-adjustment can be applied: marginal and conditional. In the marginal approach, the delta-adjustment is applied after imputation of all missing values and the adjustment at one visit does not influence imputed values at other visits. Therefore, the marginal approach with a constant delta will result in a constant departure from MAR over time.

In the conditional approach, the delta-adjustment is applied in a sequential, visit-by-visit manner. In this approach, missing values are imputed as a function of both actually observed and previously imputed delta-adjusted values. In the conditional approach with delta applied to each visit, the deltas accumulate over time, resulting in a departure from MAR that increases over time. Alternatively, delta applied to only the first missing visit results in a departure from MAR that decreases over time (O'Kelly and Ratitch 2014).

A single delta-adjustment analysis allows testing if a specific departure from MAR overturns the MAR result. However, the delta-adjustment method can also be applied repeatedly as a progressive stress test to find how extreme the delta must be to overturn the MAR result. This is the so-called tipping point approach (O'Kelly and Ratitch 2014).

To illustrate the delta-adjustment approach, consider the small example data set with dropout. The SAS code fragment to implement the delta-adjustment controlled imputation approach is listed in Section 18.5 (Code Fragment 18.1). The SAS implementation of delta-adjustment uses the conditional approach where delta-adjustment at previous imputations influences the current imputation.

The top panel of Table 18.1 summarizes results from applying a delta-adjustment of 3 points to the drug-treated arm only using several approaches. First, adjustment was applied to only the endpoint visit (Time 3). That is, delta = 0 at Time 2. Even though the SAS implementation uses the conditional method, this implementation yields the same result as a marginal approach. That is, using delta = 0 at Time 2 is equivalent to a Time 2 delta that does not influence Time 3 imputed values. The bottom panel of Table 18.1 summarizes results from assuming progressively larger values of delta applied to only the endpoint visit, which again is equivalent to a marginal approach.

TABLE 18.1

Results from Various Delta-Adjustment Approaches to the Small Example Data Set with Dropout

Delta	Endpoint Contrast	Standard Error	P	Deviation from MAR
Delta = 3				
No adjustment[a]	2.98	1.71	0.082	0.00
Time 2 only	2.70	1.73	0.119	0.28
Time 3 only	2.25	1.76	0.201	0.73
Time 2 and Time 3	1.97	1.79	0.271	1.01
Delta Applied to Endpoint Visit Only				
No adjustment[a]	2.98	1.71	0.082	0.00
Delta = 1	2.74	1.73	0.103	0.24
Delta = 2	2.49	1.74	0.152	0.49
Delta = 3	2.25	1.76	0.201	0.73
Delta = 4	2.01	1.79	0.260	0.97
Delta = 5	1.77	1.82	0.323	1.21

[a] Delta = 0, the MAR result. Results do not exactly match previous multiple imputation results due to different seed values.

In both panels of Table 18.1, results from using delta = 0, that is no adjustment, is the MAR result to which delta-adjustment results are compared. In addition, interpretation of results is further facilitated by noting the (monotone) missing data patterns of the treatment arm to which the various deltas were applied. In the drug-treated arm (trt 2), three subjects had missing values at Time 2; those same three subjects plus three additional subjects had missing values at Time 3.

The top panel illustrates that applying the same delta to the endpoint visit has greater impact on the endpoint contrast than applying that delta to missing values at Time 2 only. This stems from two reasons. First, fewer patients have missing data at Time 2 than at Time 3. Hence, delta-adjustment is applied to fewer patients. In addition, applying delta to Time 2 imputed values impacts the endpoint contrast only indirectly via the correlation implied by the imputation model between Time 2 outcomes and Time 3 outcomes. This is another example of "shrinkage estimation" that was explained in Section 5.4.

Applying delta to Time 2 and Time 3 had a greater impact on the endpoint contrast than applying delta to Time 3 only. This is because the total effect of the delta-adjustment on the endpoint contrast—in the conditional approach—is essentially the sum of the effect from directly adjusting imputed values for Time 3 and the indirect effect on Time 3 imputed values by having adjusted the Time 2 imputed values that are used as part of the Time 3 imputations.

The bottom panel of Table 18.1 illustrates that increasing the delta applied to the endpoint visit has a consistent and therefore predictable effect for a given missing data pattern. In this example, for each 1-point increment of delta, the endpoint contrast was reduced by 0.24 points. This result is intuitive in that 24% of the values were missing for Treatment 2 at Time 3. In this simple illustration of applying what is essentially a marginal delta, the effect of delta-adjustment on the endpoint contrast can be analytically determined as follows: Let π = the percentage of missing values at the endpoint visit, and Δ = the delta-adjustment applied to the endpoint visit only. The change to the endpoint contrast = $\Delta \times \pi$.

From this simple, marginal approach to delta-adjustment it is easy to appreciate several important factors. First, it shows directly the impact of the fraction of missing values on the sensitivity of the MAR result to departures from MAR. If π is cut in half, Δ must double in order for the adjustment to have the same net effect on the endpoint contrast. It is also easy to see how progressively increasing delta can be used as a stress test to ascertain how severe departures from MAR must be in order to overturn inferences from the MAR result. However, the progressive stress test is not needed here because in this small example data set, results with dropout were not significant in the MAR result.

18.4.2 Reference-Based Imputation

Reference-based imputations can be tailored to specific scenarios. One variant of reference-based imputation, termed jump to reference (J2R), is implementation such that imputed values for subjects who discontinue the active arm immediately take on the attributes of the reference arm (placebo). That is, the treatment benefit in subjects who discontinue the active arm disappears immediately upon discontinuation. In a second approach, called copy reference (CR), the imputations result in a treatment effect that gradually diminishes after dropout in accordance with the correlation structure implied by the imputation model. In a third approach, called copy increment from reference (CIR), the treatment effect after discontinuation is maintained by matching changes after withdrawal to changes in the reference arm (Carpenter et al. 2013). With regard to assessing sensitivity, J2R results in the greatest departure from MAR.

Reference-based imputations as described above can also be interpreted as estimates of certain effectiveness estimands in that they explicitly model change in or discontinuation of treatment. In the effectiveness context, the J2R approach would be useful for symptomatic treatments with short duration of action where the benefits of the drug rapidly disappear after discontinuation. The CR approach would be useful for symptomatic treatments with long duration of action. The CIR approach would be appropriate for treatments thought to alter the underlying disease process (disease modification) (Mallinckrodt 2013).

It is perhaps easiest to understand these approaches by graphically depicting what they do in comparison to traditional multiple imputation based on MAR. These depictions are in Figures 18.1 through 18.4. Additional technical details can be found in Molenberghs et al. (2015, chapter 19).

Conceptually, consider traditional MI based on MAR as involving a regression on residuals (illustrated in Figure 18.1). Each subject's deviation from their respective group mean, while that subject was observed (shown as brown vertical segments extending from the line designating the treated mean), is used to impute the missing residuals. The actual imputed value (shown as "X" placed at the end of the red vertical segments) is the sum of the imputed residual and the group mean. In MAR, the imputed value is based on the mean of the group to which the subject was originally randomized. In J2R, the regression on residuals is again applied. However, imputed values are based on adding the imputed residuals to the reference arm mean—not the arm to which the subject had been randomized.

In CR (Figure 18.3), as in J2R (Figure 18.2), the regressed residuals are again added to the reference arm. However, in CR, the residual is determined by the deviation of observed values from the reference arm (shown as the upper blue line)—not the arm to which the subject was initially randomized, as is the case for MAR-based MI and J2R. This feature has the effect of giving credit to the drug arm for any benefit resulting from the drug while the subject adhered to treatment; that benefit declines over time in accordance with the correlations implied by the imputation model.

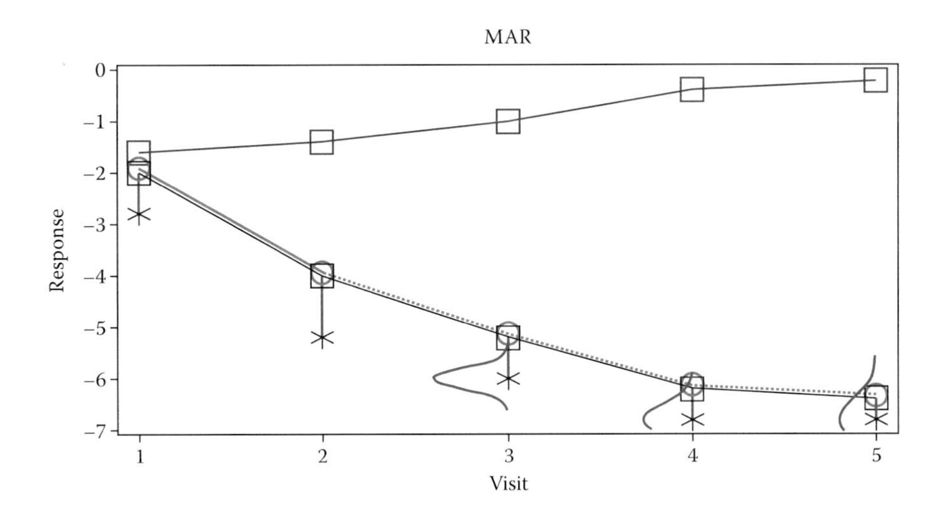

FIGURE 18.1
Illustration of multiple imputation based on MAR.

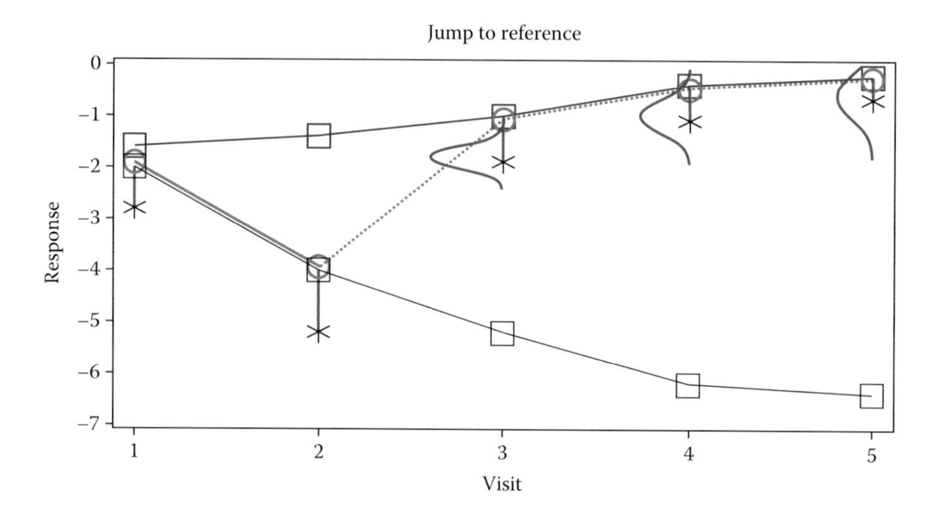

FIGURE 18.2
Illustration of jump to reference-based imputation.

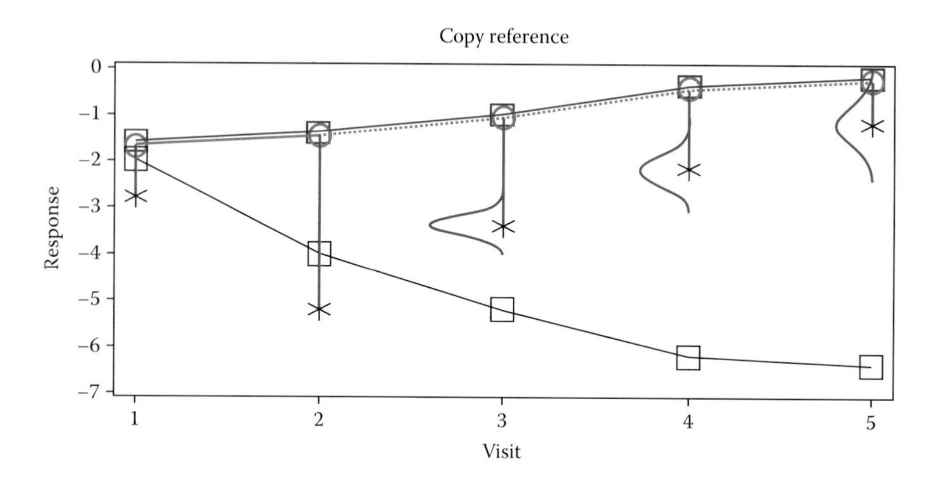

FIGURE 18.3
Illustration of copy reference-based imputation.

In CIR (Figure 18.4), residuals are determined as in MAR-based MI and J2R. However, missing values are imputed based on adding the regressed residuals to a hypothetical mean (shown as the dotted green line on the graph) that maintains the same deviation between the reference mean and the randomized group that was seen at the time of discontinuation.

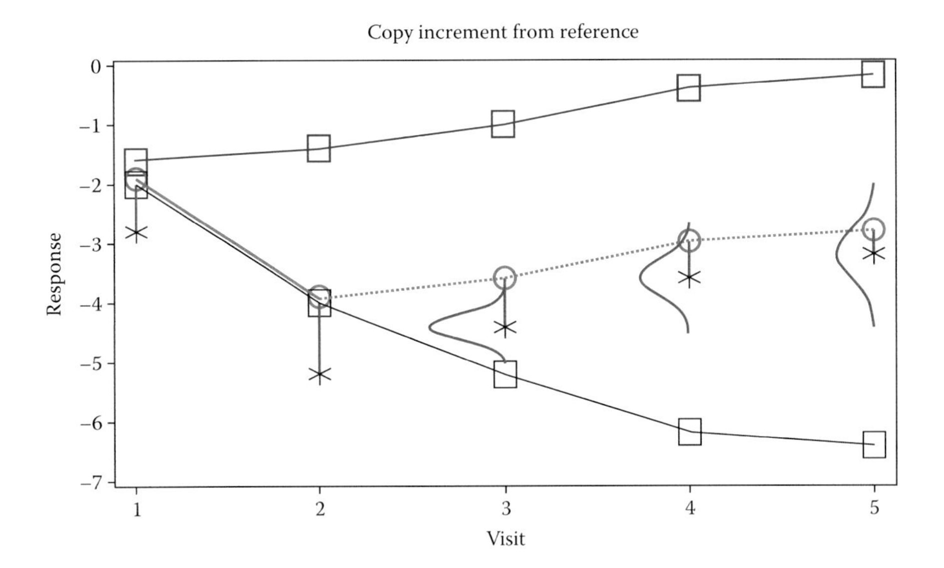

FIGURE 18.4
Illustration of copy increment from reference-based imputation.

Commercially available software to implement reference-based imputations is limited. It is possible to implement the CR approach in SAS. However, other variants must be implemented using specialty software. The Drug Information Association's (DIA) Scientific Working Group on missing data has SAS macros available at missingdata.org.uk, under the DIA working group tab, to implement a variety of reference-based imputation approaches, along with other specialty software tools. The code fragment to implement CR in SAS for the small example data set with dropout is listed in Section 18.5 (Code Fragment 18.2), and results are summarized in Table 18.2.

The deviation from MAR, based on difference in treatment contrast from the MAR analysis, when applying CR was 0.31 (2.98 versus 2.69). This deviation is smaller than would usually be the case in actual scenarios because only two post-baseline visits had missing values and these outcomes were strongly correlated.

TABLE 18.2
Results from Copy Reference Analyses of the Small Example Data Set with Dropout

Method	Endpoint Contrast	Standard Error	P	Deviation from MAR
MAR-based MI	2.98	1.71	0.082	0.00
Copy reference	2.69	1.64	0.103	0.31

18.5 Code Fragments

CODE FRAGMENT 18.1 SAS Code for Delta-Adjustment Controlled Multiple Imputation

```
/* 3 point adjustment at last visit only. No missing values
   At first post-baseline visit */
PROC MI DATA=y1 SEED=1214 OUT=outmi round=1 NIMPUTE=1000;
      by trt;
      class trt;
      monotone method=reg;
      var basval y1 y2 y3;
        mnar adjust(y2 /delta=0 adjustobs=(trt='2'));
        mnar adjust(y3 /delta=3 adjustobs=(trt='2'));
run;

ods output diffs = diffs;
proc Mixed data=finalY;
      class trt time subject;
      model y= basval trt time trt*time basval*time/ddfm=kr
         outp=check;
      repeated time / subject=subject type = un;
      by _Imputation_;
      lsmeans trt*time/diffs;
      id subject time ;
run;

data diffs2;
  set diffs;
  if time = _time and _time = 3;
run;

proc mianalyze data=diffs2;
  modeleffects estimate;
  stderr stderr;
run;
```

CODE FRAGMENT 18.2 SAS Code for the Copy Reference Method of Reference-Based Imputation

```
PROC MI DATA=y1 SEED=1214 OUT=outmi round=1 NIMPUTE=1000;
        class trt;
      monotone method=reg;
      var basval y1 y2 y3;
        mnar model (y2 / modelobs=(trt='1'));
        mnar model (y3 / modelobs=(trt='1'));
```

```
run;

ods output diffs = diffs;
proc Mixed data=finalY;
      class trt time subject;
      model y= basval trt time trt*time basval*time/ddfm=kr
         outp=check;
      repeated time / subject=subject type = un;
      by _Imputation_;
      lsmeans trt*time/diffs;
        id subject time ;
run;

data diffs2;
  set diffs;
  if time = _time and _time = 3;
run;

proc mianalyze data=diffs2;
  modeleffects estimate;
  stderr stderr;
run;
```

18.6 Summary

MNAR analyses model or otherwise take into account the missingness process and its impact on outcomes of interest. It is impossible to know if MAR is valid and it is impossible to know if any specific MNAR model is correct. Moving beyond MAR to MNAR can only be done by making (untestable) assumptions. Therefore, MNAR methods are evolving to be used as sensitivity analyses in support of an MAR-based primary analysis more so than as primary analyses.

In selection models, the joint distribution of the ith subject's outcomes (Y_i) and the missingness indicators (R_i) is factored as the marginal distribution of Y_i and the conditional distribution of R_i given Y_i. Selection models can be thought of as multivariate models, where one variable is the continuous efficacy outcome from the primary analysis and the second variable is the binary outcome for dropout modeled via logistic regression.

In a shared-parameter model, a set of latent variables, latent classes, and/or random effects is assumed to drive both the Y_i (measurement) and D_i (missingness) processes. Conditional on the latent variables, Y_i and D_i are assumed independent. A shared-parameter model can be thought of as a multivariate model, where one variable is the continuous efficacy outcome from the primary analysis and the second is (typically) a proportional hazards time to event analysis for dropout.

PMMs as originally proposed were based on the reverse factorization of the full data likelihood as for the selection model. Hence, the full data likelihood is the product of the measurement process conditional on the dropout pattern and the marginal density of the missingness process. As originally proposed, PMMs fit a response model for each pattern such that the observed data are a mixture of patterns weighted by their respective probabilities. Results are pooled over the various patterns for final inference.

It is hard to understand exactly how these methods treat missing data, especially for nonstatisticians. Therefore, as sensitivity analyses, especially for confirmatory trials in a regulatory setting, their utility is perhaps limited.

Delta-adjustment and reference-based imputations are transparent and easy to understand. These advantages are leading to a wider use of controlled imputations, especially as sensitivity analyses.

In reference-based imputation, deviations from MAR are typically created by assuming that drug-treated subjects after early discontinuation or initiation of rescue have outcomes similar to those in the reference group. In delta-adjustment, deviations from MAR are created by assuming that drug-treated patients after early discontinuation have outcomes worse than otherwise similar drug-treated patients who did not dropout by an amount equal to delta.

19

Methods for Incomplete Categorical Data

19.1 Introduction

19.1.1 Overview

In Chapter 10, it was noted that a number of issues in modeling categorical data could be handled in a similar manner as for continuous data. These similarities included modeling trends over time and accounting for within-subject correlations. In addition, the principles regarding analysis of incomplete data previously discussed for continuous outcomes also apply to categorical outcomes. For example, the missing data mechanisms (Chapter 12) apply to categorical data in essentially the same manner as for continuous data.

As such, the general methods of dealing with incomplete continuous outcomes can be considered for incomplete categorical outcomes. For the reasons detailed in Chapters 12 and 13, simple and ad hoc approaches to handling missing data are not appropriate for either continuous or categorical outcomes. Methods in the MNAR framework have an important place in the overall analysis plan, but that importance is primarily as sensitivity analyses. Therefore, as with continuous outcomes, analyses for incomplete categorical data center on likelihood-based approaches, multiple imputation and weighted generalized estimating equations (wGEE).

19.1.2 Likelihood-Based Methods

In continuous data, the linear mixed model provides a unifying analytic framework because the resulting estimates of fixed effect parameters have both a marginal and hierarchical model interpretation (Molenberghs and Kenward 2007). In other words, regardless of whether the scientific question is geared to marginal inference, where trial results are extended to the general patient population, or hierarchical inference, where trial results are conditional on the patients in the study, the same model can provide valid answers to both questions. However, this connection between the model families does not exist in nonnormal data. Therefore, analysis method must be tailored to the scientific question.

Likelihood-based methods are appealing for analyses of continuous data because of their flexible ignorability properties if missing data arise from an MAR mechanism (Chapter 14). However, Chapter 10 noted that the increased computational complexity inherent to categorical outcomes necessitate approximations. Although a full discussion of how these approximations influence results is beyond the present scope, the important implication is that the plausibility of being able to ignore the missing data in approximation-based likelihood-type analyses of categorical data is compromised over that seen with continuous data.

Therefore, analyses of incomplete categorical data may rely more on multiple imputation and wGEE than incomplete continuous data.

19.1.3 Multiple Imputation

As with continuous data, missing categorical data can be imputed by multiple imputation, followed by an analytic approach that would have been suitable had the data been complete (Schafer 2003). See Chapter 15 for details on and implementations of multiple imputation in continuous data.

Multiple imputation can be especially straightforward and useful for the analyses of dichotomized continuous variables. For example, assume, as was done in Chapter 10, that in the small example data set a change from baseline of 50% is used as the cut off to define clinically meaningful improvement. Each efficacy response on the original, continuous scale is categorized as clinically meaningful improvement: "yes"/"no."

Imputations could proceed to fill in the missing binary outcome. However, given the loss of information from dichotomizing continuous outcomes, it may be preferable to impute the missing values on the continuous scale and then categorize all outcomes, both observed and imputed, as meeting the criteria for response "yes" or "no."

19.1.4 Weighted Generalized Estimating Equations

Generalized estimating equations can circumvent the computational complexity of likelihood-based analyses of categorical data, and is therefore a viable alternative whenever interest is restricted to the mean parameters (treatment difference, time evolutions, effect of baseline covariates, etc.). In GEE, the missing data mechanism must be MCAR in order to be ignorable. Hence, similar to continuous data, weighted generalized estimating equations have been proposed to extend ignorability to both MCAR and MAR (see Chapter 16 for details of analyses in continuous data).

As detailed in Chapter 12, GEE is valid only under MCAR, and hence the interest in weighted GEE. With categorical data, as with continuous data, the idea is to weight each subject's contribution in the GEEs by the inverse probability that the subject does not drop out (i.e., remains on the assigned treatment) at a given time point (visit-wise weighting), or by the inverse probably of having observed the dropout pattern (subject level weighting).

Hence in practice, the only major modification needed for wGEE of categorical data compared with continuous data is to specify a link function for the means to account for nonlinearity and an appropriate distribution for the residuals. For binary data, the logit link is a common choice.

19.2 Examples

19.2.1 Multiple Imputation

This subsection illustrates two common analyses for categorical outcomes. The first example is a derived binary outcome (clinical response), and the second is an ordinal variable (PGI-Improvement). Similar examples were presented in Chapter 10 for analyses of complete data.

The derived binary outcome is defined as at least 50% improvement from baseline in HAMD depression score at the last scheduled evaluation. The MI analysis first imputes the underlying continuous scale data as illustrated in Code Fragment 15.1. Following imputation, the binary outcome is derived by applying the responder criterion to the observed and imputed values in each of the imputed (completed) data sets. Then, the primary analysis model is applied.

This primary analysis model is a logistic regression for responder status at Time 3, with treatment and baseline severity fitted as covariates. Finally, Rubin's combination rules are applied to produce a single estimate of treatment effect (converted to the odds ratio scale), along with the associated p-value and 95% confidence interval. A similar imputation strategy was evaluated by simulations and performed reasonably well (Lipkovich et al. 2005). The code to implement this analysis is presented in Code Fragment 19.1 (Section 19.3). Results are summarized in Table 19.1 and compared with the results from the complete data set using the same logistic model.

The second example is MI for the ordinal variable PGI Improvement (PGIIMP). To make the exercise more interesting, additional missing values resulting in nonmonotone missingness were created, similar to what was done in Section 15.3 when illustrating the MCMC method for multivariate normal data. Here, nonmonotone methods for imputing categorical data without easily specified joint distributions are illustrated. The SAS code to implement an approach using the so-called fully conditional specification (FCS) is presented in Code Fragment 19.2 (Section 19.3).

Once the completed data sets have been created, ordinal logistic regression is used to estimate the log odds ratio for the treatment effect and the associated standard errors. These results are passed to PROC MIANALYZE

TABLE 19.1

Treatment Contrasts and Least-Squares Means for Multiple Imputation of a Derived Binary Outcome Compared with Results from Complete Data Using a Logistic Model for Responder Status at Time 3[a]

	Complete Data (Logistic Model for Responder Status)		Incomplete Data (MI) (Imputing Underlying Continuous Score)	
Treatment	**LSMEANS**	**CI (95%)**	**LSMEANS**	**CI (95%)**
1	0.60	(0.38, 0.78)	0.49	(0.26, 0.71)
2	0.92	(0.72, 0.98)	0.86	(0.55, 0.97)
Endpoint Treatment Difference	7.83	(1.45, 42.3) (p=0.0167)	6.39	(1.01, 40.43) (p=0.0487)

[a] LSMEANS are on probability scale, treatment difference = odds ratio.

TABLE 19.2

Treatment Contrasts and Least-Squares Means Estimated by Multiple Imputation and from Complete Data: Ordinal Logistic Model for PGI Improvement at Time 3[a]

		Complete Data (Ordinal Logistic Model for PGIIMP Score)		Incomplete Data (MI) (Imputing PGIIMP Score Using FCS with Logistic Model)	
Treatment	**PGIIMP**	**LSMEANS**	**CI (95%)**	**LSMEANS**	**CI (95%)**
1	≤ 1	0.10	(0.04, 0.25)	0.09	(0.025, 0.29)
1	≤ 2	0.55	(0.36, 0.73)	0.56	(0.34, 0.77)
1	≤ 3	0.74	(0.55, 0.87)	0.73	(0.49, 0.88)
2	≤ 1	0.30	(0.16, 0.49)	0.34	(0.17, 0.56)
2	≤ 2	0.82	(0.64, 0.92)	0.87	(0.66, 0.96)
2	≤ 3	0.91	(0.78, 0.97)	0.93	(0.76, 0.98)
Endpoint Treatment Difference		3.64	(1.18, 11.27) (p = 0.0249)	4.93	(1.17, 20.75) (p = 0.0298)

[a] LSMEANS are probabilities PGIIMP <= level, treatment difference are = odds ratios.

to conduct combined (pooled) inference. We also obtain MI inference for the probabilities of not exceeding each level of PGIIMP by treatment arm. The results are shown in Table 19.2.

19.2.2 Weighted Generalized Estimating Equation-Based Examples

Weighted generalized estimating equations can be applied to incomplete categorical data using the methods and principles outlined in Chapter 16 for analyses of continuous incomplete data, along with an appropriate link function and error distribution as described in Chapter 10.

19.3 Code Fragments

CODE FRAGMENT 19.1 SAS Code for Multiple Imputation Analysis of Derived Binary Outcome (Responder Analysis)

```
/* perform multiple imputation of monotone data from normal
distribution */
   proc MI data = all2_transp2 out = all2_miout nimpute
   =1000 seed =123;
   by trt;
   monotone method=reg;
   var basval Yobs1 Yobs2 Yobs3;
   run;
   /* compute responder status on imputed data set */
   data all2_miout;
   set all2_miout;
   responder=(Yobs3/basval <= - 0.5);
run;

/* apply analysis model to imputed data */
   proc sort data=all2_miout ; by _Imputation_; run;
        ods output Lsmeans=Bin_ls_imp
              Estimates =bin_est_imp;
        proc genmod data=all2_miout desc;
        by _Imputation_;
        class trt ;
        model responder=trt basval/error=bin link=logit;
        estimate "trt effect at vis 3" trt -1 1;
        lsmeans trt ;
        run;

/** combine estimates using Rubin's rules **/

ods output ParameterEstimates=es_logist_mi_final;
proc mianalyze data=bin_est_imp ;
 modeleffects LBetaEstimate;
 stderr StdErr;
run;
data es_logist_mi_final;
 set es_logist_mi_final;
 OR=exp(Estimate);
 OR_upper=exp(UCLMean);
 OR_lower=exp(LCLMean);
run;

proc sort data=Bin_ls_imp ; by trt; run;
 ods output ParameterEstimates=ls_logist_mi_final;
 proc mianalyze data=Bin_ls_imp ;
```

```
  by trt ;
  modeleffects Estimate;
  stderr StdErr;
run;

  data ls_logist_mi_final;
  set ls_logist_mi_final;
  prob_est=1/(1+exp(-1*Estimate));
  prob_upper=1/(1+exp(-1*UCLMean));
  prob_lower=1/(1+exp(-1*LCLMean));
run;
```

CODE FRAGMENT 19.2 SAS Code for Multiple Imputation Analysis of PGI Improvement as Categorical Outcome Using Fully Conditional Specification Method

```
proc mi data=all3_transpA out = all4_miout_fcs nimpute =1000
seed =123;
  class trt PGIIMPGR1 PGIIMPGR2 PGIIMPGR3;
  fcs logistic(PGIIMPGR2/details)
  logistic(PGIIMPGR3/details);
 var trt basval PGIIMPGR1 PGIIMPGR2 PGIIMPGR3;
/* imputation order is specified by var statement*/
run;

ods output Estimates =es_logit_imp
      Lsmeans=ls_logit_imp;

proc genmod data=all4_miout_fcs;
 by _Imputation_;
 class trt;
 model PGIIMPGR3 =trt basval/error=mult link=clogit;
 estimate "trt effect at vis 3" trt -1 1;
 lsmeans trt;
run;

/* combine estimates using Rubin's rules */
 ods output ParameterEstimates=es_logist_mi_pooled;
 proc mianalyze data=es_logit_imp;
 modeleffects LBetaEstimate;
 stderr StdErr;
run;

data es_logist_mi_pooled;
 set es_logist_mi_pooled;
 OR=exp(Estimate);
 OR_upper=exp(UCLMean);
 OR_lower=exp(LCLMean);
```

```
run;
  proc sort data=ls_logit_imp; by trt PGIIMPGR3; run;
  ods output ParameterEstimates=ls_logist_mi_pooled;
  proc mianalyze data=ls_logit_imp;
  by trt PGIIMPGR3;
  modeleffects Estimate;
  stderr StdErr;
run;

data ls_logist_mi_pooled;
  set ls_logist_mi_pooled;
  prob_est=1/(1+exp(- 1*Estimate));
  prob_upper=1/(1+exp(- 1*UCLMean));
  prob_lower=1/(1+exp(- 1*LCLMean));
run;
```

Section IV

A Comprehensive Approach to Study Development and Analyses

The intent of Section IV is *not* to provide specific guidance on analytic approaches for specific scenarios. Rather, the intent is to illustrate how the principles for analyses of longitudinal data discussed in earlier parts of this book can be generally applied. Two example data sets are used for illustration in Section IV. These data sets were described in Chapter 4 as large data sets, one with a high rate of dropout and one with a low rate of dropout. Although these data were somewhat contrived for convenience, they maintain most of the characteristics of the original data, and are therefore realistic and convenient examples.

20

Developing Statistical Analysis Plans

20.1 Guiding Principles

Recalling the process chart for study development introduced in Chapter 2, development of analysis plans begins with considering the objectives of the trial, which are determined from the decisions to be made from the trial. Estimands are chosen to address the objectives. A design is chosen to focus on the primary objective, and to also address key secondary objectives to the degree feasible. With clarity on objectives, estimands and design, analyses and sensitivity analyses can be chosen. It is important to appreciate the benefits from this being an iterative process, essentially then jointly considering all aspects of the process. Iteration can lead to objectives, estimands, and designs that are more relevant given the circumstances, and analyses that are aligned with the design, estimands, and objectives.

To illustrate, reconsider the example introduced in Section 2.6: a short-term, acute phase clinical trial is conducted where it is anticipated that the extensive efforts to maximize adherence will result in 95% of patients remaining on the initially assigned study medication. With this level of adherence, plausible departures from MAR are unlikely to overturn positive findings for a de jure estimand. Given this strong compliance and the highly-controlled study conditions, a de jure primary estimand may be most relevant. However, in a long-term trial in the same setting but with a design more similar to clinical practice, the more pragmatic nature of the trial and the inevitable loss of adherence over time may result in a de facto primary estimand being most relevant.

No single estimand is likely to meet the needs of all stakeholders. De jure and de facto estimands each have strengths and limitations, and more fully understanding a drug's effects requires understanding results from both families of estimands. Therefore, analysis plans need to address multiple estimands. Therefore, it is especially important that the analysis plans make clear which analyses address which estimands.

Choosing and specifying an analytic approach for a particular situation requires clarity on the data to be used, the method of estimation, and the model. A key aspect of choosing data is whether or not assessments after discontinuation of the initially randomized intervention and/or initiation of rescue medication should be included in the analysis. This is of course contingent on the estimand. However, including versus not including post-rescue data can have an important impact on results and therefore sample size implications must be considered.

For example, consider a scenario where estimand 1 from Table 2.1 (de facto estimand for effects of treatment regimen, post-rescue data is included) is of scientific interest. However, the medical condition addressed by the intervention is rare and patients are hard to enroll. Given that assessing pragmatic effectiveness via estimand 1 may require considerably more patients and therefore delay results of the trial for years, another estimand may be chosen as primary with estimand 1 evaluated secondarily.

Decisions regarding method of estimation are inherently tied to the model to be used. For continuous data, likelihood-based estimation in mixed-effect models provides a unifying framework for addressing marginal and random effect inference. With continuous data, the flexible ignorability property of likelihood-based estimation with regard to missing data is appealing. However, multiple imputation and weighted GEE analyses are very useful, especially for more inclusive modeling where additional covariates can be included to help account for missing data. Multiple imputation can also be useful when covariates are missing.

It is important to appreciate, however, that multiple imputation is, as the name denotes, an imputation technique, not a method of estimation. Even if the imputation step is valid and implemented via a principled likelihood-based model, the analysis model could be misspecified, resulting in invalid inference. The analyst must choose therefore also choose an appropriate method and model to analyze the data.

For categorical data, the elegant properties of the linear mixed-effects models with normal errors no longer hold and different analyses are needed for marginal inference versus hierarchical (random effects) inference. Often, interest in clinical trials will be more so on marginal inference that applies to the entire population as opposed to random effects inference that is specific to the subjects in the trial.

Moreover, the lack of simple specifications for multivariate distributions with categorical data leads to additional analytic complexity, which necessitates approximations for likelihood-based estimation. These approximations mean that missing data arising from an MAR mechanism are no longer ignorable and, as with GEE, the more restrictive requirement of MCAR is needed for ignorability. Therefore, for categorical data, multiple imputation and weighted GEE are particularly useful.

An overarching consideration regarding objectives is whether the study is considered exploratory (e.g., phase I or phase 2) or confirmatory (phase 3). The ICH E9 guidance (http://www.ich.org/fileadmin/Public_Web_Site/ICH_Products/Guidelines/Efficacy/E9/Step4/E9_Guideline.pdf) outlines the need for and benefit from pre-specification of statistical analyses.

These benefits include objectivity and avoidance of result-guided analytic choices that could bias inferences. Compared with confirmatory studies, analytic plans for exploratory studies can have greater flexibility, thereby relying more on methods and models developed from the data in the study. Confirmatory studies generally rely more on pre-specification of analyses. The basic idea is to exploit flexibility of exploratory studies to learn as much as possible, and then confirm those learnings in subsequent studies.

However, regardless of scenario, pre-specification of analyses to the degree appropriate is useful. The fundamental purpose of statistical analysis plans is to pre-specify analyses in order to provide the necessary scientific rigor and objectivity sought in the E9 guidance. Although pre-specification avoids bias from result-guided analyses, it also means that assumptions about the data must be made. It is therefore important to understand the characteristics of the anticipated data. Previous experience, especially results from earlier phase studies of the same intervention, can be extremely valuable in anticipating future data.

Consequently, exploratory phase analysis plans can be developed to help inform the decisions needed for pre-specification of analyses in confirmatory trials. To that end, there is a clear connection between exploratory and confirmatory analyses plans. Some of the same basic approaches to model building that are used in exploratory studies can be used to assess the appropriateness of pre-specified methods in confirmatory studies. Therefore, analysis plans will typically either employ several analytic approaches in order to test which one is best (exploratory studies), or use several analytic approaches to evaluate the validity of assumptions in the pre-specified primary analytic approach (confirmatory studies).

20.2 Choosing the Primary Analysis

20.2.1 Observed Data Considerations

In considering primary analyses it can be useful to divide the decision into two parts: how to model the observed data, and how to account for the missing data. Regarding the observed data, the general principles outlined in Part II of this book can be used to help inform choice of primary endpoint (change, percent change, etc.) along with how to model means over time, how to model the covariance between repeated measurements, and how to account for covariates.

Clinical trials typically have a pre-determined number of assessment times that are fixed within narrow intervals. The number of assessment times relative to the number of patients is typically small. These attributes suggest that unstructured modeling of mean trends over time (i.e., time is a categorical covariate) and unstructured modeling of within-patient covariance (the so-called full multivariate normal model) is possible. This is important, especially in confirmatory studies, because an unstructured model for the means requires no assumption about the time trend and models with fewer assumptions are preferred.

The number of parameters to describe the means over time from an unstructured model increases linearly with the number of assessment times. The number of parameters to be estimated for unstructured modeling of covariance increases by $n(n + 1)/2$, where n is the number of assessment times. Although convergence of the full multivariate normal model has been a consideration (Mallinckrodt et al. 2008), these models virtually always converge in practice. However, convergence should still be considered, especially if separate unstructured covariance matrices are fit by treatment or by some other demographic or prognostic factor.

Primary analyses in clinical trials typically have models with a few covariates at most. Additional covariates (subgroups) are assessed in secondary analyses. When a covariate is fit, including the covariate-by-time interaction should also be considered. Fitting just the main covariate effect imposes the restriction that the covariate has the same effect at all assessment times. If a covariate has many levels, such as investigative site, fitting the site-by-time interaction could require estimation of a large number of parameters, thereby inducing potential convergence issues. In exploratory studies that are often smaller and more limited in the number of parameters that can be estimated, analysis plans can specify methods for determining the model with the best fit.

Choice of the dependent variable, such as percent change versus actual change, and choice of the test statistic (endpoint contrast, main effect, etc.) are often driven by convention in confirmatory trials. However, analysts should always understand the alternatives and be willing to propose the most appropriate test and endpoint given the estimand and characteristics of the data.

20.2.2 Considerations for Missing Data

As noted in Chapter 2, choice of estimand influences what data are included in an analysis and whether or not data are considered missing. This section concerns those situations where some of the data that was intended to be collected to evaluate the particular estimand are indeed missing.

Fundamental issues exist in selecting a model and assessing its fit to incomplete data that do not apply to complete data. It was previously noted in Chapter 12 and elsewhere that the assumption of MCAR is unlikely to hold in most clinical trial scenarios. The validity of MCAR can be assessed using logistic regression analysis of probability of dropout. If the outcome variable being analyzed is associated with the probability of dropout, there is evidence to reject MCAR for that outcome. Tests for MCAR can also be based on comparing visit-wise means for patients that dropped out versus patients that continued. If means differ, there is evidence to reject MCAR (Mallinckrodt 2013).

These tests are geared toward assessing the association of observed outcomes with probability of dropout. Finding an association rejects MCAR. However, not finding an association isn't proof MCAR is valid. For MCAR to hold there must also be no association between the unobserved values and the probability of dropout, which as for testing validity of MAR, cannot be assessed from the observed data. Therefore, it is possible to prove MCAR doesn't hold, but it is not possible to prove MCAR is valid.

Given the implausibility of MCAR, analyses assuming MCAR are difficult to justify a priori and are therefore generally not appropriate choices for the primary analysis (Mallinckrodt et al. 2008; NRC 2010; Permutt 2015b). Ad hoc, single imputation methods, such as LOCF and BOCF, entail strong and restrictive assumptions that are unlikely to hold in practice. Therefore, these methods are also generally not suitable for the primary analysis in clinical trials (Molenberghs and Kenward 2007; Mallinckrodt et al. 2008; NRC 2010).

The assumption of MAR can never be confirmed in a clinical trial. However, MNAR methods also entail assumptions that cannot be verified. Both approaches are making assumptions about the missing data, which again cannot be verified (Verbeke and Molenberghs 2000). However, the difficulties in model selection and the consequences of model misspecification are generally greater for MNAR methods (Verbeke and Molenberghs 2000). In addition, departures from assumed distributions can be more problematic in MNAR models (Verbeke and Molenberghs 2000).

Therefore, assuming MAR in the primary analysis can be a reasonable starting point in many clinical trial scenarios. However, the possibility of MNAR can never be excluded. With an MAR primary analysis, sensitivity analyses are needed to understand how strongly inferences are influenced by departures from MAR (Verbeke and Molenberghs 2000; Molenberghs and Kenward 2007; Mallinckrodt et al. 2008; Siddiqui, Hong, and O'Neill 2009; Permutt 2015b). Sensitivity analyses are discussed in Section 20.4.

20.2.3 Choosing between MAR Approaches

When implemented in a similar fashion, likelihood-based, multiple imputation-based, and weighted GEE analyses tend to yield similar results, with the degree of similarity increasing with size of the data set, and in the case of MI, the number of imputations.

Likelihood-based methods tend to be more efficient. Hence, in situations where restrictive models that include only the design factors of the experiment are to be used, likelihood-based methods may be somewhat preferred. However, when more flexibility is desired in accounting for missingness, such as whenever inclusive modeling is used, MI and wGEE are generally preferred. When an appreciable number of covariate values are missing,

MI would be preferred over likelihood-based methods. When covariates to be included in the analysis are missing, wGEE and direct-likelihood exclude the entire record. However, multiple imputation can be used to impute the missing covariate values. A special case of the covariate considerations is for baseline severity. In this case baseline could be considered as part of the response vector for the likelihood analysis, as illustrated in Chapter 9. This avoids the need to discard the entire record, but entails further considerations.

20.3 Assessing Model Fit

20.3.1 Means

If an unstructured modeling of means over time is used, there are no assumptions to test. However, it may still be useful to evaluate more parsimonious models, especially in exploratory studies where the enhanced precision from a more parsimonious model could be especially beneficial. If a structured form of the mean trends is pre-specified, model fit should be compared with an unstructured model. Given that these models are nested (i.e., sub-models of each other), standard likelihood ratio tests can be used.

20.3.2 Covariances

Standard practice has evolved to use unstructured covariance/correlation matrices for modeling the within-subject errors. This helps avoid misspecification (Mallinckrodt et al. 2008). However, this approach does not guarantee validity. Structures more general than unstructured are possible, such as separate unstructured matrices by group (treatment).

Use of the sandwich estimator for standard errors in place of the model-based approach provides valid inference when the correlation structure is misspecified (Verbeke and Molenberghs 2000). Therefore, use of the sandwich estimator as the default approach would protect against correlation misspecification. However, when the sandwich estimator is used in SAS PROC MIXED, only the between-within method for estimating denominator degrees of freedom is available, an approach that is known to be biased, especially in small samples (SAS 2013). Moreover, the sandwich estimator assumes MCAR, which is difficult to justify a priori (Mallinckrodt 2013).

Therefore, a correlation structure deemed to be appropriate based on prior experience can be pre-specified as the primary analysis. Often this will be an unstructured covariance matrix. Model fit statistics and treatment contrasts from more general (separate unstructured matrices by treatment or other group) and more parsimonious structures can be compared to the primary analysis. If the primary analysis yields the best fit then the primary analysis can be considered appropriate. If the primary analysis does not provide the best fit but treatment contrasts or other relevant inferences do not differ between the primary analysis and the structure that yielded better fit, then the inferences from the primary analysis are robust to choice of covariance structure. Examples of fitting alternate covariance structures for the small example data sets were provided in Chapters 7 and 8. An example of assessing sensitivity to covariance assumptions is provided in Chapter 21.

20.3.3 Residual Diagnostics

Important assumptions required for valid regression-type analyses of continuous outcomes include linearity, normality, and independence (Wonnacott and Winacott 1981). These assumptions are in regards to the residuals (difference between observed and predicted values) not on the actual observations. An illustration of residual diagnostics from the small example data set was provided in Chapter 11 and an example from real clinical trial data is provided in Chapter 21. It is good practice to include residual diagnostics for the primary analysis in the clinical study report.

Diagnostics can reveal patterns in the residuals suggesting that the model is misspecified. Therefore, residual diagnostics can be an iterative process wherein residuals are rechecked after alterations to the model based on the first set of residual diagnostics. The focus of residual diagnostics is not as much on whether or not deviations from assumptions existed, but rather on how much departure from assumptions influenced results. For example, if the residuals were not normally distributed, but this lack of normality had a trivial impact on the primary treatment contrast, then the result would be useful, even if not entirely valid in the strictest sense, because inferences were not contingent on this assumption.

20.3.4 Influence Diagnostics

Influence diagnostics (and residual diagnostics) can be thought of conceptually as warning lights. These methods can flag data points or clusters of data that are unusual. Understanding to what degree study results are changed by the unusual data is important in understanding the overall robustness of results.

Although methods to test for the existence and impact of outlier (influential) observations have been around for decades, new methods have been developed for use in MNAR analyses. To this end, interest has grown in local influence approaches (Molenberghs et al. 2015, chapter 16). Local influence provides an objective approach to identifying and examining the impact of influential observations and clusters of observations on various aspects of the analysis, including the missing-data mechanisms and treatment effects (Mallinckrodt 2013).

However, given the newness and complexity of such methods, and that the methods are geared to the MNAR setting, the simpler influence diagnostics introduced in Chapter 11 are often appropriate. The basic idea is again not to simply identify whether or not influential observations or clusters (patients, investigative sites) were present, but rather to assess how the most influential observations affected the parameters of interest. It is good practice to include influence diagnostics for the primary analysis in the clinical study report.

20.4 Assessing Sensitivity to Missing Data Assumptions

20.4.1 Introduction

Assumptions about the missingness mechanism cannot be verified from the observed data, and therefore sensitivity analyses are needed to assess how departures from the assumed conditions influence inferences. In a broad sense, sensitivity analyses can be defined as several statistical models considered simultaneously, or further scrutiny of statistical models using specialized tools, such as diagnostic measures (NRC 2010).

One approach to assessing sensitivity is to fit a selected number of models, all of which are deemed plausible. A second approach is varying assumptions in a systematic manner within a particular analysis. This approach is often implemented by setting certain parameters, especially those that quantify the departure from MAR towards MNAR, at various levels within a plausible range. Unlike model parameters, sensitivity parameters by their very nature are not estimable from available data and represent the "untestable" portion of the model assumptions. The degree to which conclusions (inferences) are stable across such analyses provides an indication of the confidence that inferences are not contingent on assumptions.

The focus of sensitivity analyses, at least initially, should be more so on comparing the magnitude of the primary treatment contrast from the primary analysis with results from the sensitivity analysis (analyses). Initially, emphasis should not be placed too heavily on statistical significance. For example, if MAR was entirely valid and the primary result from an MAR analysis yielded a P value just under the pre-chosen significance level, sensitivity analyses may yield nonsignificant results despite the fact that estimated treatment contrasts would be similar to the primary result (Mallinckrodt 2013).

In addition, the focus of sensitivity analyses should be on sensitivity to assumptions, not sensitivity to methods. Many methods (e.g., likelihood-based mixed models, multiple imputation, EM algorithm, …) rely on the same assumption that data are MAR. Therefore, comparing results from these methods does not assess sensitivity to the assumption of MAR and could lead to a misleadingly optimistic view of the robustness of the conclusions (Mallinckrodt 2013; Permutt 2015b).

20.4.2 Inference and Decision Making

In the previous section it was emphasized that the initial focus of sensitivity analyses is often based on estimation—how the magnitude of the treatment effect is influenced by departures from assumptions. However, ultimately the results of most trials are used to inform a "yes"/"no" decision as to whether the trial met its primary objective. In exploratory studies, this decision may be used to determine if development of the drug continues or is terminated. In confirmatory trials to be evaluated by regulatory agencies, the regulators must determine if the study provided confirmatory evidence of drug benefit. This need for a "yes/no" decision provides motivation for simple approaches to sensitivity analyses that focus on systematic changes to the primary analysis (Permutt 2015b).

Conducting a series of analyses that rely on different assumptions is useful for showing how much results are contingent on the assumptions, but this information is not all that useful in fostering the "yes"/"no" decisions made by regulators (Permutt 2015b). The problem is that if the results differ, it may be difficult to say why. Results could differ because the assumptions of one model are satisfied and the assumptions of the other are not. Alternatively, it could be that the assumptions of both models are satisfied and the difference is random. Finally, it could be that the assumptions of neither model are satisfied so that neither analysis is valid (Permutt 2015b).

Therefore, systematically varying the assumptions of the primary (often MAR-based) analysis may be more useful in supporting yes/no decisions than comparing results from a series of different analyses. To this end, the controlled imputation approaches described in Chapter 18 are particularly well-suited. Reference-based controlled imputation can be used to formulate a plausible worst-case scenario. The delta-adjustment approach can be used similarly by specifying a specific delta as the worst plausible cause, or deltas can be progressively increased as a stress test (Ratitch and O'Kelly 2014). This stress-testing format has been termed a tipping point analysis because it identifies the point at which results tip from significant to nonsignificant.

If a plausible worst-case scenario can be specified a priori, this can reduce the problem of sensitivity to a single analysis. If the results of the plausible worst case agree with the primary result, then inferences were not contingent on the assumptions. In cases where a plausible worst case cannot be identified, the delta-adjustment tipping point approach can be employed. However, the tipping point approach does not necessarily avoid the need to understand plausibility of departures from MAR. Inference from the tipping point approach is contingent upon whether or not the delta required to overturn the primary result is plausible or not. If the delta needed to overturn the primary result is not a plausible departure, then results are robust to plausible departures.

In providing specific advice on sensitivity analyses for confirmatory studies in a regulatory environment, Permutt (2015b) advocated the tipping point approach and noted that the decision problem then becomes a matter of judgment about the plausibility of values of delta. He suggested that protocols should address the question of what deviations might be considered plausible so that this may form the basis of discussion, and sometimes even of agreement, with regulatory agencies before results are known.

Such discussions and agreements can also inform planning of trials, especially with respect to sample size (Permutt 2015b). The crucial question is whether the plausible range of deviations from MAR lies entirely within the range of statistical significance. It is important to appreciate the regulator's perspective. In practice, an effect may confidently be considered significant only if it remains significant at the outer limit of a plausible range of deviations from MAR. The best estimates might be those based on MAR. However, binary decisions are needed in the regulatory setting. As a practical matter, regulators will need to act on the analyses at the unfavorable end of the plausible range, and applicants will need to anticipate and plan accordingly (Permutt 2015b).

For example, it might be best to power studies not on the anticipated magnitude of the treatment effect, but on the treatment effect minus the worst plausible departure from MAR. This regulatory perspective reinforces the need for the iterative study development process described in Chapter 2. It especially reinforces the benefits from minimizing missing data.

See Chapter 21 for examples of applying sensitivity analyses and drawing inference.

20.5 Other Considerations

20.5.1 Convergence

Failure of analytic algorithms to converge almost always results from improperly preparing the data (e.g., two observations on the same patient at the same time point) or from overspecified fixed effects models. Failure to converge almost never results from the pre-specified covariance matrix being too general. However, nonconvergence is possible with separate unstructured covariance matrices for groups, very high rates of dropout and/or need to estimate a large number of fixed effect parameters (such as when the time-by-site interaction is fit when there are many sites and frequent assessments).

If data are prepared correctly and the analysis fails to converge, convergence can be enhanced by using software features such as inputting starting values for parameter estimates, or the use in the initial round(s) (but not final rounds) of iteration algorithms such as Fisher's scoring rather than the Newton–Raphson algorithm, which is the default algorithm in many software packages.

Rescaling and/or centering of the data (e.g., using orthogonal polynomials to model time trends) are also options. If outcomes and covariates are made to fall in ranges in the order of magnitude of unity, interpretations and conclusions will not be changed; but, avoiding manipulation of large or small numbers from a numerical analysis perspective reduces the risk of ill-conditioned matrices, and ultimately, overflow or underflow (Mallinckrodt et al. 2008).

If all else fails, the protocol can envision one of several model-fitting approaches for determining the covariance structure. A set of structures can be specified. The structure converging to the best fit as assessed by standard model-fitting criteria is considered the primary analysis. Alternatively, a series of structures can be pre-specified in a fixed sequence, and the first correlation structure to yield convergence is considered the primary analysis. For example, unstructured could be specified as the structure for the primary analysis; but if it failed to converge, a series of ever more parsimonious structures appropriate to the situation at hand could be fit until one converges, which would then be considered the primary analysis.

Again, it is important to emphasize that in practical situations it is almost always possible to gain convergence from an unstructured covariance matrix. However, in instances when correctness of the covariance structure is a concern, standard errors and the associated inferences from maximum likelihood analyses can be based on the so-called sandwich estimator, which does not require correct specification of the correlation structure in order to yield valid inferences (Lu and Mehrotra 2009). However, as detailed in Section 20.3.2, the sandwich estimator requires MCAR. Therefore, specification of model-based standard errors as the primary approach is often preferable in likelihood-based analyses.

20.5.2 Computational Time

Mixed-effects models can be computationally intensive, and execution times can be long. Computational intensity stems from solving the mixed model equations and considerable CPU time is often required to compute the likelihood function and its derivatives. These latter computations are performed for each round of Newton–Raphson iteration (SAS 2013).

The following suggestions from the SAS on line documentation (SAS 2013) can be helpful when dealing with a model that has excessive compute time. Each of these factors could also be considered as means of aiding convergence:

- Examine the number of columns in the X and Z matrices. A large number of columns in either matrix can greatly increase computing time. Eliminating higher-order effects can markedly reduce the computational burden.
- In general, specify random effects with many levels in the REPEATED statement and those with a few levels in the RANDOM statement.

- Use the parms statement to specify plausible starting values for parameters.
- If the Z matrix has many columns (e.g., many subjects), consider using the between-within method to estimate denominator degrees of freedom in order to eliminate the time required for the containment method.
- If possible, "factor out" a common effect from the effects in the RANDOM statement and make it the SUBJECT = effect. This creates a block-diagonal G matrix and can often speed calculations.
- If possible, use the same or nested SUBJECT = effects in all RANDOM and REPEATED statements.
- The LOGNOTE option in the PROC MIXED statement writes periodic messages to the SAS log concerning the status of the calculations, which can help diagnose where the slowdown is occurring.

20.6 Specifying Analyses—Example Wording

20.6.1 Introduction

To fully specify an analysis, the method of estimation, the analytic model, and the choice of data must be made clear. Perhaps most importantly, it must also be clear what estimand the analysis is addressing.

A key principle of pre-specification is that analysts independently following the specifications arrive at the same results. For method of estimation, the primary options covered in this book include likelihood-based (maximum or restricted), generalized estimated equations, or least squares. Choice of data must include any imputation of missing data (e.g., multiple imputation) and whether or not data after discontinuation of initially randomized medication and/or initiation of rescue medication are to be included in the analysis.

All aspects of the analytic model should be pre-specified. Although there is no standard approach for model specification, a useful place to begin is in describing the dependent variable. Such specification should include the outcome variable and whether it is the actual values, change from baseline, percent change, etc., that is to be analyzed. In addition, any transformations or link functions that are utilized to account for nonnormality should be specified.

Concise and clear specification of covariates (independent variables) in the model is also essential. Such specification includes the variables themselves, interactions between variables, whether or not each variable is considered a categorical or continuous effect, and whether or not each variable is considered a fixed or random effect.

In addition, it is also necessary to specify what inferential tests will be the primary basis for evaluation (e.g., treatment main effect, endpoint contrast). In addition, it is also necessary to specify other details about the inferential test, such as the type of sums of squares (type I, type II, type III, etc.) and how denominator degrees of freedom are estimated.

20.6.2 Example Language for Direct Likelihood

The following example text illustrates one way to specify a priori all the details of a likelihood-based analysis such that independent analysts will arrive at exactly the same results. This particular wording specifies the full multivariate approach for an analysis of mean change from baseline with an unstructured modeling of treatment effects over time and within-patient error correlations.

Mean changes from baseline will be analyzed using a restricted maximum likelihood (REML)-based repeated measures approach. Analyses will include the fixed, categorical effects of treatment, investigative site, visit, and treatment-by-visit interaction, as well as the continuous, fixed covariates of baseline score and baseline score-by-visit-interaction. An unstructured (co)variance structure will be used to model the within-subject errors. The Kenward–Roger approximation will be used to estimate denominator degrees of freedom and adjust standard errors. Significance tests will be based on least-squares means using a two-sided $\alpha = 0.05$ (two-sided 95% confidence intervals). Analyses will be implemented using (insert software package). The primary treatment comparisons will be the contrast between treatments at the endpoint Visit.

20.6.3 Example Language for Multiple Imputation

The following example text is for an MI-based approach, assuming MAR, with sequential imputation for monotone missing data and multivariate Gaussian model/partial MCMC imputation for nonmonotone missing data. This model uses MCMC for partial imputation of nonmonotone data under MAR followed by sequential MI regression for monotone data. If desired, MCMC can be used for all missing data, both monotone and nonmonotone. Alternatively, a two-step process can be followed where only nonmonotone data is imputed first with the MCMC method, followed by a second step using the sequential MI regression to impute the remaining monotone missing data. This may be desirable if, for example, the primary outcome or other post-baseline auxiliary outcomes are categorical and would be better modeled with a logistic regression imputation model. In that case, sequential MI for monotone data can use regular regression models for continuous variables and logistic regression models for categorical variables that need to be imputed. In the example text that follows, measure1 is the dependent variable in the primary analysis.

Mean changes from baseline in measure1 will be analyzed based on data observed while the subject remains on study as well as data imputed using multiple imputation (MI) methodology for time points at which no value is observed. Multiple imputation will be performed under the assumption of missing-at-random (MAR) and will be implemented in two steps using {software, version}.

First, partial imputation will be carried out to impute intermittent (non-monotone) missing data based on a multivariate joint Gaussian imputation model using the Markov chain Monte Carlo (MCMC) method. A separate imputation model will be used for each treatment arm. The imputation models will include {list of baseline covariates}, measure1 assessments at each time point {Baseline, Visit x,…,y}. The MCMC method will be used with multiple chains, 200 burn-in iterations, and a noninformative prior. In case of nonconvergence or nonestimability issues, a ridge prior and a single model will be considered with treatment arm added as an explanatory variable to the model.

The remaining monotone missing data will be imputed using sequential regression multiple imputation, where a separate regression model is estimated for imputation of each variable (i.e., measurement at each time point). Each regression model will include explanatory variables for {list of baseline covariates}, treatment and all previous (Baseline, Visit x,…,y) values of measure1. No rounding or range restrictions will be applied to imputed continuous values.

Imputed data will consist of {MM} (e.g., 500) imputed data sets. The random seed number for partial imputation with the MCMC method will be {XXXXX}, and the random seed number for the sequential regression multiple imputation will be {YYYYYY}.

Each imputed data set will be analyzed using the following analysis method. Change in measure1 from baseline to each post-baseline visit will be based on observed and imputed data. {Insert description of analysis model/method, e.g., direct likelihood MMRM as described above, or ANCOVA.} Treatment group comparison at Visit T will be based on the least squares mean (LSM) difference between treatment groups in change from baseline in measure1 estimated by the analysis model in each of the imputed data sets. Results from analysis of each imputed data set, that is, LSM treatment differences and their standard errors, will be combined using Rubin's imputation rules to produce a pooled LSM estimate of treatment difference, its 95% confidence interval, and a pooled P-value for the test of null hypothesis of no treatment effect.

20.7 Power and Sample Size Considerations

Chapter 5 included a subsection illustrating how changes in variance components of a mixed-effects model influence parameter estimates and their uncertainty. A key implication of those illustrations was that variance components need to be considered when assessing power in planning longitudinal studies. Other key considerations in powering studies include the rate of missing data. It is intuitively easy to appreciate that the more missing data, the lower the power. Therefore, the impact to power and sample size from missing data should be considered in the protocol and some degree of protection against unexpectedly higher rates of dropout may be warranted.

Although a wide array of commercial software for power and sample size determination exist, simulation studies are fairly easy to conduct and often more useful. With fairly simple coding and reasonable compute times, flexible programs can be tailored to the specific circumstances at hand. The impact of correlation structure and missing data can be easily evaluated by changing the relevant input parameters. The need to maintain robustness to plausible departures from MAR could be addressed by including, for example, a delta-adjusted power/sample size. Results can be used to compare power for treatment main effects, interaction effects, or visit-wise contrasts. The impact of fitting versus not fitting a covariate can be assessed.

Clinical development in general relies increasingly on simulation studies to inform plans. Clinical trial simulation to inform power/sample size can be seen as simply one specific aspect of the general trend.

21

Example Analyses of Clinical Trial Data

21.1 Introduction

This chapter illustrates the analyses of longitudinal clinical trial data using the principles and recommendations outlined in previous chapters. The analyses conducted here are for illustration and should not be considered universal recommendations for similar situations. Data for these analyses are the so-called high and low dropout (large) data sets described in Chapter 4. Recall, these data are somewhat contrived for convenience, but were extracted from two real clinical trials and thus provide a useful illustration of analyses, model verification procedures, and sensitivity analyses. Parts of this example were previously reported in Molenberghs et al. (2015, chapter 22).

For this example, the primary objective was to compare treatment versus control in mean change from baseline to Week 8 on the Hamilton 17-item depression rating scale (Hamilton 1960). The primary analysis targeted a de jure (efficacy) estimand—the effects of the initially randomized medication if taken as directed; that is, estimand 3 described in Table 2.1. Effectiveness was assessed secondarily as the effects of the drug as actually taken; that is, estimand 2 described in Table 2.1. Post-rescue data were not collected in these studies. Therefore, it was not possible to assess the de facto treatment regimen estimand (estimand 1 in Table 2.1). Had post-rescue data been available, estimand 1 could have been evaluated using the same methods as for estimand 3. Additional details on descriptive, primary, and sensitivity analyses are provided below.

21.2 Descriptive Analyses

The number of observations by assessment time is summarized in Table 21.1.

Visit-wise mean changes for patients who completed the trials versus those who discontinued early were summarized by visit in Figures 4.1 and 4.2 for the low and high dropout data sets, respectively. In the high dropout

TABLE 21.1

Number of Observations by Week in the High and Low Dropout Data Sets

	High Dropout					Low Dropout				
Week	1	2	4	6	8	1	2	4	6	8
Placebo	100	92	85	73	60	100	98	98	95	92
Drug	100	91	85	75	70	100	98	95	93	92

data set, visit-wise mean changes for patients who discontinued early were less than for completers, suggesting that patients with poorer response were more likely to drop out; therefore, the missingness mechanism was unlikely MCAR. With only a few dropouts at each visit in the low dropout data set, trends were not readily identifiable.

21.3 Primary Analyses

To assess the primary de jure estimand, mean changes from baseline were analyzed using a restricted maximum likelihood (REML)-based repeated measures approach. The analysis included the fixed, categorical effects of treatment, investigative site (site), visit, treatment-by-visit interaction, and site-by-visit interaction, along with the continuous, fixed covariates of baseline score and baseline score-by-visit-interaction. An unstructured (co)variance structure was used to model the within-patient errors. The Kenward–Roger approximation was used to estimate denominator degrees of freedom. Significance tests were based on least-squares means using a two-sided $\alpha = 0.05$ (two-sided 95% confidence intervals). Analyses were implemented using SAS PROC MIXED (SAS 2013). The primary comparison was the contrast between treatments at Week 8.

Results from the primary analyses are summarized in Table 21.2. In the high dropout data set, the advantage of drug over placebo in mean change from baseline to Week 8 was 2.29 (SE = 1.00, P = 0.024). The corresponding results in the low dropout data set were 1.82 (SE = 0.70, P = 0.010). The standard error for the difference in lsmeans at Week 8 in the high dropout data set was nearly 50% larger than in the low dropout data set. This was partly due to the lower variability in the low dropout data set (see Table 21.4). The larger variability in the high dropout data set accounted for a 32% increase in standard error on its own. The additional increase in standard error in the high dropout data set came from the additional quantity of missing data.

The secondary, de facto estimand was assessed based on treatment success or failure. Treatment success was defined as improvement greater than or equal to 50% of the baseline severity and completion of the acute treatment phase. Any patient that discontinued study medication was considered

TABLE 21.2

Visit-Wise LSMEANS and Contrasts for $HAMD_{17}$ from the Primary Analyses of the High and Low Dropout Data Sets

	LSMEANS				
	Placebo	**Drug**	**LSMEAN Difference**[a]	**Standard Error**	**P**
High Dropout					
Week 1	−1.89	−1.80	−0.09	0.64	0.890
Week 2	−3.55	−4.07	0.52	0.81	0.518
Week 4	−4.87	−6.20	1.32	0.86	0.125
Week 6	−5.51	−7.73	2.22	0.93	0.019
Week 8	−5.94	−8.24	2.29	1.00	0.024
Low Dropout					
Week 1	−2.22	−1.76	−0.45	0.38	0.235
Week 2	−4.93	−4.89	−0.04	0.56	0.943
Week 6	−7.79	−8.31	0.52	0.61	0.392
Week 4	−9.45	−10.69	1.25	0.66	0.060
Week 8	−10.57	−12.39	1.82	0.70	0.010

[a] Advantage of drug over placebo. Negative values indicate an advantage for placebo.

TABLE 21.3

Percent Treatment Success for the De Facto Secondary Estimand in the High and Low Dropout Data Sets

High Dropout Treatment Success (%)				Low Dropout Treatment Success (%)			
Placebo	**Drug**	**Difference**	**P**	**Placebo**	**Drug**	**Difference**	**P**
25	39	14	0.034	50	68	18	0.001

a treatment failure regardless of outcome. Treatment groups were compared using Fisher's exact test. Results are summarized in Table 21.3.

Both trials yielded significant advantages of drug over control in percent treatment success. The definition of the treatment success included completion, so there was no missing data and no need to assess sensitivity to missing data assumptions, per se. However, generalizability results should be considered and it is still advisable to understand how changes in the rates of dropout influence outcomes. The low dropout data set had greater within-group mean changes in addition to greater adherence. It is unclear if or how design differences may have influenced the within-group mean changes and adherence. However, the two trials give different views of effectiveness. The percent treatment success on placebo in the low dropout data set was two-fold greater than in the high dropout data set.

21.4 Evaluating Testable Assumptions of the Primary Analysis

21.4.1 Sensitivity to Covariance Assumptions

Unstructured covariance matrices were used for the primary analyses. Correlations and (co)variances from the primary analyses of the high and low dropout data sets are summarized in Table 21.4.

Treatment contrasts from more general and more parsimonious covariance structures, with and without use of the sandwich estimator, are summarized in Table 21.5. In the high dropout data set, an unstructured matrix common to both treatment groups that was used as the primary analysis provided the best fit, thereby supporting results from the primary analysis as valid. However, the potential importance of choice of covariance structure with this high rate of dropout can be seen in the comparatively large range in treatment contrasts (1.69–2.29), standard errors and P-values across the covariance structures.

In the low dropout data set, the range in treatment contrasts across the covariance structures (1.76–1.85) was approximately six-fold smaller than in the high dropout data set, and all structures yielded a significant treatment contrast. Separate unstructured matrices by treatment group yielded the best fit, with the second best fit being from a single unstructured matrix that was specified as the primary analysis. The consistency of results across covariance structures indicates conclusions were not sensitive to correlation structure, thereby supporting validity of the primary analysis.

21.4.2 Residual and Influence Diagnostics—High Dropout Data Set

Given the comparatively small number of sites in these contrived data, influence of each site was investigated by removing sites one at a time and repeating the primary analysis on the data subsets. In scenarios with more sites, influence diagnostics as presented in Chapter 11 could be implemented to first identify influential sites and then repeat analyses deleting only the influential sites.

The influence option in the model statement of SAS PROC MIXED (SAS 2013) was used to determine which patients had the greatest influence on various aspects of the model. Results based on restricted likelihood distance (RLD) are discussed below. The RLD is a measure of influence on the objective function; that is, a measure of overall influence not specific to any particular model parameter. In addition, residual diagnostics were used to further identify unusual patients or individual observations.

Residual plots from the high dropout data set are shown in Figure 21.1. The upper left panel shows no association between magnitude of residual and magnitude of prediction, and no clear increase in variance across predicted values. The upper right and lower left panels suggest residuals satisfied normality assumptions.

Box plots of residuals for each treatment-by-time combination in the high dropout data set are shown in Figure 21.2. These plots suggest aberrant residuals

TABLE 21.4

Covariance and Correlation Matrices from the Primary Analyses of the High and Low Dropout Data Sets

	High Dropout					Low Dropout				
Week	**1**	**2**	**4**	**6**	**8**	**1**	**2**	**4**	**6**	**8**
(Co) variances										
1	20.16					7.22				
2	14.05	29.86				4.79	15.50			
4	11.55	19.74	32.09			3.87	11.54	18.07		
6	10.7	18.56	25.27	35.10		3.74	9.96	14.65	20.59	
8	11.51	17.67	22.57	30.88	39.55	2.23	7.03	10.73	16.61	22.82
Correlations										
1	1.000					1.000				
2	0.573	1.000				0.453	1.000			
4	0.454	0.638	1.000			0.339	0.689	1.000		
6	0.402	0.573	0.753	1.000		0.307	0.558	0.760	1.000	
8	0.408	0.514	0.634	0.829	1.000	0.174	0.374	0.528	0.766	1.000

TABLE 21.5

Treatment Contrasts from Alternative Covariance Matrices from the Primary Analyses

Structure[a]	AIC	Endpoint Contrasts	Standard Error	P
High Dropout				
UN	4679.82	2.29	1.00	0.024
UN EMPIRICAL	4679.82	2.29	0.97	0.020
TOEPH	4684.44	2.10	0.91	0.023
TOEPH EMPIRICAL	4684.44	2.10	0.92	0.023
TOEPH GROUP = TRT	4689.88	1.82	0.91	0.048
UN GROUP = TRT	4692.05	1.96	1.00	0.053
CSH	4735.81	1.86	0.93	0.047
CSH EMPIRICAL	4735.81	1.86	0.91	0.041
CSH GROUP = TRT	4739.34	1.69	0.93	0.070
Low Dropout				
UN GROUP = TRT	4861.70	1.85	0.703	0.009
UN	4867.68	1.82	0.699	0.010
UN EMPIRICAL	4867.68	1.82	0.666	0.007
TOEPH GROUP = TRT	4888.93	1.82	0.647	0.005
TOEPH	4897.89	1.79	0.649	0.006
TOEPH EMPIRICAL	4897.89	1.79	0.662	0.006
CSH	5030.40	1.76	0.705	0.013
CSH EMPIRICAL	5030.40	1.76	0.667	0.008
CSH GROUP = TRT	5031.92	1.80	0.708	0.011

[a] UN, unstructured; TOEPH, heterogeneous toeplitz; CSH, heterogeneous compound symmetric; GROUP = TRT means that separate structures were fit for each treatment group; Empirical means that empirical (sandwich-based) estimators of the standard error were used rather than the model-based standard errors.

were relatively rare compared to the total number of observations and that there was no systematic trend in the residuals, suggesting the model was appropriate.

RLDs for each patient in the high dropout data set are shown in Figure 21.3. The largest RLD values were approximately 2.0. Values of this magnitude generally suggest no individual patient had a large influence on the overall model.

Additional measures of influence (not presented here) include case deletion metrics based on Cook's D, as described in Chapter 11, to assess the influence of individual patients on each specific model parameter, including fixed effects and covariance parameters. No individual patient was found to have a large influence on any individual parameter.

21.4.3 Residual and Influence Diagnostics—Low Dropout Data Set

Residual and influence diagnostics for the low dropout data set were conducted as previously described for the high dropout data set. Residual plots

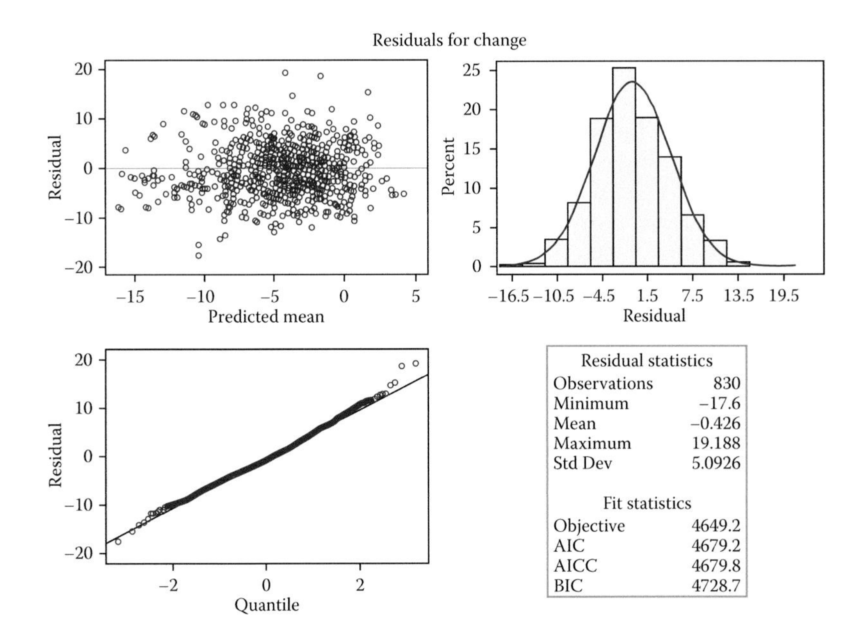

FIGURE 21.1
Residual plots for the high dropout data set.

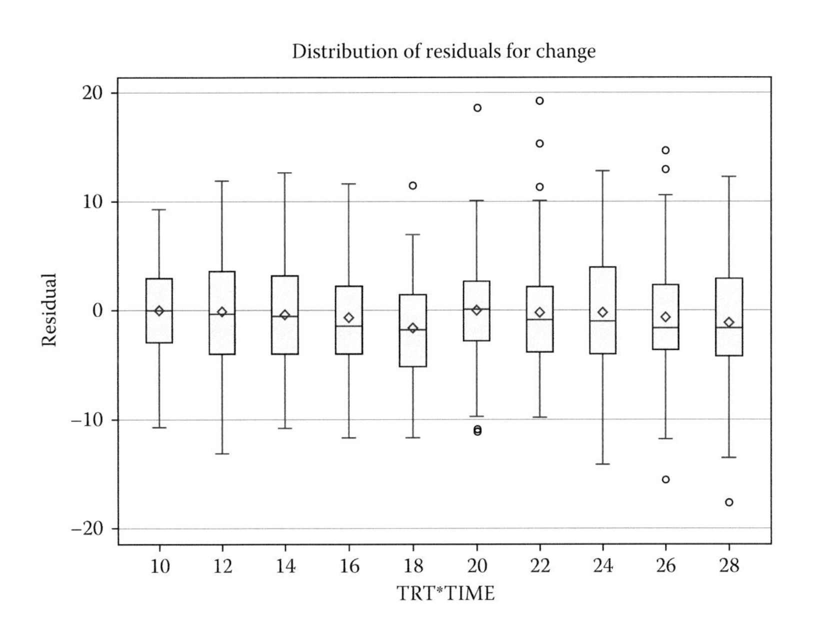

FIGURE 21.2
Box plots of residuals by treatment and time in the high dropout data set.

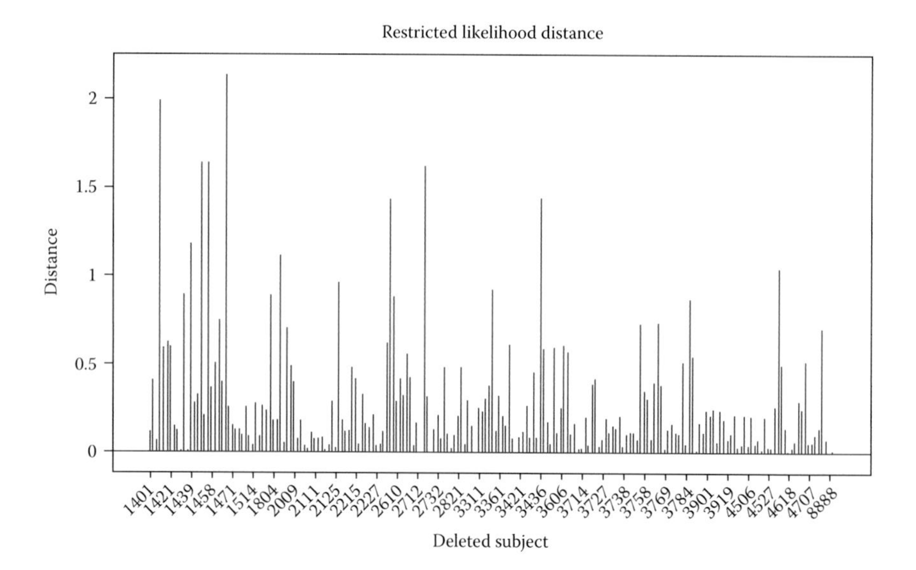

FIGURE 21.3
RLDs for influence of patients in the high dropout data set.

from the low dropout data set are shown in Figure 21.4. These figures show an unusual observation with a large residual. This value is seen in the upper left corner of the upper left panel, the residual–predicted value plot. This outlier is also seen in the far right tail of the residual histogram in the upper right panel, and in the upper right corner of the Q–Q plot in the lower left panel.

Box plots of residuals for each treatment-by-time combination in the low dropout data set are shown in Figure 21.5. These plots show the aberrant residual was in Treatment 2 at Week 8, an especially important finding because the primary analysis was the treatment contrast at Week 8. The magnitude of the aberrant residual was approximately twice that of the next largest residual.

RLDs for each patient in the low dropout data set are shown in Figure 21.6. The largest RLD value was, not surprisingly, from the same patient with the aberrant residual. This patient had an RLD of nearly 40, which was five-fold greater than the next largest RLD.

Additional measures of influence (not presented here) include case deletion metrics based on Cook's D, as described in Chapter 11, to assess the influence of individual patients on each specific model parameter, including fixed effects and covariance parameters. The influential patient identified above was influential on a number of fixed effect and covariance parameters, especially those involving Week 8.

The visit-wise data for the most influential patient is listed in Table 21.6. The data were unusual in several regards. The baseline HAMD score of 35

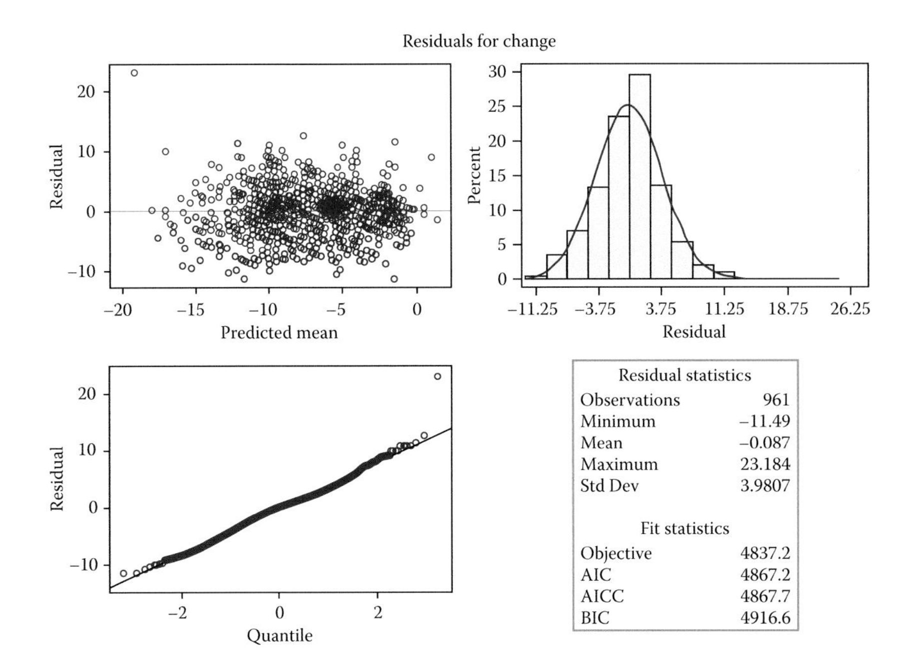

FIGURE 21.4
Residual plots for the low dropout data set.

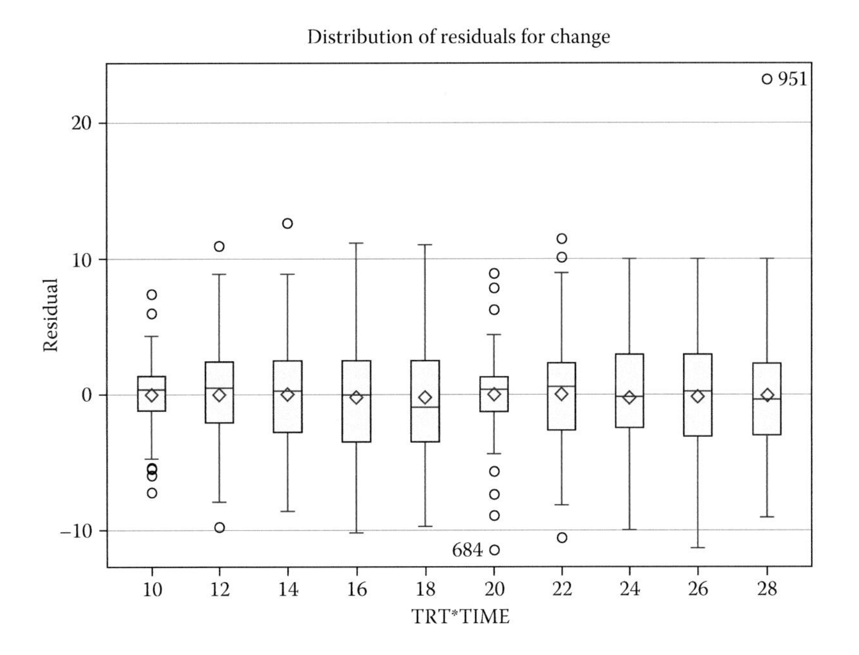

FIGURE 21.5
Box plots of residuals by treatment and time in the low drop out data set.

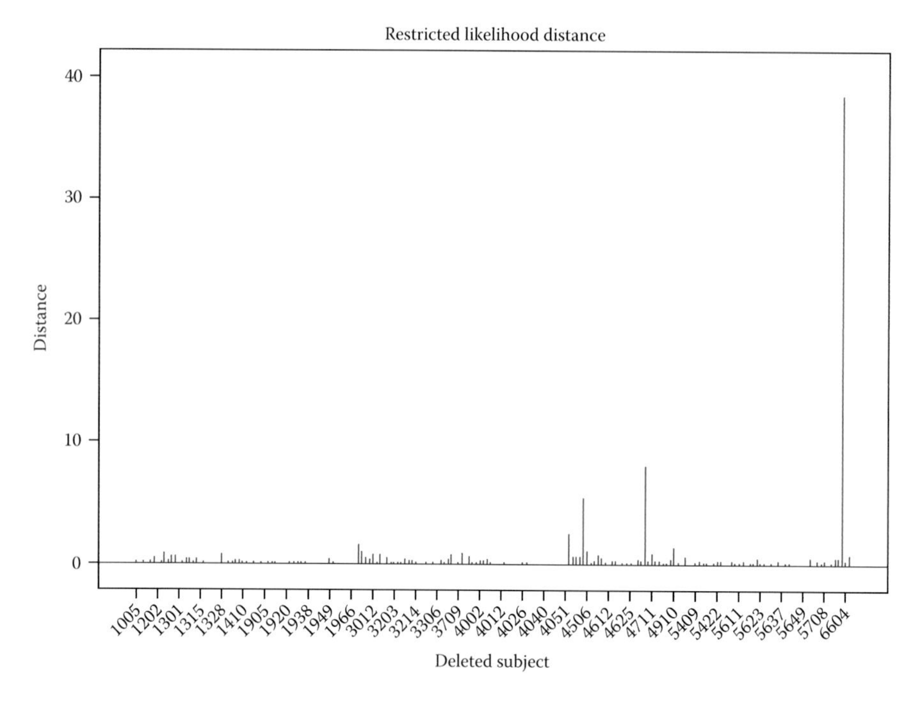

FIGURE 21.6
RLDs for the influence of each patient in the high dropout data set.

TABLE 21.6
Visit-Wise Data for the Most Influential Patient in the Low Dropout Data Set

Treatment	Site	Baseline HAMD	Time	HAMD Change	PGIIMP
2	141	35	1	–6	3
			2	– 7	5
			4	– 13	7
			6	– 18	7
			8	4	.

indicated this was one of the most severely ill patients. The patient had improvements at Weeks 1 through 6 that were greater than the group means. However, from Weeks 6 to 8 that patient had a marked worsening in condition, going from an improvement of 18 points to a worsening of 4 points. This 22-point change was the largest visit-to-visit change in the data set and was opposite in direction of other large changes. Interestingly, the patient-rated PGIIMP scores for this patient at Weeks 4 and 6 were 7, indicating a marked worsening; whereas, the corresponding clinician-rated HAMD scores showed improvement at those assessment times. At Week 8, the clinician-rated

HAMD scores reflected the worsening, and the PGIIMP score was missing. This unusual profile and the conflict between the clinician-rated HAMD scores and the patient-rated PGIIMP scores should trigger additional investigation. Entries in comment fields of case report forms and/or other site documentation could help lend insight into the situation.

21.4.4 Analyses with Influential Patients and Sites Removed

As previously noted, given the small number of sites, influence of each site was investigated by removing each site one at a time and repeating the primary analysis on the data subsets. In situations with more sites, influence diagnostics would be used to identify influential sites and the primary analysis repeated after removing each influential site. Emphasis was placed on the magnitude of change in the treatment contrasts rather than maintenance of statistical significance because of the markedly smaller sample size when a site was deleted. Results for this case deletion of sites are summarized in Table 21.7.

In the high dropout data set, deleting sites 003 and 028 decreased the treatment contrasts slightly. Deleting sites 005 and 001 increased the treatment contrasts slightly. Although statistical significance was lost when deleting site 003, this was due to the decreased sample size (nearly 300 observations removed) rather than a smaller treatment contrast. In the low dropout data set, deleting site 121 had the greatest effect on the treatment contrast. However, the treatment contrast remained significant. Therefore, statistical significance was not driven by a single site in either of these two data sets.

TABLE 21.7

Influence of Sites on Endpoint Contrasts in the High and Low Dropout Data Sets

	Numbers of			
Data Set	**Patients**	**Observations**	**Endpoint Contrast**	**P**
High Dropout				
All Data	200	830	2.37	0.021
Drop Site 005	175	723	2.96	0.008
Drop Site 001	165	684	2.78	0.013
Drop Site 028	159	677	2.18	0.049
Drop Site 003	132	536	2.27	0.079
Low Dropout				
All Data	200	961	1.85	0.008
Drop Site 121	167	801	1.56	0.047
Drop Site 131	145	694	1.82	0.028
Drop Site 141	147	710	2.10	0.005
Drop Site 101	141	678	1.77	0.044

The impact of influential patients was also assessed using a case deletion approach. However, all patients identified as influential were deleted by treatment group rather than one at a time, except for the most influential patient in the low dropout data set. In that instance results were repeated after removing just that one patient. Results from analyses of the primary outcome excluding influential patients are summarized in Table 21.8.

In the high dropout data set, the five most influential patients were investigated; two were randomized to the drug arm and three to placebo. Dropping placebo-treated influential patients decreased the endpoint contrast slightly. Dropping drug-treated influential patients increased the endpoint contrast slightly, as did dropping all influential patients.

In the low dropout data set, the six most influential patients were investigated; two were randomized to the drug arm and four to placebo. Dropping all placebo-treated influential patients decreased the endpoint contrast. Dropping all drug-treated influential patients increased the endpoint contrast, as did dropping all influential patients. Dropping only patient 6602, the most influential patient, resulted in a comparatively large increase in the treatment contrast and a decrease in the standard error. Patient 6602 had a very unusual response profile, which resulted in noticeable reductions in magnitude and precision of the estimated treatment contrast.

Observations with a studentized residual ≥ 2.0 or ≤ – 2.0 were considered aberrant. The primary analysis was repeated with all observations from drug-treated patients having aberrant residuals removed, with all observations from placebo-treated patients having aberrant residuals removed, and deleting all the observations having aberrant residuals. Results are summarized in Table 21.9.

TABLE 21.8

Endpoint Contrasts for All Data and for Data with Influential Patients Removed from the High and Low Dropout Data Sets

	Numbers of			
Data Set	**Patients**	**Observations**	**Endpoint Contrast**	**P**
High Dropout				
All Data	200	830	2.29	0.024
Drop All	195	808	2.50	0.015
Drop Drug	198	823	2.59	0.010
Drop Placebo	197	815	2.21	0.032
Low Dropout				
All Data	200	961	1.82	0.010
DROP 6602	199	956	2.07	0.002
Drop All	194	931	1.97	0.003
Drop Drug	196	941	1.97	0.003
Drop Placebo	198	951	1.80	0.011

TABLE 21.9

Endpoint Contrasts for All Data and Data with Subjects Having Aberrant Residuals Removed from the High and Low Dropout Data Sets

	Number of Observations	Endpoint Contrast	P
High Dropout			
All Data	830	2.29	0.024
Drop All	796	2.42	0.009
Drop Drug	809	2.57	0.006
Drop Placebo	817	2.13	0.035
Low Dropout			
All Data	961	1.82	0.010
Drop All	915	1.92	0.002
Drop Drug	938	2.16	0.001
Drop Placebo	938	1.59	0.019

In both the high dropout and low dropout data sets, excluding all placebo-treated patients with aberrant residuals decreased the endpoint contrast. Excluding drug-treated patients and all patients with aberrant residuals increased the endpoint contrast. However, changes in the treatment contrasts were small. Given the decrease in sample size due to excluding patients, influence on the treatment contrast is best judged by changes in magnitude rather than statistical significance. However, preservation of statistical significance for the treatment effect provided an extra level of assurance that outlier patients did not influence inferences.

21.5 Sensitivity to Missing Data Assumptions

21.5.1 Introduction

In this section, a variety of MNAR approaches are implemented to assess the sensitivity of results from the primary analysis to departures from MAR. In practice, not all these approaches would be needed. As illustrated in Chapter 18, controlled imputation approaches to sensitivity analyses are easy to understand and implement. For this reanalysis, the marginal delta-adjustment approach was chosen as the primary basis upon which sensitivity was assessed. Results from other MNAR approaches are included for illustration.

The intent is not to imply that delta adjustment is always the best choice for assessing sensitivity. Rather, the intent is to illustrate the general attributes of a variety in methods while also implementing a decision-making framework that would be useful in realistic scenarios.

21.5.2 Marginal Delta Adjustment

The marginal delta adjustment approach was implemented similar to the approach utilized in Code Fragment 18.1. In the present application, $m = 100$ imputations was shown to stabilize results and therefore each delta adjustment analysis used 100 imputed data sets. Results from applying marginal delta-adjustment to the high and low dropout data sets are summarized in Table 21.10. In the marginal approach, the delta adjustment at one visit does not influence imputed values at other visits. Results from using delta = 0 (i.e., no adjustment, the MAR result) are included for reference. The MAR (delta = 0) results differ slightly from the primary results in Table 21.2 because the primary result was generated using direct likelihood and the delta = 0 results in Table 21.10 are based on multiple imputation.

Deltas were progressively increased in the tipping-point format to identify the magnitude of delta needed to overturn the primary results. Delta = 2 was a particularly informative choice because that delta was approximately equal to the treatment effect and therefore is a useful reference point in gauging plausibility of a departure from MAR (Permutt 2015b). Specifically, a delta equal to the average treatment effect would typically be considered a plausible departure, but perhaps the largest plausible departure.

Using delta = 2, the endpoint contrast was significant in the low dropout data set, but significance was lost in the high dropout data set. In fact, delta = 1 was sufficient to overturn significance in the high dropout data set. In the low dropout data set, delta = 7 was required to overturn significance.

TABLE 21.10

Results from Marginal Delta-Adjustment Multiple Imputation—Delta Applied on Last Visit to Active Arm Only

	Low Dropout Data Set			High Dropout Data Set		
Value of Delta Adj	Endpoint Contrast	Standard Error	P	Endpoint Contrast	Standard Error	P
0	1.86	0.70	0.008	2.27	1.12	0.042
1	1.79	0.70	0.011	1.96	1.13	0.083
2	1.71	0.70	0.015	1.64	1.14	0.151
3	1.64	0.71	0.201			
4	1.57	0.71	0.027			
5	1.50	0.72	0.037			
6	1.42	0.72	0.049			
7	1.35	0.73	0.065			

Increasing the delta applied to the endpoint visit had a consistent and therefore predictable effect on the endpoint contrasts. For each 1-point increase in delta, the endpoint contrast was decreased by approximately 0.08 points in the low dropout data set and by approximately 0.30 points in the high dropout data set. As discussed in Chapter 18, this systematic change is intuitive in that 8% of the values were missing for Treatment 2 at endpoint in the low dropout data set, and 30% of the values were missing for Treatment 2 in the high dropout data set.

As discussed in Chapter 18, the effect of a marginal delta adjustment on the endpoint contrast can be analytically determined as follows:

$$\text{Change to the endpoint contrast} = \Delta \times \pi$$

where π = the percentage of missing values and Δ = the marginal delta adjustment

These results help reinforce the straightforward and easy to understand nature of marginal delta adjustment. First, there is a direct correspondence between the fraction of missing values and the sensitivity of results to departures from MAR. If π is cut in half, Δ will have half the effect on the endpoint contrast. In addition, progressively increasing delta results in predictable and easy to understand changes in the endpoint contrasts that make for a useful stress test to ascertain how severe departures from MAR must be in order to overturn inferences from the MAR result.

21.5.3 Conditional (Sequential) Delta Adjustment

Results from conditional (sequential) delta adjustment are summarized in Table 21.11. In conditional delta adjustment, imputations are done sequentially, visit-by-visit, with patients' delta-adjusted imputed data contributing to imputed values at subsequent visits. The net effect of sequential imputation is that when deltas are applied to each visit, they have an accumulating effect such that patients who drop out earlier have larger "net" deltas (indicating a more severe departure from MAR) than patients who drop out later.

TABLE 21.11

Results from Delta-Adjustment Multiple Imputation—Delta Applied on All Visits After Discontinuation to Active Arm Only

	Low Dropout Data Set			High Dropout Data Set		
Value of Delta Adj	**Endpoint Contrast**	**Standard Error**	**P**	**Endpoint Contrast**	**Standard Error**	**P**
0	1.85	0.71	0.009	2.31	1.02	0.024
0.5	1.77	0.71	0.013	2.00	1.03	0.051
2.0	1.52	0.73	0.037			
2.5	1.44	0.74	0.051			

In the high dropout data set, the delta = 0.5 points on the $HAMD_{17}$ overturned the primary result ($P > 0.05$). The endpoint contrast changed 0.62 for each 1-point change in delta. The corresponding tipping point in the low dropout data set was 2.5 points, with the endpoint contrast changing 0.16 for each 1-point change in delta.

In the conditional approach, the impact of delta for a patient in the drug group withdrawing at Week 2 was the accumulation of an increment of approximately delta × 1 + the sum of the correlations between Week 2 and subsequent visits. That is, delta × (1 + 0.51 + 0.63 + 0.83) = 2.97 in the high dropout data set. An early dropout therefore had a nearly threefold greater accumulation—and therefore larger impact—than missing data at the last visit only.

In the conditional approach, it is still possible to analytically derive the impact of a particular delta, but the calculations are more involved. The net effect of a conditional delta can be approximately explained using the accumulations described above, as applied to each assessment week, and the number of subjects discontinuing at each week, divided by the total number of subjects: $0.5 \times (9 \times 2.97 + 6 \times 2.46 + 10 \times 1.83 + 5 \times 1)/100 = 0.32$. The corresponding tipping point in the low dropout data set was 2.5 points with a shift of 0.41, which is approximately explained as $2.5 \times (2 \times 2.66 + 3 \times 2.29 + 2 \times 1.77 + 1 \times 1)/100 = 0.42$.

In marginal delta adjustment, each patient has the same impact on the endpoint contrast and it is therefore easier to understand the impact of any particular delta. In conditional delta adjustment, the impact on the endpoint contrast is not the same for each patient—it varies by time of dropout. If the same delta is applied at each visit in the conditional approach, patients dropping out earlier have a greater impact on the endpoint contrast because the "net" delta has a greater accumulation over visits.

21.5.4 Reference-Based Controlled Imputation

Results from reference-based imputation analyses are summarized in Table 21.12. Recall that the jump to reference approach (J2R) assumes the benefit of the drug immediately disappears after discontinuation or rescue; copy reference (CR) assumes a decaying benefit; and copy increment from reference (CIR) assumes a constant benefit. For these data, J2R is a reasonable worst plausible case sensitivity analysis. That is, if results from J2R were significant, then results from the primary analysis could be declared robust to plausible departures from MAR. Results were also assessed using CR and CIR for illustration. Analyses were conducted using the SAS macros made available freely to the public by the Drug Information Association's (DIA) Scientific Working Group for missing data at www.missingdata.org.uk.

As expected, treatment contrasts from J2R were smaller than from CR, and the treatment contrasts from CR were smaller than CIR. Also as expected, the J2R results closely mirror results from marginal delta-adjustment when delta is approximately equal to the mean difference between treatments.

TABLE 21.12

Results from Reference-Based Multiple Imputation of the High and Low Dropout Data Sets

	LSMEAN Changes		Endpoint	Standard	
	Placebo	Drug	Contrast	Error	P
High Dropout					
MAR	−5.95	−8.24	2.29	1.00	0.024
J2R	−5.97	−7.57	1.60	0.99	0.110
CR	−5.96	−7.71	1.75	0.98	0.075
CIR	−5.95	−7.78	1.83	0.97	0.040
Low Dropout					
MAR	−10.56	−12.40	1.84	0.70	0.009
J2R	−10.55	−12.26	1.71	0.70	0.016
CR	−10.55	−12.27	1.72	0.70	0.015
CIR	−10.55	−12.27	1.72	0.70	0.015

In the high dropout data set, the endpoint contrast from J2R was 1.60 (SE = 0.99, P = 0.110). In the low dropout data set, the endpoint contrast from J2R was 1.71 (SE = 0.70, P = 0.016). The difference from MAR was approximately sixfold smaller in the low dropout data set than in the high dropout data set. Statistical significance was preserved in the low dropout data set, but not for the high dropout data set.

21.5.5 Selection Model Analyses

A selection model was fit in which the parameters describing the MNAR part of the model were varied. The primary outcome was assessed using a repeated measures model similar to the primary analysis, and the probability of dropout was simultaneously modeled using a logistic regression that fit the log odds of dropout as a function of visit, separate intercepts (Ψ_1, Ψ_2) for each treatment group, and separate linear regression coefficients for previous (Ψ_3, Ψ_4) and current (possibly unobserved) efficacy outcomes (Ψ_5, Ψ_6). Hence, the outcome variable from the measurement model was a covariate in the dropout model. Fitting separate missingness models for each treatment allowed for different departures from MAR for drug and placebo groups. Analyses were implemented using macros made available freely to the public by the DIA Scientific Working Group for missing data at www.missingdata.org.uk.

The parameters Ψ_5 and Ψ_6 were of particular interest because they were the "MNAR" part of the model. These values assess the change in log odds for withdrawal per unit increase in the outcome measure. A value of 0.2 indicated that the odds of withdrawal increased by a factor 1.22 ($e^{0.2}$) for each 1-point change on the $HAMD_{17}$. Setting Ψ_5 and $\Psi_6 = 0$ was important

TABLE 21.13

Results from Selection Model Analyses of High Dropout Data Set

Input Values		Week 8 LSMEANS		Endpoint	Standard	
Ψ_5[a]	Ψ_6[a]	Placebo	Drug	Contrast	Error	P
0.2	0.2	4.87	7.33	2.46	1.09	0.023
0.0	0.2	5.60	7.38	1.78	1.05	0.091
−0.2	0.2	6.28	7.41	1.18	1.05	0.282
−0.4	0.2	6.76	7.42	0.66	1.06	0.527
0.2	0.0	4.94	7.97	3.03	1.07	0.005
0.0[b]	0.0	5.63	8.00	2.37	1.04	0.022
−0.2	0.0	6.29	8.04	1.75	1.02	0.087
−0.4	0.0	6.75	8.05	1.30	1.02	0.204
0.2	−0.2	4.97	8.57	3.60	1.06	0.001
0.0	−0.2	5.67	8.57	2.89	1.03	0.004
−0.2	−0.2	6.31	8.59	2.29	1.01	0.024
−0.4	−0.2	6.76	8.63	1.86	1.01	0.064
0.2	−0.4	4.97	8.97	4.01	1.07	<0.001
0.0	−0.4	5.68	8.96	3.28	1.03	0.002
−0.2	−0.4	6.33	8.98	2.64	1.01	0.009
−0.4	−0.4	6.78	9.01	2.22	1.01	0.027

[a] Ψ_5 and Ψ_6 are the regression coefficients (placebo and drug, respectively) for the association between the current, possibly missing efficacy scores and the logit for probability of dropout.

[b] Results differ from the primary result because the baseline value by site interaction was not fit in the selection model.

because the missingness and outcome models become independent and the model reduces to the MAR model in the primary analysis.

Results from selection model analyses of the high dropout data set with varying levels of both Ψ_5 and Ψ_6 are summarized in Table 21.13. These results are used to illustrate general aspects of selection model results. Subsequently, selection models are implemented in a tipping point approach for both the high dropout and low dropout data sets.

As expected, when $\Psi_5 = \Psi_6 = 0$, results matched results from the primary direct likelihood analysis. With negative values for Ψ_5 and Ψ_6, the within-group mean changes were greater than the mean changes when assuming MAR ($\Psi_5 = \Psi_6 = 0$). Conversely, positive values for Ψ_5 and Ψ_6 led to smaller within-group mean changes. A positive Ψ value implied that patients with negative residuals were more likely to drop out, leading to greater mean changes observed in the remaining data, with the selection model compensating for this by reducing the lsmean.

When there is more dropout in the placebo group and $\Psi_5 = \Psi_6 < 0$, the within-group mean change increased more in the placebo group than the drug group and the endpoint contrast was reduced. Conversely with $\Psi_5 = \Psi_6 > 0$, the endpoint contrast was increased. However, it is important to notice that whenever $\Psi_5 = \Psi_6$, that is, when the same MNAR model is assumed for both treatment arms, the impact of MNAR on the treatment contrast was fairly small.

When the input values for Ψ_5 and Ψ_6 differed, between-group differences (endpoint contrasts) followed a consistent pattern dictated by the within-group changes previously noted. Whenever Ψ_6 (the regression coefficient for the drug group) was less than Ψ_5 (the regression coefficient for the placebo group), the treatment contrast was greater than from the MAR primary analysis. When Ψ_5 was greater than Ψ_6, the treatment contrast was smaller than in MAR.

An understanding of these relationships can be used to systematically vary Ψ_5 and Ψ_6 in a selection model to generate departures from MAR in a tipping point approach. Results from a selection model tipping point sensitivity analyses are summarized in Table 21.14. A value of $\Psi_5 = 0$ was used to assume MAR for the placebo group. Recall that standard implementations of delta-adjustment and reference-based controlled imputations assume MAR for placebo. Values of Ψ_6 were progressively changed to create increasing departures from MAR that reduced the treatment contrasts. In the high dropout data set, $\Psi_6 = 0.2$ overturned the primary result. In the low dropout data set, $\Psi_6 > 1.0$ was required to overturn the primary result.

Although selection models can be used in a tipping point approach much the same way as delta-adjustment, judging the plausibility of departures from MAR is more complex in selection models. The regression coefficients (Ψ) in selection models are on the log odds scale. Judging plausibility therefore requires judging plausibility of changes in log odds per unit change in the (possibly unobserved) outcome measure.

TABLE 21.14

Results from Tipping Point Selection Model Analyses of High Dropout and Low Dropout Data Sets

Input Values		Low Dropout Data Set		High Dropout Data Set	
Ψ_5[a]	Ψ_6[a]	Endpoint Contrast	P	Endpoint Contrast	P
0	0.0	1.81	0.008	2.29	0.019
0	0.2	1.72	0.012	1.62	0.114
0	0.4	1.64	0.018	–	–
0	0.6	1.54	0.028	–	–
0	0.8	1.48	0.036	–	–
0	1.0	1.41	0.047	–	–

[a] Ψ_5 and Ψ_6 are the regression coefficients (placebo and drug, respectively) for the association between the current, possibly missing efficacy scores and the logit for probability of dropout.

For example, the value of Ψ that was sufficient to overturn the primary result in the high dropout data set was 0.2. This result indicated that if the odds of dropout increased by a factor 1.22 for each 1-point change on the current, possibly missing $HAMD_{17}$ score, the primary result would be overturned. The value of Ψ that was needed to overturn the primary result in the low dropout data set (>1.0) indicated that the odds of dropout had to increase approximately three-fold for each 1-point change in the current, possibly missing $HAMD_{17}$ in order to overturn the primary results.

With mean baseline scores of 20 and standard deviations >5, a 1-point change in HAMD is a small change. Therefore, the three-fold increase in odds of withdrawal per 1-point change in HAMD needed to overturn results in the low dropout data set doesn't seem plausible. Results in the low dropout data set appear to be robust to plausible departures from MAR.

In the high dropout data set, results are less clear. The key question is whether it is plausible that the odds of withdrawal could increase by a factor of 1.22 for each 1-point change in HAMD. This setup is less intuitive and transparent than in delta adjustment, where plausibility simply requires judging the magnitude of delta.

21.5.6 Pattern Mixture Model Analyses

Results from pattern-mixture model (PMM) analyses under various identifying restrictions are summarized in Table 21.15. Analyses were conducted using the macros made available freely to the public by the DIA Scientific Working Group for missing data at www.missingdata.org.uk.

Three identifying restrictions were implemented. The ACMV restriction assumed MAR, whereas CCMV and NCMV assumed MNAR. Therefore, comparing results from ACMV with those from other restrictions assessed the impact of departures from MAR.

Pattern mixture model analysis requires that all parameters are estimable in all patterns of dropouts. For analysis of the high dropout data set, sites had to be pooled into two grouped sites. Analysis of the low dropout data

TABLE 21.15

Results from Pattern-Mixture Model Analyses of High Dropout Data Set

Identifying Restriction	Endpoint Contrast	Standard Error	P
ACMV	2.67	1.17	0.022
CCMV	2.51	1.05	0.016
NCMV	2.87	1.69	0.089

Note: ACMV = available case missing values, CCMV = complete case missing values, NCMV = neighboring case missing values.

set was not feasible because, with so few missing observations, the treatment effect was not estimable in all dropout patterns.

Compared with ACMV, the endpoint contrast and standard error in the high dropout data set were slightly smaller in CCMV and larger in NCMV. Notice the large standard error for the NCMV result. Even with a high rate of dropout, the number of patients in certain patterns was limited, which in turn reduced precision of results, leading to a nonsignificant contrast even though the point estimate was larger than in ACMV.

21.6 Summary and Drawing Conclusions

21.6.1 Overview

The preceding examples from the high and low dropout data sets illustrated some fundamental points in analyzing longitudinal data. The primary analysis focused on a precisely defined estimand, in this instance a de jure estimand. Aspects of the model that could be evaluated from observed data were checked. Sensitivity analyses were used to aid understanding of the degree to which departures from MAR for the unobserved data could alter inferences from the primary analysis. A secondary estimand from the de facto family was also evaluated.

These illustrations were not intended to be general prescriptions or specific recommendations. The intent was to illustrate general approaches and considerations. Certainly, other approaches could be considered in these situations. And other situations could require different approaches.

Perhaps the most important aspect of these illustrations was the benefit from lower rates of missing data. Although this chapter in particular—and this book in general—focuses on analytic methods, the inescapable conclusion is that analyses can only assess sensitivity. Preventing missing data is the only way to improve sensitivity to missing data assumptions.

Importantly, the greater variability in results across various model assumptions from the high dropout data set was not limited to sensitivity analyses for plausible MNAR scenarios. Results from some of the standard diagnostics, such as choice of covariance structure, also showed greater variability with higher dropout.

21.6.2 Conclusions from the High Dropout Data Set

The primary analysis yielded a statistically significant result. Residual diagnostics showed no evidence that nonnormality or nonlinearity had an appreciable influence on results, thereby suggesting the model was appropriate. No patients or sites were found to have had a strong influence on results. The unstructured covariance specified in the primary analysis provided the best fit to the data.

However, the possibility of plausible departures from MAR overturning the primary result could not be entirely ruled out. Evidence for a treatment effect was supported by significance on the secondary de facto estimand.

The decision we would make from these analyses is that treatment was significantly better than placebo. However, we recognize the difficulty in making black and white decisions, and that others could come to a different decision. Again, the most important aspect of the illustration is not the decision itself, but rather the process for arriving at it.

21.6.3 Conclusions from the Low Dropout Data Set

The primary analysis yielded a statistically significant result. Residual diagnostics showed one clear outlier but no evidence that nonnormality or nonlinearity systematically influenced results, thereby suggesting the model was appropriate. Influence diagnostics also noted the aberrant patient with a very large residual. The RLD for this patient suggested it had an appreciable influence on results. However, that patient had an unfavorable outcome in the treatment group and therefore deleting data from that patient increased the magnitude and significance of the primary result. No one site had an undue influence on results. The unstructured covariance specified in the primary analysis provided one of the best fits to the data and significance of the primary result was insensitive to choice of covariance structure. Inferences from the primary analysis were robust to even the largest plausible departures from MAR.

Model diagnostics and sensitivity analyses, combined with a low rate of missing data, confirm the robustness of these results. Therefore, the decision we would make from these analyses is that treatment was significantly better than placebo.

References

Agresti A. (2002). *Categorical Data Analysis*. 2nd edition. New York: Wiley.

Alosh M, Kathleen F, Mohammad H, et al. (2015). Statistical considerations on subgroup analysis in clinical trials. *Statistics in Biopharmaceutical Research*, 7(4): 1–68. DOI: 10.1080/19466315.2015.1077726.

Ayele B, Lipkovich I, Molenberghs G, et al. (2014). A multiple-imputation-based approach to sensitivity analyses and effectiveness assessments in longitudinal clinical trials. *Journal of Biopharmaceutical Statistics*, 24(2):211–228.

Barnes SA, Carter K, Lindborg SR, et al. (2008). The impact of missing data and how it is handled on the rate of false positive results in drug development. *Pharmaceutical Statistics*, 7:215–225.

Buncher C. Ralph, Tsay J-Y. (2005). *Statistics in the Pharmaceutical Industry*. 3rd edition. New York: Chapman Hall.

Cao W, Tsiatis AA, Davidian M. (2009). Improving efficiency and robustness of the doubly robust estimator for a population mean with incomplete data. *Biometrika*, 96:723–734.

Carpenter JR, Kenward MG. (2007). Missing data in clinical trials|a practical guide. Birmingham: National Health Service Coordinating Centre for Research Methodology. Freely downloadable from http://www.pcpoh.bham.ac.uk/publichealth/methodology/projects/RM03 JH17 MK.shtml (accessed 28 May 2009).

Carpenter JR, Kenward MG, Vansteelandt S. (2006). A comparison of multiple imputation and doubly robust estimation for analyses with missing data. *Journal of the Royal Statistical Society, Series A*, 169:571–584.

Carpenter JR, Roger J, Kenward M. (2013). Analysis of longitudinal trials with protocol deviation: A framework for relevant, accessible assumptions, and inference via multiple imputation. *Journal of Biopharmaceutical Statistics*, 23(6):1352–1371.

Collins LM, Schafer JL, Kam CM. (2001). A comparison of inclusive and restrictive strategies in modern missing data procedures. *Psychological Methods*, 6(4):330–351.

Committee for Medicinal Products for Human Use (CHMP). (2010). Guideline on missing data in confirmatory clinical trials. EMA/CPMP/EWP/1776/99 Rev. 1.

Crowe B, Lipkovich I, Wang O. (2009). Comparison of several imputation methods for missing baseline data in propensity scores analysis of binary outcome. *Pharmaceutical Statistics*, 9:269–279.

Crump SL. (1947). *The Estimation of Variance in Multiple Classification*, PhD thesis, Department of Statistics, Iowa State University.

Daniel RM, Kenward MG. (2012). A method for increasing the robustness of multiple imputation. *Computational Statistics & Data Analysis*, 56(6):1624–1643. ISSN 0167-9473.

Detke MJ, Wiltse CG, Mallinckrodt CH, et al. (2004). Duloxetine in the acute and long-term treatment of major depressive disorder: A placebo- and paroxetine-controlled trial. *European Neuropsychopharmacology*, 14(6):457–470.

Diggle PD, Kenward MG. (1994). Informative dropout in longitudinal data analysis (with discussion). *Applied Statistics*, 43:49–93.

Diggle PJ, Heagerty P, Liang KY, et al. (2002). *The Analysis of Longitudinal Data*. 2nd edition. Oxford, England: Oxford University Press.

Efron B. (1994). Missing data, imputation, and the bootstrap. *Journal of the American Statistical Association*, 89(426):463–475.

Fedorov VV, Liu T. (2007). Enrichment Design, in *Wiley Encyclopedia of Clinical Trials*. Ralph D'Agostino, Lisa Sullivan, and Joe Massaro (eds.), Hoboken: John Wiley & Sons, Inc. pp. 1–8.

Firth D. (1993). Bias reduction of maximum likelihood estimates. *Biometrika*, 80:27–38.

Fisher RA. (1925). *Statistical Methods for Research Workers*. London: Oliver and Boyd. Gallant.

Fitzmaurice GM, Laird NM, Ware JH. (2004). *Applied Longitudinal Analysis*. Hoboken, NJ: Wiley Interscience.

Fitzmaurice GM, Molenberghs G, Lipsitz SR. (1995). Regression models for longitudinal binary responses with informative dropouts. *Journal of the Royal Statistical Society, Series B*, 57:691–704.

Flemming TR. (2011). Addressing missing data in clinical trials. *Annals of Internal Medicine*, 154:113–117.

Garrett A. (2015). Choosing appropriate estimands in clinical trials (Leuchs et al.): Letter to the editor. *Therapeutic Innovation & Regulatory Science*, 49(4):601.

Goldstein DJ, Lu Y, Detke MJ, et al. (2004). Duloxetine in the treatment of depression: A double-blind placebo-controlled comparison with paroxetine. *Journal of Clinical Psychopharmacology*, 24:389–399.

Graham JW, Olchowski AE, Gilreath TD. (2007). How many imputations are really needed? Some practical clarifications of multiple imputation theory. *Prevention Science*, 8:206–213.

Guy W. (1976). *ECDEU Assessment Manual for Psychopharmacology*. Rockville, MD: National Institute of Mental Health. pp. 217–222, 313–331.

Hamilton M. (1960). A rating scale for depression. *Journal of Neurology, Neurosurgery & Psychiatry*, 23:56–61.

Hartley HO, Rao JNK. (1967). Maximum-likelihood estimation for the mixed analysis of variance model. *Biometrika*, 54:93–108.

Harville DA. (1977). Maximum likelihood approaches to variance component estimation and to related problems. *Journal of the American Statistical Association*, 72:320–338.

Harville DA. (1988). Mixed-model methodology: Theoretical justifications and future directions, Proceedings of the Statistical Computing Section, American Statistical Association, New Orleans, 41–49.

Harville DA. (1990), BLUP (Best Linear Unbiased Prediction), and Beyond, in *Advances in Statistical Methods for Genetic Improvement of Livestock*, D. Gianola (eds.). Berlin: Heidelberg, Springer-Verlag. pp. 239–276.

Henderson CR. (1953). Estimation of variance and covariance components. *Biometrics*, 9:226–252.

Henderson CR. (1984). *Applications of Linear Models in Animal Breeding*. University of Guelph, Ont: University of Guelph.

Henning Z. (2011). Paracetamol and the placebo effect in osteoarthritis trials: A missing link? *Pain Research and Treatment*. Article ID 696791, 6, DOI: 10.1155/2011/696791.

Hogan JW, Laird NM. (1997). Mixture models for the joint distribution of repeated measures and event times. *Statistics in Medicine*, 16:239–258.

Holubkov R1, Dean JM, Berger J, et al. (2009). Is "rescue" therapy ethical in randomized controlled trials? *Pediatric Critical Care Medicine*, 10(4):431–438. DOI: 10.1097/PCC.0b013e318198bd13.

Horvitz DG, Thompson DJ. (1952). A generalization of sampling without replacement from a finite universe. *Journal of the American Statistical Association*, 47:663–685.

Hughes S, Harris J, Flack N, et al. (2012). The statistician's role in the prevention of missing data. *Pharmaceutical Statistics*, 11:410–416.

Hurvich CM, Tsai C-L. (1989), Regression and time series model selection in small samples. *Biometrika*, 76:297–307.

ICH guidelines. Available at: http://www.ich.org/fileadmin/Public_Web_Site/ICH_Products/Guidelines/Efficacy/E9/Step4/E9_Guideline.pdf, Accessed on July 14, 2015.

ICH guidelines. Available at: http://www.ich.org/fileadmin/Public_Web_Site/ICH_Products/Guidelines/Efficacy/E10/Step4/E10_Guideline.pdf, Accessed on July 14, 2015.

Jansen I, Beunckens C, Molenberghs G, et al. (2006). Analyzing incomplete binary longitudinal clinical trial data. *Statistical Science*, 21(1):52–69.

Jennrich RI, Schluchter MD. (1986). Unbalanced repeated measures models with structural covariance matrices. *Biometrics*, 42(4):805–820.

Kang DY, Schafer JL. (2007). Demystifying double robustness: A comparison of alternative strategies for estimating a population mean from incomplete data (with discussion and rejoinder). *Statistical Science*, 22:523–539.

Kenward MG, Molenberghs G. (2009). Last observation carried forward: A crystal ball? *Journal of Biopharmaceutical Statistics*, 19:872–888.

Laird NM. (1994). Discussion to Diggle PJ, Kenward MG. Informative dropout in longitudinal data analysis. *Applied Statistics*, 43:84.

Laird NM, Ware JH. (1982). Random-effects models for longitudinal data. *Biometrics*, 38:963–974.

Lane PW. (2007). Handling drop-out in longitudinal clinical trials: A comparison of the LOCF and MMRM approaches. *Pharmaceutical Statistics*, 7(2):93–106. (early view) DOI: 10.1002/pst.267.

Langley RG, Ellis CN. (2004). Evaluating psoriasis with Psoriasis area and severity index, Psoriasis Global Assessment, and Lattice System Physician's Global Assessment. *Journal of American Academy of Dermatology*, 51:563–569.

LaVange LM. Permutt T. (2015). A regulatory perspective on missing data in the aftermath of the NRC report. *Statistics in Medicine*, 35(17):2853–2864. DOI: 10.1002/sim.6840.

Leuchs AK, Zinserling J, Brandt A, et al. (2015). Choosing appropriate estimands in clinical trials. *Therapeutic Innovation and Regulatory Science*, 49(4):584–592.

Liang KY, Zeger SL. (1986). Longitudinal data analysis using generalized linear models. *Biometrika*, 73:13–22.

Liang KY, Zeger SL. (2000). Longitudinal data analysis of continuous and discrete responses for pre-post designs. *Sankhya: The Indian Journal of Statistics*, 62(Series B):134–148.

Lindstrom MJ, Bates DM. (1988). Newton–Raphson and EM algorithms for linear mixed-effects models for repeated-measures data. *Journal of the American Statistical Association*, 83:1014–1022.

Lipkovich I, Duan Y, Ahmed S. (2005). Multiple imputation compared with REPL and GEE for analysis of binary repeated measures in clinical studies. *Pharmaceutical Statistics*, 4:267–285.

Lipkovich I, Kadziola Z, Xu L, et al. (2014). Comparison of several multiple imputation strategies for repeated measures analysis of clinical scales: Truncate or not to? *Journal of Biopharmaceutical Statistics*, 24:924–943.

Lipkovich I, Ratitch B, O'Kelly M. (2016). Sensitivity to censored-at-random assumption in the analysis of time-to-event endpoints. *Pharmaceutical Statistics*, 15:216–229.

Little RJA. (1993). Pattern-mixture models for multivariate incomplete data. *Journal of American Statistical Association*, 88(421):125–134.

Little RJA. (1994). A class of pattern-mixture models for normal incomplete data. *Biometrika*, 81(3):471–483.

Little RJA. (1995). Modeling the drop-out mechanism in repeated measures studies. *Journal of American Statistical Association*, 90(431):1112–1121.

Little RJA, Rubin DB. (1987). *Statistical Analysis with Missing Data*. 1st edition. New York: Wiley.

Little RJA, Rubin DB. (2002). *Statistical Analysis with Missing Data*. 2nd edition. New York: Wiley.

Little R, Yau L. (1996). Intent-to-treat analysis for longitudinal studies with dropouts. *Biometrics*, 52(4):1324–1333.

Liu GF, Kaifeng L, Robin M, et al. (2009). Mehrotra. Should baseline be a covariate or dependent variable in analyses of change from baseline in clinical trials? *Statistics in Medicine*, 28:2509–2530.

Mallinckrodt CH. (2013). *Preventing and Treating Missing Data in Longitudinal Clinical Trials: A Practical Guide*. New York: Cambridge University Press.

Mallinckrodt CH, Clark WS, Carroll RJ, et al. (2003). Assessing response profiles from incomplete longitudinal clinical trial data under regulatory conditions. *Journal of BioPharmaceutical Statistics*, 13(2):179–190.

Mallinckrodt CH, Kenward MG. (2009). Conceptual considerations regarding choice of endpoints, hypotheses, and analyses in longitudinal clinical trials. *Drug Information Journal*, 43(4):449–458.

Mallinckrodt CH, Lane PW, Schnell D, et al. (2008). Recommendations for the primary analysis of continuous endpoints in longitudinal clinical trials. *Drug Information Journal*, 42:305–319.

Mallinckrodt CH, Lin Q, Lipkovich I, et al. (2012). Structured approach to choosing estimands and estimators in longitudinal clinical trials. *Pharmaceutical Statistics*, 11:456–461.

Mallinckrodt CH, Rathmann S, Molenberghs G. (2016). Choosing estimands in clinical trials with missing data. *Pharmaceutical Statistics*. DOI: 10.1002/pst.

Mallinckrodt CH, Roger J, Chuang-Stein C, et al. (2014). Recent developments in the prevention and treatment of missing data. *Therapeutic Innovation and Regulatory Science*, 48(1):68–80.

McCullagh P, Nelder JA. (1989). *Generalized Linear Models*. 2nd edition. London: Chapman and Hall.

McLean RA, Sanders WL. (1988). Approximating degrees of freedom for standard errors in mixed linear models, Proceedings of the Statistical Computing Section, American Statistical Association, New Orleans, 50–59.

Meng XL. (1994). Multiple imputation with uncongenial sources of input (with discussions). *Statistical Science*, 9:538–574.
Molenberghs G, Fitzmaurice G, Kenward M, et al. (2015). *Handbook of Missing Data Methodology*. Boca Raton, FL: CRC Press.
Molenberghs G, Kenward MG. (2007). *Missing Data in Clinical Studies*. Chichester: Wiley.
Molenberghs G, Kenward MG, Lesaffre E. (1997). The analysis of longitudinal ordinal data with nonrandom dropout. *Biometrika*, 84(1):33–44.
Molenberghs G, Thijs H, Jansen I, et al. (2004). Analyzing incomplete longitudinal clinical trial data. *Biostatistics*, 5(3):445–464.
Molenberghs G, Verbeke G. (2005). *Models for Discrete Longitudinal Data*. New York: Springer.
National Research Council (2010). *The Prevention and Treatment of Missing Data in Clinical Trials*. Panel on Handling Missing Data in Clinical Trials. Committee on National Statistics, Division of Behavioural and Social Sciences and Education. Washington, DC: The National Academies Press.
O'Kelly M, Ratitch B. (2014). Clinical trials with missing data. Chichester: Wiley.
O'Neill RT, Temple R. (2012). The prevention and treatment of missing data in clinical trials: An FDA perspective on the importance of dealing with it. *Clinical Pharmacology and Therapeutics*, 91(3):550–554.
Patterson HD, Thompson R. (1971). Recovery of inter-block information when block sizes are unequal. *Biometrika*, 58:545–554.
Permutt T. (2015a). A taxonomy of estimands for regulatory clinical trials with discontinuations. *Statistics Med*. DOI: 10.1002/sim.6841.
Permutt T. (2015b). Sensitivity analysis for missing data in regulatory submissions. *Statistics Med*. DOI: 10.1002/sim.6753.
Phillips A, Abellan-Andres J, Andersen S. et al. (2016). Pharmaceutical Statistics, accepted. Estimands: Discussion Points from the PSI Estimands and Sensitivity Expert Group.
Piantadosi S. (2005). *Clinical Trials: A Methodologic Perspective*. New York: Wiley.
Prasad NGN, Rao JNK. (1990). The estimation of mean squared error of small-area estimators. *Journal of the American Statistical Association*, 85:163–171.
Ratitch B, O'Kelly M. (2011). Implementation of pattern-mixture models using standard SAS/STAT Procedures. PharmaSUG. Available at http://pharmasug.org/proceedings/2011/SP/PharmaSUG-2011-SP04.pdf, (accessed 4 October 2011).
Robins JM, Rotnitzky A. (1995). Semiparametric efficiency in multivariate regression models with missing data. *Journal of American Statistical Association*, 90:122–129.
Robins JM, Rotnitzky A, Zhao LP. (1995). Analysis of semiparametric regression models for repeated outcomes in the presence of missing data. *Journal of the American Statistical Association*, 90:106–121.
Robins JM, Wang N. (2000). Inference for imputation estimators. *Biometrika*, 87:113–124.
Robinson GK. (1991). That BLUP is a good thing: The estimation of random effects. *Statistical Science*, 6: 15–51.
Rubin DB. (1976). Inference and missing data. *Biometrika*, 63(3):581–592.
Rubin DB. (1978). Multiple imputations in sample surveys—a phenomenological Bayesian approach to nonresponse. In: *Imputation and Editing of Faulty or Missing Survey Data*. Washington, DC: U.S. Department of Commerce, pp. 1–2.
Rubin DB. (1987). *Multiple Imputation for Nonresponse in Surveys*. New York: Wiley.

SAS Institute Inc. 2013. *SAS/STAT® 9.4* User's Guide. Cary, NC: SAS Institute Inc.
Schafer JL. (1997). *Analysis of Incomplete Multivariate Data*. New York: Chapman & Hall.
Schafer JL. (2003). Multiple imputation in multivariate problems when the imputation and analysis models differ. *Statistica Neerlandica*, 57:19–35.
Seaman S, Copas A. (2009). Doubly robust generalized estimating equations for longitudinal data. *Statistics in Medicine*, 28:937–955.
Searle SR. (1971). *Linear Models*. New York: Wiley.
Siddiqui O, Hung HM, O'Neill RO. (2009). MMRM vs. LOCF: A comprehensive comparison based on simulation study and 25 NDA Datasets. *Journal of Biopharmaceutical Statistics*, 19(2):227–246.
Snedecor GW, Cochran WG. (1980). *Statistical Methods*. Ames, IO: Iowa State University Press.
Stroup WW. (1989). Predictable functions and prediction space in the mixed model procedure, in *Applications of Mixed Models in Agriculture and Related Disciplines*, Southern Cooperative Series Bulletin No. 343, Louisiana Agricultural Experiment Station, Baton Rouge, pp. 39–48.
Tanner MA, Wong WH. (1987). The calculation of posterior distributions by data augmentation. *Journal of the American Statistical Association*, 82:528–540.
Temple R. (2005). Enrichment designs: Efficiency in development of cancer treatments. *Journal of Clinical Oncology*, 23(22):4838–4839.
Thompson WA. (1962). The problem of negative estimates of variance components. *Annals of Mathematical Statistics*, 33:273–289.
Tsiatis AA. (2006). *Semiparametric Theory and Missing Data*. New York: Springer.
Tsiatis AA, Davidian M, Cao W. (2011). Improved doubly robust estimation when data are monotonely coarsened, with application to longitudinal studies with dropout. *Biometrics*, 67:536–545.
Van Buuren S. (2007). Multiple imputation of discrete and continuous data by fully conditional specification. *Statistical Methods in Medical Research*, 16:219–242.
Van Buuren S. (2012). *Flexible imputation of missing data*. Boca Raton, FL: CRC Press.
Van Buuren S, Groothuis-Oudshoorn K. (2011). mice: Multivariate imputation by chained equations in R. *Journal of Statistical Software*, 45(3):1–67.
Vansteelandt S, Carpenter J, Kenward MG. (2010). Analysis of incomplete data using inverse probability weighting and doubly robust estimators. *Methodology: European Journal of Research Methods for the Behavioral and Social Sciences*, 6(1):37–48.
Verbeke G, Molenberghs G. (2000). *Linear Mixed Models for Longitudinal Data*. New York: Springer.
Verbeke G, Molenberghs G, Thijs H, et al. (2001). Sensitivity analysis for nonrandom dropout: A local influence approach. *Biometrics*, 57(1):7–14.
Wang N, Robins JM. (1998). Large-sample theory for parametric multiple imputation procedures. *Biometrika*, 85:935–948.
Wonnacott TH, Wonnacott RJ. (1981). *Regression: A Second Course in Statistics*. New York: Wiley.
Wu MC, Bailey KR. (1989). Estimation and comparison of changes in the presence of informative right censoring: Conditional linear model. *Biometrics*, 45(3):939–955.
Wu MC, Carroll RJ. (1988). Estimation and comparison of changes in the presence of informative right censoring by modeling the censoring process. *Biometrics*, 44:175–188.

Index